A Strategy To & Worked Practice For the
MRCP PACES

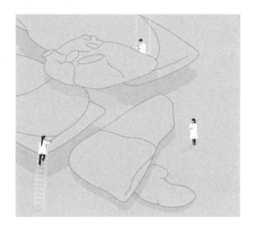

A Strategy To & Worked Practice For the
MRCP PACES

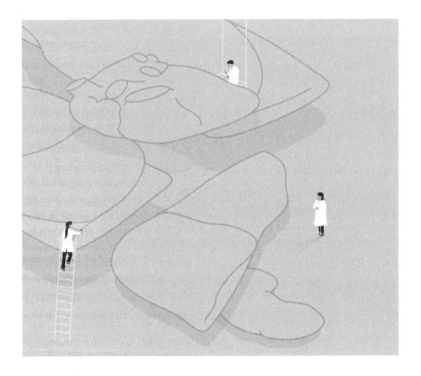

Dr. Nigel Fong
Dr. Marianne Tsang
Singapore General Hospital, Singapore

World Scientific

NEW JERSEY • LONDON • SINGAPORE • BEIJING • SHANGHAI • HONG KONG • TAIPEI • CHENNAI • TOKYO

Published by

World Scientific Publishing Co. Pte. Ltd.
5 Toh Tuck Link, Singapore 596224
USA office: 27 Warren Street, Suite 401-402, Hackensack, NJ 07601
UK office: 57 Shelton Street, Covent Garden, London WC2H 9HE

British Library Cataloguing-in-Publication Data
A catalogue record for this book is available from the British Library.

A STRATEGY TO AND WORKED PRACTICE FOR THE MRCP PACES

Copyright © 2023 by World Scientific Publishing Co. Pte. Ltd.

All rights reserved. This book, or parts thereof, may not be reproduced in any form or by any means, electronic or mechanical, including photocopying, recording or any information storage and retrieval system now known or to be invented, without written permission from the publisher.

For photocopying of material in this volume, please pay a copying fee through the Copyright Clearance Center, Inc., 222 Rosewood Drive, Danvers, MA 01923, USA. In this case permission to photocopy is not required from the publisher.

ISBN 978-981-125-039-2 (hardcover)
ISBN 978-981-126-308-8 (paperback)
ISBN 978-981-126-198-5 (ebook for institutions)
ISBN 978-981-126-199-2 (ebook for individuals)

For any available supplementary material, please visit
https://www.worldscientific.com/worldscibooks/10.1142/12669#t=suppl

Printed in Singapore by Mainland Press Pte Ltd.

MRCP PACES was the first examination in my life that I failed — not once, but thrice. I stumbled because of difficult cases (lithium toxicity, Takayasu arteritis, pulmonary stenosis with regurgitation), exacting examiners (who docked marks for not performing four-limb blood pressure), and my own imprecision in eliciting physical signs. It felt like a journey in the wilderness, but it taught me to wait on God and made me a sharper, wiser, and humbler physician.*

Nigel

As a family physician, MRCP is not required for training and promotion, but it is still relevant. I took PACES out of a desire to sharpen myself clinically. I had bread and butter cases, cooperative patients, reasonable examiners, and passed on the first attempt — it was entirely by God's grace. The lessons and skills learnt from the PACES preparation and exam still serve me well today.

Marianne

---

*Ryder's legendary *An Aid to the MRCP PACES*, currently in its fourth edition, was born out of his similar experience of having failed thrice.

Preface

The rigour of PACES ensures that generations of physicians retain bedside clinical skills — and rightly so, for the loss of bedside skills will make medicine costlier and more impersonal[1]. However, the outcome of the examination depends not just on the candidate's clinical ability, but also on examiner stringency[2] as well as patient and external factors. Pass rates vary wildly across test centres and diets, as do the difficulty of cases. Our PACES journeys (preceding page) illustrate this reality.

While some of these factors are outside of the candidate's control, what the candidate must do is develop the requisite clinical knowledge, skills, and habits of mind, and also learn specific strategies to tackle the PACES format (at best an approximation of clinical practice) and nuances in marking. This book is written to help you hone these clinical skills and gain from the various tips and strategies that we have picked up.

Section A provides a strategy to the Physical Examination stations. Many candidates with reasonable knowledge and technique falter due to inaccuracy in identifying physical signs and difficulty interpreting signs in the heat of the examination. Therefore, this section discusses techniques to optimise the identification of physical signs, provides advice on common pitfalls and areas of difficulty, and suggests a step-by-step approach to interpret and integrate physical signs that reduces cognitive load while under pressure.

Sections B and C provide 50 Consultation and 20 Communication worked practices respectively, each covering an important condition or diagnostic approach. For maximal learning value, do not simply read through the scenarios; rather, attempt the scenarios as mock stations with a colleague or tutor simulating the patient's role. Fully dialogued patient briefs are provided for this purpose. Each scenario is followed by a short tutorial on the clinical reasoning approach, sample responses to the patient's concerns, and a suggested discussion with examiners. The index will allow quick identification of a particular approach or condition for revision.

---

[1] Grady D. Scientist at work – Dr Abraham Verghese: Physician Revives a Dying Art: The Physical. *The New York Times*, 11 Oct 2010, retrieved 1 Jan 2021, www.nytimes.com/2010/10/12/health/12profile.html

[2] McManus IC, Thomson M, Mollon J. Assessment of examiner leniency and stringency ('hawk-dove effect') in the MRCP(UK) clinical examination (PACES) using multi-facet Rasch modelling. *BMC Med Educ* 2006 18(6):42

The material in this book is intentionally more difficult than average. This may be unnecessary for kinder examination circuits, but it will be wise to be aware of less straightforward diagnoses. Most of the uncommon conditions covered in this book have previously appeared in the exam.

Finally, remember that there is no substitute for bedside practice with patients. In fact, the best way to prepare for PACES is to deploy these history, examination, and communication skills in your daily practice[3]. We wish you the very best in your PACES examination, and in your growth as a clinician.

Nigel Fong and Marianne Tsang

---

[3] And equally importantly, remove bad habits incompatible with PACES from your daily practice!

Reviewers

Subspecialty Reviewers:

CARDIOLOGY
Dr Hong Rilong
Senior Resident, Cardiology,
National Heart Centre Singapore

DERMATOLOGY
Dr Dawn Oh Ai Qun
Senior Resident, Dermatology,
National Skin Centre Singapore

ENDOCRINOLOGY
Dr Sarah Tan Ying Tse
Associate Consultant, Endocrinology,
Singapore General Hospital

HAEMATOLOGY
Dr Denise Tan Yan
Consultant, Haematology,
Sengkang General Hospital, Singapore

INFECTIOUS DISEASE
Dr Sophie Tan Seine Xuan
Senior Resident, Infectious Diseases,
Singapore General Hospital

NEPHROLOGY
Dr Kog Zheng Xi
Senior Resident, Renal Medicine,
Singapore General Hospital

NEUROLOGY
Dr Tan You Jiang
Consultant, Neurology,
National Neuroscience Institute, Singapore

Dr Rebecca Hoe Hui Min
Associate Consultant, Neurology,
National Neuroscience Institute, Singapore

Dr Shawn Lin Zhi Zheng
Senior Resident, Neurology,
National Neuroscience Institute, Singapore

ONCOLOGY
Dr Kennedy Ng Yao Yi
Associate Consultant, Medical Oncology,
National Cancer Centre Singapore

OPHTHALMOLOGY	**Dr Chan Shu Wen Nicole** (co-author for ophthalmology chapters) *Senior Resident, Ophthalmology, National University Hospital, Singapore*
PALLIATIVE MEDICINE	**Dr Sara Ho Wei Fen** *Associate Consultant, Palliative Care, National University Cancer Institute, Singapore*
	Dr Jamie Zhou Xuelian *Consultant, Supportive & Palliative Care, National Cancer Centre Singapore*
RESPIRATORY	**Dr Marcus Sim Jin Hui** *Associate Consultant, Respiratory Medicine, Changi General Hospital*
RHEUMATOLOGY	**Dr Jon Yoong Kah Choun** *Senior Consultant, Rheumatology, Singapore General Hospital*
GASTROENTEROLOGY	*The reviewer for Gastroenterology wishes to remain anonymous.*

PACES candidate reviewers:

Dr Angel Tan	Dr Khaing Zin	Dr Samuel Koh
Dr Ashley Leong	Dr Lai Hsuan	Dr Sarah Too
Dr Cheney Wong	Dr Lau Wei Ren	Dr Shermain Chia
Dr Cheryl Ma	Dr Lee Kin Min	Dr Sim Meng Ying
Dr David Ang	Dr Lim Ying Huey	Dr Song Yang
Dr Grace Tan	Dr Louis Wang	Dr Stella Setiawan
Dr Jason Liew	Dr Natasha Fay Anthony	Dr Tan Sher Yin
Dr Joy Ong	Dr Paul Tern	Dr Wilnard Tan
Dr Kenneth Yong	Dr Samantha Koh	Dr Xiong Jiaqing

Acknowledgements

We thank God for His grace in sustaining us each day. We remember that every gift or ability we enjoy and exercise is from Him. To Him be all glory.

We are indebted to our many tutors who have taught us in preparation for our PACES exams, and the many before us who have prepared PACES resources (published or informal). We must also thank our study buddies, with whom many of the strategies in this book were ironed out.

We are very grateful to the physicians who have generously provided clinical photos for this work (below). We also greatly thank the subspecialty reviewers (previous page) whose feedback have improved this text and corrected numerous errors, as well as the PACES candidates who have commented on pilot versions of this text.

Finally, we thank the publishing team at World Scientific, in particular our editor Sook Cheng, for putting this book together. We also thank Jonathan Lim, a dear friend and artist, who provided the cover illustration.

Photo Credits:

Dr Chan Shu Wen Nicole	*Senior Resident, Ophthalmology, National University Hospital, Singapore*
Assoc Prof Derrick Aw Chen Wee	*Senior Consultant, Sengkang General Hospital*
Dr Jay Siak	*Consultant, Singapore National Eye Centre*
Dr Jon Yoong Kah Choun	*Senior Consultant, Rheumatology, Singapore General Hospital*
Dr Lie Jia Ling Cheryl	*Resident Physician, Dermatology, KK Women's and Children's Hospital*
Dr Loh Lih Ming	*Senior Consultant, Endocrinology, Singapore General Hospital*
Assoc Prof Mark Koh Jean Aan	*Senior Consultant, Dermatology, KK Women's and Children's Hospital*
Clin Assoc Prof Sharon Tow	*Senior Consultant, Singapore National Eye Centre*
Dr Stanley Angkodjojo	*Consultant, Rheumatology, Sengkang General Hospital*
Assoc Prof Tan Ju Le	*Senior Consultant, Cardiology, National Heart Centre Singapore*

Contents

Preface — vii

Reviewers — ix

Acknowledgements — xi

The New PACES Format — 1

Section A: Physical Exam

1 Strategy — 9

2 Neurology (Limbs) — 17
- 2.1 Bilateral UMN Signs — 30
- 2.2 Unilateral UMN Signs — 39
- 2.3 Mixed UMN and LMN Signs — 42
- 2.4 LMN Signs + Normal Sensation — 45
- 2.5 LMN Signs + Distal Numbness — 52
- 2.6 Foot Drop — 57
- 2.7 Finger/Wrist Drop — 61
- 2.8 Unilateral Weak/Wasted/Claw Hand — 64
- 2.9 Cerebellar Signs Only — 67
- 2.10 Parkinsonism — 70
- 2.11 Discussion Framework — 73

3 Neurology (Cranial Nerves) — 77
- 3.1 Multiple Cranial Nerve Palsy — 83
- 3.2 Ophthalmoplegia — 88

3.3	Ptosis	93
3.4	Facial Droop	97
3.5	Speech Abnormality	100
3.6	Discussion Framework	105

4 Cardiology 109

4.1	Systolic Murmur	115
4.2	Diastolic Murmur	122
4.3	Systolic + Diastolic Murmur	125
4.4	Prosthetic Valves	128
4.5	Cyanosis/Clubbing	131
4.6	Dextrocardia	134
4.7	Discussion Framework	135

5 Abdomen 141

5.1	Hepatosplenomegaly/Splenomegaly (*or splenectomy scar*)	148
5.2	Isolated Hepatomegaly	153
5.3	Ascites Only	156
5.4	Ballotable Kidney(s)	158
5.5	Transplant Kidney	162
5.6	Discussion Framework	166

6 Respiratory 171

6.1	Interstitial Lung Disease	178
6.2	Bronchiectasis	181
6.3	Pleural Effusion	184
6.4	Lung Resection	186
6.5	Collapse	188
6.6	Consolidation	191
6.7	Chronic Obstructive Pulmonary Disease	193
6.8	Discussion Framework	195

Section B: Consultations

Practice these cases with a colleague or tutor! The pull-out booklet contains the Candidate's Information.

1 Introduction and Walk-Through — 201

2 Same Presentation, Different Conditions — 209

    Case 01: Mdm Ruby Toh (Dyspnoea) — 210

    Case 02: Mrs Puff (Dyspnoea) — 216

    Case 03: Ms G. Mao (Dyspnoea) — 221

    Case 04: Mdm Miles (Dyspnoea) — 226

    Case 05: Ms Chuan (Dyspnoea) — 231

    Case 06: Mr Freddie (Dyspnoea) — 237

    Case 07: Mr Nafas (Dyspnoea) — 243

3 Same Condition, Different Presentations — 249

4 Worked Practice — 255

    Case 08: Mr Ee Chee (Rash) — 257

    Case 09: Mrs Lump (Rash) — 263

    Case 10: Mrs Sweet (Rash) — 268

    Case 11: Ms McDonald (Weight Gain) — 273

    Case 12: Mdm Grumps (Headache) — 279

    Case 13: Ms Ache (Painful Hands) — 285

    Case 14: Mrs Potts (Back Pain) — 291

    Case 15: Mr Pop (Chest Pain) — 296

    Case 16: Ms Slim (Weight Loss) — 301

    Case 17: Mr Bocelli (Difficulty Seeing) — 307

    Case 18: Mdm Kant Xi (Difficulty Seeing) — 315

    Case 19: Ms See (Difficulty Seeing) — 323

    Case 20: Mr Hong Yan (Red Eye) — 328

    Case 21: Mr Pei (Haematuria) — 334

    Case 22: Mrs Childless (Amenorrhoea) — 340

Case 23: Ms Liu B. Xue (Epistaxis) — 346
Case 24: Mr A. M. Indra (Hyperlipidaemia) — 352
Case 25: Mdm Hashi (Fatigue) — 357
Case 26: Mr Rachmaninoff (Numbness) — 364
Case 27: Ms Kat (Hypertension) — 371
Case 28: Mr Kay (Blackout) — 377
Case 29: Ms Oh (Blackout) — 382
Case 30: Mr H. Dumpty (Falls) — 388
Case 31: Ms Alice (Muscle Cramps) — 393
Case 32: Mr White (Anaemia) — 398
Case 33: Mdm Na (Hyponatraemia) — 403
Case 34: Mr Choke (Dysphagia) — 409
Case 35: Mr Philippe (Painful Hands) — 414
Case 36: Ms S. L. Ee (Mouth Ulcers) — 420
Case 37: Mdm Yang (Itch) — 425
Case 38: Ms Poo (Diarrhoea) — 430
Case 39: Ms L. Sai (Abdominal Pain) — 436
Case 40: Ms Jackson (Abnormal Movement) — 441
Case 41: Ms Mabok (Giddiness) — 446
Case 42: Ms Campbell (Giddiness) — 452
Case 43: Mrs Drowsy (Confusion) — 458
Case 44: Ms Claudia (Leg Pain) — 464
Case 45: Mr Pee (Frequent Urination) — 469
Case 46: Mr Kuning (Deranged Liver Enzymes) — 474
Case 47: Ms Fairchild (Raised aPTT) — 479
Case 48: Ms Clot (Low Platelets) — 484

5 How Examiners Grade — 489

Case 49: Mr Beer (Acute Kidney Injury) — 492
Case 50: Mr Ezekiel (Fractures) — 498

Colour Plates for Consultation Stations — 505

Section C: Communications

Practice these cases with a colleague or tutor! The pull-out booklet contains the Candidate's Information.

1 Introduction and Walk-Through   **523**

2 Worked Practice   **531**

Case 01: Missed Bleed	533
Case 02: Brain Dead	538
Case 03: Discussing Anticoagulation	542
Case 04: Still Hypertensive	548
Case 05: Still Seizing	552
Case 06: Still Coughing	556
Case 07: Indeterminate Western Blot	561
Case 08: HIV Positive	566
Case 09: Needlestick Injury	570
Case 10: Ascitic Drain	573
Case 11: Chronic Pain I	577
Case 12: Chronic Pain II	581
Case 13: Drug Overdose	585
Case 14: Withdrawal of Dialysis	589
Case 15: Supratentorial	594
Case 16: BRCA Testing	598
Case 17: Doctor Dangerous	601
Case 18: Send Her Home	605
Case 19: Sacral Sores	609
Case 20: A Right to Know?	613

Index to Worked Cases   **617**

Introduction
The New PACES Format

A brief history of the PACES format

The Membership examination has existed since the nineteenth century, and has undergone many transformations in syllabus and format over the years. Prior to the introduction of PACES, candidates underwent a long case and were essentially led around a large room to examine any number and combination of short cases, at the examiner's fancy. The implementation of PACES in 2001 sought to improve the validity and reliability of the examination. Its key features included the use of standardised marking rubrics, a 'carousel' in which all candidates in the same circuit encountered the same patients, and independent marking of each station by different examiners so as to improve objectivity.

PACES was revamped in 2009, when the four five-minute short examinations covering the endocrine, rheumatology, dermatology, and ophthalmology systems were replaced with a new *Brief Clinical Consult* (BCC) station that integrated history-taking, examination, and communication with the patient in a single encounter (Table 1). This change sought to address the concern that candidates either spoke to the patient but did not examine them or vice versa, which was felt to be dissociative and artificial. Additionally, it was desired that the scope of PACES be broadened to include topics such as acute medicine or geriatrics, which could not be tested in the 2001 format. The marking scheme was also amended to move away from an overall judgement mark for each station, towards individual marking of seven 'core clinical skills'. Passing PACES now requires a minimum score in each of the seven skills, along with a minimum overall mark.

The third iteration of the PACES format was due to be launched in 2020, but was postponed due to the COVID-19 pandemic. It makes two key changes to address the deficiencies identified with the 2009 format. Firstly, while the 2009 BCC was very real-life, it was also very rushed. Conversely, the history-taking station was too long and testing history-taking in isolation felt artificial. Therefore, the BCC and history stations were combined into two 20-minute Consultation stations combining history-taking, examination, and communication with the patient. One could say that we have come full circle to the pre-PACES 'long case' format.

The second change was to split the communications station into two separate 10-minute encounters, each paired with a physical examination task. Additionally, it was determined that the five-minute question and answer with examiners added little to the assessment and was therefore removed. Going from one to two communications stations also means that the mark weightage of communications is now doubled.

Table 1. Comparison of PACES 2001, 2009, and current formats.

Station	PACES 2001	PACES 2009	New (current)
Physical Exam - Cardiac - Abdominal - Respiratory - Neurology	10 min each (6 min examination + 4 min Q&A). Respiratory + abdominal paired to form a 20-min station; similarly for neurology and cardiovascular.	No change from 2001 format.	Retains basic format. Abdominal and respiratory stations now paired with communications task.
Communications and Ethics	One 20-min station (14 min with the patient, 1 min reflection, 5 min Q&A).	No change from 2001 format.	Split into two 10-min encounters. Q&A removed.
History-taking	One 20-min station (14 min with the patient, 1 min reflection, 5 min Q&A).	No change from 2001 format.	History-taking and *Brief Clinical Consult* combined into two 20-min *Consultation* stations that integrate history and physical examination (15 min with patient, 5 min Q&A).
"Station 5"	One 20-min station with four 5-min cases: endocrine, joints, skin, and eyes. Focus is on physical signs, often with 'spot diagnosis' type cases.	One 20-min station with two 10-min *Brief Clinical Consult*; integrated history and examination (8 min with patient, 2 min Q&A).	

Q&A: Question and answer with examiners.

The New PACES format

The New PACES format involves five 20-minute stations, three of which are divided into two 10-minute tasks.

Station 1:	Communication A	10 min: 10 min with patient.
	Respiratory	10 min: 6 min examination + 4 min Q&A
Station 2:	Consultation A	20 min: 15 min with patient + 5 min Q&A
Station 3:	Cardiovascular	10 min: 6 min examination + 4 min Q&A
	Neurology	10 min: 6 min examination + 4 min Q&A
Station 4:	Communication B	10 min: 10 min with patient.
	Abdominal	10 min: 6 min examination + 4 min Q&A
Station 5:	Consultation B	20 min: 15 min with patient + 5 min Q&A

Candidates may start at any station and proceed in a 'round-robin' fashion (i.e., Station 4 → Station 5 → Station 1 and so on). There is a 5-minute interval between stations, which gives candidates time to read the 'Candidate's information' for the subsequent station and plan a strategy.

The specifics of each station (physical examination, consultation, or communication) and its appropriate strategy are discussed in detail in the rest of this book.

Marking Scheme

The Marking Scheme is in flux at present and readers are advised to refer to www.nigelfong.net, where updates to this chapter will be periodically published.

Page intentionally left blank, pending confirmation of marking scheme. Refer to www.nigelfong.net for updated chapter.

Section A: Physical Exam

Physical Examination

1 | Strategy

The physical examination stations have changed little since PACES was introduced in the early 2000s. You have six minutes to read an opening stem and examine the patient. A timekeeping reminder is given when there is one minute left. In the remaining four minutes, you present your findings, state your differential diagnoses, and answer the examiner's questions, which typically revolve around underlying aetiology, complications, investigations, and management of the patient. The contents of the discussion is at the examiner's discretion — occasionally you may also be asked about the pathophysiological basis of the condition or physical signs.

A limited variety of conditions appear in the physical exam stations. Patients have to be well and not in pain — this rules out many acute conditions such as a pneumothorax. As patients are usually recruited 4–6 weeks ahead of the examination, those whose signs may disappear are typically not listed. Therefore, each station can be reduced to a small number of clinical syndromes, each with a defined list of conditions.

This is an exam that can be prepared for. The most common reason that candidates fails PACES is failure at the "Physical Signs" skill (See 'Pitfall' below). This book focuses on addressing the modifiable factors that one can work on.

Pitfall: How "physical signs" marks are lost

> **Modifiable factors – skill and strategy:**
> - Poor examination technique: Candidate performs correct steps but has reduced sensitivity and specificity due to suboptimal technique. This is particularly critical when signs are not obvious.
> - Examining but not actively looking for signs: Going through the motions of the examination steps without a high index of suspicion of signs that are present. We advise a mental checklist of critical signs and key decision points to mitigate this.
> - Poor time management: Inability to complete the examination or having to rush at the end.
> - Suboptimal presentation strategy: Failure to present positive signs that were identified, convoluted presentations that make the candidate appear unconfident to the examiner, blindly following memorised scripts that include signs that are not present.

(Cont'd)

Modifiable factors – cognitive and emotional:

- Cognitive overload: Difficulty 'piecing the signs together' whilst examining causes a mental fog that predisposes the candidate to confusion and doubt over signs identified. Prior preparation in having thought through possible signs and their interpretation helps.
- Premature closure: trying to pigeonhole the patient into a known diagnosis script leads to presentation of signs that are not present. Sometimes the signs simply do not fit! We once had a patient with a lobectomy whose trachea unexpectedly deviated to the opposite side from the lobectomy due to scoliosis — most candidates said that the trachea was deviated to the side of the lobectomy!
- Exam anxiety: Some nerves are inevitable, but this must be managed so as not to cloud thinking. Should examiners pick up the lack of confidence and ask 'are you sure', anxious candidates often undermine themselves by retracting correct signs presented or guessing signs that are not present.

Non-modifiable factors – out of candidate's control:

- Patient factors: subtle or debatable signs, uncooperative patient (for signs that require patient cooperation to elicit, particularly in neurology).
- Examiner factors: some examiners are stricter than others. Calibration errors also occur, both Type 1 (examiner picking up a sign that is not evident, often because of prior knowledge of the diagnosis) and Type 2 (examiner missing a sign that is present).

Marking Scheme

Begin with the end in mind — our strategy must start from an understanding of how the stations are marked. Each station is marked according to individual skills, and each skill is graded satisfactory (2 points), borderline (1 point), or unsatisfactory (0 points). Both examiners mark independently. Therefore, the physical examination station, containing 5 skills and 2 points per skill per examiner, is marked out of a total of 20 marks (5 skills × 2 points per skill × 2 examiners). The candidate must pass not just the overall score, but also each individual skill.

A process of 'calibration' precedes every PACES carousel. This entails the pair of examiners assigned to each station examining the patient independently, verifying the physical signs present, and agreeing on a marking rubric (Table A1.1). In theory, examiners should examine the patient 'blind' (without knowing the diagnosis in advance); signs identified and differentials considered by only one examiner but not both should not be included as mandatory signs. In practice, some examiners may be unduly influenced by reading the diagnosis before examining the patient, or by knowing the supposed signs present on the basis of CT scans or echocardiography findings.

From the examiner's perspective, the candidate's task is to perform a smooth and professional examination, state the physical signs agreed to be present, and hit the required differentials, investigations, and management. Skills C and D are 'linked skills', meaning that if Skill B is unsatisfactory, a maximum of a borderline mark can be awarded for Skills C and D.

Table A1.1. Example of a post-calibration marking rubric.

Skill	A satisfactory candidate should consider...	Comment
A: Physical examination	See marksheet	Examiners expect standard steps, no further calibration done.
B: Identifying physical signs	Collapsing pulse Elevated JVP Displaced apex beat Early diastolic murmur	Typically 3–4 mandatory signs. 'Borderline' awarded if one sign is missed. Presenting signs that are not present (make up signs) is typically unsatisfactory.
C: Differential diagnosis	Aortic regurgitation	Must include the correct diagnosis.
D: Clinical judgement	Echocardiogram Aortic valve replacement Diuretics	Can include investigation, management, and others.
E: Maintaining patient welfare	See marksheet	Awarded unless the candidate causes distress to the patient or is unsafe.

The nature of this marking system — that the candidate must hit certain pre-specified points to attain a satisfactory score — has significant implications:

- Candidates must not only get the correct diagnosis, but also mention all relevant physical signs (in the above example, it is easy to forget to mention that the apex beat is displaced, especially if the diagnosis is clear-cut).
- No additional marks are awarded for presenting negatives (e.g., no stigmata of infective endocarditis) or signs that the examiners do not happen to include in the rubric.
- Negative marking applies — the penalty for presenting signs that are not present is severe.
- The points required under clinical judgement are typically basic and written in broad terms. No marks for nitty-gritty ward management (e.g., parameters monitoring), motherhood statements, or subspecialist-level advanced discussions (you must first cover the basics for which marks are awarded).

Examination and Picking Up Signs

The candidate's role in the six minutes allocated for uninterrupted physical examination is to:

(1) Demonstrate a practiced, professional, and smooth examination technique.
(2) Pick up the correct physical signs.
(3) Interpret the signs and be ready to present.

It is important that (1)–(3) happen simultaneously, beginning from inspection at the foot of the bed. Shortlisting diagnostic possibilities early will allow you to (a) look out for specific signs associated with the diagnosis so as not to miss them, and (b) modify the examination routine to pick up additional features that will distinguish between diagnostic possibilities (for example, if you have found lower motor neuron foot drop, you will need to check hip abduction, which is otherwise not a routine part of the lower limb examination).

How to prepare?

(1) **Examination technique**. This should be second nature — aim for full marks for the Physical Examination skill. Practice in groups, simulate the exam setting, and critique each other's examination. Avoid taking shortcuts when you practice — it is far harder to unlearn a bad habit that had been picked up. Aim to complete the examination in five minutes — allowing one minute's grace to enter the room, read the stem, undress the patient, and so on. The specifics for each station are discussed in subsequent sections.

(2) **Picking up signs**. There is no substitute for seeing many patients. You must practice not only on patients with florid signs, but also on those with more subtle findings that require careful technique to elicit, as well as on patients who are less than optimally cooperative. It is helpful to prime yourself to look out for specific signs (what the mind does not think, of the eye does not see), which thinking about differential diagnoses as you examine will allow you to do.

(3) **Interpreting signs**. This is a common struggle especially for candidates who are less familiar with the range of conditions that commonly appear in PACES. The 'Clinical Syndromes' sections will suggest a thought process to interpret and integrate findings, and hence reduce the cognitive load faced during physical examination.

Presenting Findings and Differentials

Presentation styles:

Thank the patient and turn to the examiners to present. Two presentation formats are possible — either (1) diagnosis upfront, or (2) positive signs first.

(1) Diagnosis upfront

Diagnosis: This gentleman has a prosthetic aortic valve.

Justification: I say this because he has a midline sternotomy scar without saphenous vein graft scar, audible prosthetic clicks that occur after the

(2) Positive signs first

My positive signs are:
– Midline sternotomy without saphenous vein graft scar.
– Metallic click audible at bedside, occurring after carotid pulse.
– Implanted cardiac device in situ.

(Cont'd)

carotid pulse, and a prosthetic second heart sound.

Aetiology: The underlying aetiology is likely aortic regurgitation as the apex beat is deviated.

Complications: The valve sounds are crisp. There is a short grade 2/6 ejection systolic murmur best heard in the aortic position with no radiation, likely a flow murmur. I also note that he is in atrial fibrillation, and there is an implanted cardiac device. There is no evidence of congestive cardiac failure, pulmonary hypertension, stigmata of infective endocarditis, or overanticoagulation.

In summary, this gentleman has a prosthetic aortic valve which is well-functioning.

– Irregularly irregular pulse.
– Prosthetic second heart sound which is crisp.
– Grade 2 ejection systolic murmur best heard in aortic position with no radiation.

Significant negatives: There is no evidence of cardiac failure, pulmonary hypertension, or infective endocarditis.

Do not present a long list of negatives, only the major ones.

Diagnosis: This patient has a prosthetic aortic valve which is well-functioning. The underlying aetiology may be aortic regurgitation as the apex beat is deviated.

Our Recommendation:

We generally recommend presenting positive signs first (i.e., option 2). Presenting the diagnosis upfront (option 1) is slicker but no additional marks are awarded for being slick. Conversely, presenting the diagnosis upfront opens up potential dangers that have led to the downfall of many candidates. These include:

- Leaving out positive signs. In this example, it is easy to forget to mention the sternotomy scar (because the diagnosis is so obvious), or the presence of an implanted cardiac device (because it is not directly relevant to the prosthetic valve). Such signs are likely to be in the calibration rubric and failure to mention them will certainly lead to loss of marks.

- Incorrect upfront diagnosis will lead examiners to pay little heed to the rest of your presentation.

- Committing to an overly specific diagnosis upfront, for instance, 'myeloproliferative disease' instead of 'hepatosplenomegaly' when there is no indisputable sign that excludes other causes of hepatosplenomegaly. In cases where not every sign fits nicely into a single picture, discuss the possible differentials, explaining what is consistent and what is not. Examiners look for evidence of clinical reasoning rather than misplaced confidence in overly narrow differentials.

- Following a memorised diagnosis script without tailoring this to the patient, for instance, rattling off the signs of chronic liver disease, including those that the patient does not have! 'Making up signs' is definitely penalised.

- Doing a long and meandering presentation – there is simply no time for this. Leaving important signs to the later part of the presentation is also risky should the examiner interrupt your presentation to rush you along.

The exception is the obvious and straightforward case you are very confident about – presenting the diagnosis upfront is not an issue here.

What if you are unsure about a sign?

Do all you can to optimise your examination technique and convince yourself one way or the other. If you are still unsure, several pieces of advice apply:

- Be aware of what signs are reliable and which are often soft. For instance, if plantars are upgoing but reflexes only just slightly brisk, the patient almost certainly has an upper motor neuron lesion. Similarly, if you thought that the pulse was possibly slow rising, but the murmur was best heard over the lower left sternal edge and did not radiate to the carotid, the pulse is probably not slow-rising.
- Consider whether the unclear sign is consistent with the overall clinical picture. You can explain that some signs were equivocal and make a call based on the overall picture. For example: "My patient has bilateral lower limb proximal and distal weakness. He has increased tone which goes in favour of an upper motor neuron lesion, however the reflexes did not seem brisk and his plantars were equivocal."
- It is generally better not to present an unclear sign. Examiners look far more harshly on presenting signs that are not present (for which the marking scheme mandates an 'unsatisfactory' mark), than on missing signs that are present (for which you may be awarded a 'borderline' mark).
- Conversely, there are some scenarios in which taking the gamble of presenting the unclear sign pays off. The typical situation is a cardiology patient who has atrial fibrillation, an undisplaced apex, and a loud first heart sound, but you could not hear any murmurs no matter how hard you tried. Mitral stenosis remains the most likely diagnosis – it is notoriously soft – and it would be quite clear that other differentials are unlikely.

Further Discussion

Investigations and management should be presented in broad principles as you only have 4 minutes. Tailor your discussion to the patient and to the stem given. For example, if the diagnosis is aortic stenosis and the stem provides a history of breathlessness, then state that valve replacement is almost certainly indicated assuming that his breathlessness is due to valvular heart disease and you will first exclude other causes of breathlessness. Similarly, if the stem is abdominal pain and the patient has polycystic kidneys, explain that you will take further history and do further examination to explore general causes of abdominal pain, and specifically consider the complications of polycystic kidney disease that present with abdominal pain.

Interaction with the examiner is often a cause of anxiety. Unlike medical school examinations where one might get reaffirming nods and smiles, examiners in PACES are instructed to be stoic and expressionless. Do not take this to mean that you are on the wrong track. Similarly, the PACES examiner who asks 'did you find anything else' or 'are you sure it is a liver' is not necessarily giving you a cue to change your diagnosis and contradict yourself — if you did not find anything else, say so rather than make up signs! Examiners may be curt and rushed, but if they do so it is often to help you cover ground and quickly tick off the marking points.

Physical Examination

2 | Neurology (Limbs)

The neurological examination appears daunting, but in trained hands it is actually the most reliable system with very reliable signs and clear localisation algorithms. The main struggles candidates face are: (a) neurophobia, (b) inability to elicit signs accurately due to poor examination technique, (c) inability to elicit patient cooperation due to poor communication, and (d) cognitive overload when deciding on additional localisation steps or in 'piecing it all together'. It is the aim of this chapter to assist you to overcome these challenges by providing advice on examination technique and systematic localisation algorithms that can be used even in complicated or unfamiliar cases.

This is, of course, no substitute for having seen many cases. Regular practice shortens the standard examination sequence to 4–5 minutes, leaving the remaining 1–2 minutes for additional manoeuvres (such as checking for fatigability) that help to clinch the diagnosis.

Acronyms used in this section:

UMN	Upper motor neuron		CN	Cranial nerve
LMN	Lower motor neuron			

Walk-Through and Tips: Upper Limbs

Listen to the stem

In the neurology station the stem can be exceptionally helpful. For example:

- "Patient has longstanding weakness." → Be alert for congenital causes and muscular dystrophies.
- "Patient has weakness and numbness." → Prioritise a differential of neuropathy (which can lead to numbness) over myopathy or neuromuscular junction disease (in which sensation is normal).
- "Patient has weakness of fingers." → Be alert for median, ulnar, and radial nerve palsies; C7 and C8 lesions, and myotonic dystrophy.

- "... Examine as appropriate." (instead of examine upper or lower limbs) → Hint that this is a movement disorder or cerebellar disease, and you might be expected to examine more than one region.

Inspection

Approach the patient with a warm greeting, smile, and handshake. This immediately reveals dysarthria, hypophonia, facial droop, and grip myotonia. Step back and inspect the patient as a whole — not just the upper limbs. Look around the patient for walking aids, urinary catheters, motorised aids, limb splints, and other devices. Look at the face for any facial droop (stroke?), facial diplegia (myopathy?), mask-like facies (Parkinsonism?), or ptosis (various causes). Look at the posture of the limbs — is there tremor, chorea, contractures, or upper motor neuron posturing (flexion at the elbow and wrist)?

Now go closer to the patient. Ensure adequate exposure — the shirt should be removed so that the overriding scapula of facioscapulohumeral dystrophy is immediately revealed. Observe wasting particularly by comparing left and right, looking at the dorsal interossi of the fingers, and for any clawing of the toes. Look for scars over the limbs, neck, and head. Fasciculations are best observed at this stage (and again in the tongue). Do not flick for fasciculations; flicking does not make fasciculations appear. Although inspection alone can sometimes yield the diagnosis, avoid jumping to a 'spot diagnosis' based on the presence of a few signs (e.g., pes cavus = Charcot-Marie-Tooth, fasciculation = motor neuron disease). You can be misled, and even if you are right, you need to show evidence of a robust thought process rather than lucky 'guessing'.

Screening tests. (1) is an expected part of the upper limb examination, while (2) and (3) are our recommendations given how commonly myotonic dystrophy appears in PACES, as well as the possibility of mononeuropathies which can confuse you during power testing:

(1) **Pronator drift**: Ask the patient to hold both arms outstretched in front, with palms upwards and eyes closed. To improve sensitivity, ensure full forearm supination and finger adduction. Look for a pronator drift; i.e., pronation and downward drift (upper motor neuron weakness), claw hand (ulnar claw), or finger escape sign (cervical myelopathy). Push both palms downwards and look for an overshoot rebound (cerebellar disease).

(2) **Wrist and fingers cocked up**: Next, ask the patient to hold both hands outstretched with wrist in dorsiflexion, as if testing for asterixes. Look for wrist or finger drop (radial nerve palsy). In this position, walk behind the patient, looking for any winging of scapula (e.g., facioscapulohumeral dystrophy) or neck scars.

(3) **Make a tight fist and open quickly**: Look for any benediction sign (median nerve palsy), grip myotonia (myotonic dystrophy), or slow grip and release (Parkinsonism). If Parkinsonism is suspected, check rapid alternating movements (e.g., repeatedly make a fist and open).

Pitfall: Common errors in inspection

> The inspection step is very important — missing some diagnoses here can be an unsalvageable calamity. Common flops include:
> - Missing a diagnosis of myotonic dystrophy. This is usually due to a failure to recognise characteristic facial features (facial diplegia, ptosis, frontal balding) and therefore a failure to screen for grip and percussion myotonia. The tale is also told of the patient with myotonic dystrophy who always wears a cap at exams — so as not to give away obvious frontal balding to the candidate who fails to hunt for it. This can be circumvented by screening for grip myotonia in *all* upper limb cases.
> - Missing a diagnosis of Parkinsonism. This can occur in patients with only a subtle rest tremor, if the candidate fails to examine tone carefully or fails to distinguish spasticity (velocity dependant — UMN) from rigidity (velocity independent — Parkinsonism). Therefore it is important to look out for hypophonia and mask-like facies.
> - Missing a diagnosis of facioscapularhumeral dystrophy. Its classic features — overriding scapula, polyhill sign, winged scapula — are obvious on inspection, but will be missed if exposure is inadequate. If you opt not to remove the patient's shirt right from the start, you must certainly remove it later should the patient have proximal weakness with lower motor neuron signs and normal sensation.
> - Using the "OK sign" as a screen. This has little value because it tests only the anterior interosseous nerve and is completely normal in a median nerve lesion at the carpal tunnel (which is also the most common median nerve lesion).

Be prepared to modify the examination routine or perform additional steps based on the suspected diagnosis. For example, if you notice mask-like facies, the next step is to demonstrate the signs of Parkinsonism and distinguish between idiopathic Parkinson's disease vs. Parkinson-plus syndromes. Completing the sensory exam takes a back seat. This is discussed further in the relevant clinical syndromes.

Determine UMN vs. LMN lesion

Tone. Before beginning, check if the patient has any pain. Explain, *"Sir, I will now like to see how relaxed you can be. Rest completely and let me move your hands."* Assess tone over one joint at a time, isolating the joint tested. The usual sequence is elbow flexion/extension, forearm pronation/supination, and wrist flexion/extension; compare left and right at each step. In each joint, begin with large, slow movements to look for rigidity (Parkinsonism — velocity independent), then perform rapid extension/supination movements to catch spastic flexors (UMN — velocity dependant). Recall that a UMN lesion in the upper limbs results in greater spasticity and power in flexors (i.e., antigravity muscles) than in extensors; therefore rapid elbow extension, forearm supination, or wrist extension will best allow you to catch spasticity. Apart from UMN spasticity, be alert for the leadpipe rigidity and cogwheeling of Parkinsonism — this may be the last chance to catch Parkinsonism if you did not notice any tremor or mask-like facies.

Reflexes. Rest the patient's elbows on the bed/armrests, ensuring that he/she is completely relaxed, and fold both hands in front of the patient such that elbows are slightly flexed and left and right are symmetrical. In this position, test biceps and supinator jerks. Next, holding the patient's forearm so as to support its weight, test the triceps jerk. If there is hyporeflexia, reinforce by asking the patient to clench his/her jaw on the count of three. If there is hyperreflexia, additional reflexes (e.g., pectoral, finger) can be performed, but are not necessary and do not add additional localisation value.

Pitfall: Common errors in reflex testing

> Reflex testing is a skill acquired from years of deliberate practice. Try to have a neurology consultant observe your technique at least once. Even at the PACES level, it is not uncommon to see candidates hold or swing the tendon hammer incorrectly. Some common errors include:
>
> 1. Failing to ensure that the arm is completely relaxed (i.e., its weight completely rests on another surface), which leads to artificially depressed reflexes. Ideally, the arm should be resting on a surface and not lifted up; if lifting the patient's arm is necessary (e.g., for the triceps jerk), instruct the patient to rest the weight of his/her arm completely on yours. The upper limb examination can be done with the patient either sitting in a chair or lying in a bed propped up at 45 degrees; you should be familiar with the necessary positioning in both circumstances.
> 2. Testing reflexes with the tendon in an over-stretched position (e.g., testing biceps and supinator jerk with elbow fully extended) or over-relaxed position (e.g., testing ankle jerk without first slightly flexing the knee and ankle). The elbow, knee, and ankle should all be slightly flexed when testing reflexes.
> 3. Asymmetry of left and right arm when eliciting reflexes. Both arms should be positioned symmetrically for accurate comparison.

The inverted supinator reflex

> The inverted supinator reflex has specific localisation value. It is seen in a cord lesion at C5/6, when tapping the brachioradialis tendon leads to brisk finger flexion (C8) but minimal elbow flexion (C5/6). With a C5/6 lesion, the triceps reflex (C7) will be brisk and the biceps reflex (C5/6) will be depressed. Therefore, you should only ever call a supinator reflex inverted when the biceps reflex is depressed and the triceps reflex is brisk.

Decision point. By this stage, you must be able to identify if there are (1) UMN signs (hypertonia, brisk reflexes), (2) LMN signs, or (3) evidence of extrapyramidal dysfunction. Frank hyporeflexia and hypotonia may not always be present in LMN disorders (e.g., reflexes and tone are normal in myasthenia gravis); rather, the absence of UMN signs plus the presence of wasting or fasciculations will point towards a LMN pathology.

Neurology (Limbs)

Power

Explain to the patient that you will like to see how strong he/she is. Isolate each joint and do not test at a mechanical disadvantage. The usual muscles tested are listed in Table A2.1. Identify the presence and distribution of weakness (i.e., symmetrical vs. asymmetrical, proximal vs. distal), grading power on the Medical Research Council scale out of 5. If there is any suggestion of a mononeuropathy or distal wasting/weakness, do specific tests for the medial, ulnar, and radial nerve (see Syndrome 2.8).

Table A2.1. Power testing, upper limb.

Action	Root	Nerve	Notes
Shoulder abduction	C5	Axillary	
Elbow flexion (in supination)	C6	Musculocutaneous	Elbow flexion in mid-pronation tests brachioradialis (C6, radial nerve), which is useful to distinguish C7 vs. radial nerve lesion.
Elbow extension	C7	Radial	Do not put patient at a mechanical disadvantage; test elbow flexion/extension at 90 degrees of flexion.
Wrist flexion	C6	Median, Ulnar	Do not put patient at a mechanical disadvantage; test wrist flexion/extension at neutral position.
Wrist extension	C7	Radial	
Finger flexion	C8	Median, Ulnar	Get the patient to curl his/her fingers around yours, and attempt to uncurl their fingers (this is better than 'squeeze my fingers' which does not impose resistance).
Index finger abduction	T1	Ulnar	Test the patient's first dorsal interossei against yours by placing the lateral border of your index finger's proximal phalanx against the patient's, and asking the patient to abduct his/her index finger. Repeat with little finger against little finger. Keep the wrist in slight extension, or the patient will be at a mechanical disadvantage.

Sensation

Spinothalamic tracts. Test pinprick sensation using either a neurotip or the sharp end of a bamboo skewer or toothpick. Using the forehead as a reference point, explain what you will do: *"Sir/Mdm, I will now like to test the feeling on your arms. This is a neurotip/toothpick. I am going to test this against your forehead, it should feel sharp. I am now going to test your arms. Each time I touch you, please let me know whether it feels equally sharp, or if it feels blunt or simply abnormal."* Try to exert a consistent amount of pressure — a bamboo skewer is favourable because you can gently grasp its

Table A2.2. Sensory test points, upper limb.

Location	Root	Nerve	Notes
Outer arm	C5	Axillary	
Radial forearm	C6	Musculocutaneous	
Thumb	C6	Median	If suspecting ulnar or median neuropathy, test thenar and hypothenar eminence and for a split ring finger.
Middle finger	C7	Median	
Little finger	C8	Ulnar	
Ulnar forearm	C8	Medial cutaneous of forearm	These nerves come directly from the brachial plexus
Inner arm	T1	Medial cutaneous of arm	

sides and slide your thumb and finger down. You would usually use the standard dermatomal test points (Table A2.2), but if peripheral neuropathy is suspected, it would be more impressive to test from distal to proximal to identify a glove and stocking distribution of numbness.

Dorsal columns. Test either proprioception or vibration sense. Test proprioception at the thumb, grasping the sides of the thumb (so as not to give a clue from pressure sensation), using small deflections of approximately 5–10°. Instruct the patient to tell you whether the direction of movement is up, down, or if they are not sure. Test vibration sense using a 128 Hz (not 512 Hz) tuning fork, using the forehead as reference point, and beginning at the bony prominence of the interphalangeal joint of the thumb. There are several acceptable ways to test vibration, such as placing the tuning fork for ≥8 seconds (normal if able to sense vibration after 8 seconds) or stopping the vibration with your fingers and asking the patient if the tuning fork is still vibrating (should be able to discern that vibration has stopped). If vibration sense at the thumb is impaired, it is ideal to move proximally to the next bony prominence (wrist, elbow, clavicle); however, this is not essential as the decision point is whether vibration/proprioception is affected, rather than the severity of dorsal column dysfunction.

Pitfall: Common errors in sensory testing

A number of common errors arise during sensory testing:
1. Do not use the sternum as a reference point when testing upper limb sensation. The sternum (T2-3) has a lower dermatome value than the upper limbs (C5-T1). A high cervical cord lesion leads to reduced sensation in both the sternum and upper limbs. In this situation, using the sternum as a reference point can give erroneously 'normal' sensation.
2. Communicate clearly to the patient that your intent is to check if there is any reduced sensation. An instruction of "please let me know whether you can feel it," taken literally by the patient, invites binary answers (i.e., "yes, I can feel it" or "no, I cannot feel anything"), and you will miss areas of diminished, but not absent, sensation.

(Cont'd)

3. Always test two sensory modalities. Neglecting to test dorsal columns when pinprick sensation is normal can lead to misdiagnosis, for instance, of subacute combined degeneration as simple spastic paraparesis.
4. When testing proprioception, use small deflections (5–10° is adequate). Proprioception is actually very sensitive — try it on a friend! Using overly large deflections will reduce the sensitivity of proprioception testing and lead to falsely 'normal' proprioception.

Cerebellar

Omit cerebellar testing if the patient has poor vision, or if power is less than grade 3. When testing dysmetria (past-pointing), stress the cerebellar system by ensuring that the patient's arm is fully extended to touch your finger. Look not just at whether the patient is able to accurately touch your finger, but also whether he/she misses his/her nose. When testing dysdiadochokinesia, ensure that the moving hand is lifted a good distance above the stationary palm, and *tap lightly* on the stationary palm (i.e., demonstrate smooth acceleration and deceleration). Patients with cerebellar dysfunction are not able to gauge the 'stopping point' and tend to 'overshoot', leading to a hard slap on the stationary palm — some attempt to slap hard all the time to mask this 'overshooting'.

Subsequent steps in the upper limb examination may be performed to further localise the pathology (e.g., testing for fatigability in suspected myasthenia, demonstration of additional features of Parkinsonism). This has to be tailored to pathology found so far, and is discussed in the specific clinical syndromes.

Walk-Through and Tips: Lower Limbs

Key principles of neurological testing, discussed in the upper limb section, apply here. Only additional salient points are highlighted.

Listen to the stem

As in the upper limbs, the stem can be exceptionally helpful — for example:
- Patient has longstanding weakness" → Be alert for congenital/childhood causes (e.g., hereditary motor sensory neuropathy (Charcot-Marie-Tooth), old polio, or muscular dystrophies).
- "Patient has weakness and numbness" → Prioritise a differential of neuropathy (which can lead to numbness) over myopathy or neuromuscular junction disease (in which sensation is normal).
- "Patient has stiffness. Please examine lower limbs" → this is a giveaway for spastic paraparesis.
- "Patient has unsteady gait/frequent falls" → Cerebellar dysfunction, Parkinsonism, or sensory ataxia is more likely than spastic gait.

Inspection

As with the upper limb examination, approach the patient with a warm greeting, smile, and handshake. Inspect from the foot of the bed, looking for walking aids or wheelchairs, limb splints, urinary catheters, and devices. Expose both upper and lower limbs. Look at the lower limbs for any asymmetry (shortened leg in polio), wasting, pes cavus, clawed toes, and a champagne-bottle appearance (Charcot-Marie-Tooth); observe for contractures and surgical scars (e.g., tendon release). Look at the upper limbs for wasting, fasciculation, and abnormal posturing (e.g., overt hemiparesis). Look at the face for facial droop and ptosis.

Screening tests. Ask the patient to dorsiflex both ankles. This quick screen for foot drop is valuable—unilateral foot drop will prompt you to test power in additional muscles (particularly hip abduction). We recommend assessing gait at the end because gait is tricky to interpret without a prior idea of pathology, and walking takes too long in a weak patient.

Determine UMN vs. LMN lesion

Tone. Check if the patient has any pain and explain what you are doing. Assess internal and external rotation of the hip by rolling the legs on the bed, checking knee flexion and extension slowly, then lifting the knee rapidly to catch spastic knee extensors (in a UMN lesion, lower limb extensors are more spastic than flexors). Be careful when doing this manoeuvre—previous PACES candidates have been kicked in the face by spastic lower limbs. Equally, be wary of flaccid legs that can flop back and hit the patient's gluteal region—be prepared to catch the patient's leg if so.

Clonus. Flex the knee and ankle slightly, before firmly dorsiflexing the ankle. Up to 3 beats of clonus is normal.

Reflexes. Place your arm under the patient's knee and ask the patient to put the weight of his leg on your arm. Check the knee jerk, comparing left and right. Flexing the knee and ankle slightly so as to stretch the soleus and gastrocnemius tendons (but do not over-flex), check the ankle jerk. Reinforce if reflexes are depressed.

Plantar (or Babinski) reflex. Warn the patient beforehand—"*Sir this is the blunt end of a stick, I will be using it to scratch the bottom of your foot. It may be slightly uncomfortable but should not be painful. If it is too uncomfortable tell me and I will stop.*" As you go up the lateral border of the foot, begin with only light pressure, and increase the amount of pressure as tolerated to elicit a response. A positive (abnormal) Babinski sign is an extensor or upgoing plantar response, fanning out of the toes ± ankle dorsiflexion. This is a very reliable sign of a UMN lesion, but must be distinguished from a withdrawal response (i.e., extension of all toes/ankle, especially even before you cross the forefoot).

Neurology (Limbs)

Pitfall: Plantars vs. patient welfare

> Plantar testing is uncomfortable for the patient, so aim to test plantars just once or, at most, twice. Adjust the amount of pressure applied as you go up the lateral border of the foot: decrease pressure if the patient starts to withdraw, increase if patient does not respond. Aim to cross the forefoot with the right amount of pressure to elicit a response, but not too much pressure so as to lead to a withdrawal reaction. If you can elicit neither flexor nor extensor responses after 3 or more attempts, know when to move on. Some patients simply have equivocal plantars. A candidate who makes 'too many' attempts risks being penalised for patient welfare.

At this stage, decide if there are (1) UMN signs (hypertonia, brisk reflexes, upgoing plantar response, clonus), (2) LMN signs (hypotonia, hyporeflexia), or (3) neither.

Power

Explain to the patient that you will like to see how strong he/she is. Identify the presence and distribution of weakness (Table A2.3). Always test power against gravity first (e.g., ask the patient to extend the knee) before testing against resistance. Be particularly alert to an UMN pattern of weakness; i.e., relative preservation of power in antigravity muscles (extensors in the lower limbs, compared to the flexors), which may indicate UMN pathology even if tone and reflexes are equivocal.

Table A2.3. Power testing, lower limb.

Action	Root	Nerve	Notes
Hip flexion	L2	Femoral	
Hip extension	L4-5	Inferior gluteal	Ask the patient to press his/her heel into the bed. The gluteus maximus is normally strong enough to lift the buttock off the bed.
Knee extension	L3-4	Femoral	Ensure to test with knees flexed at 90°.
Knee flexion	L5, S1	Sciatic	
Ankle dorsiflexion	L4-5	Deep peroneal	These muscles are normally very strong (as they act against a person's body weight). You should not be able to overcome them easily with your upper limbs.
Ankle plantarflexion	S1	Tibial (from sciatic)	
Toe dorsiflexion	L5	Deep peroneal	
Hip abduction	L5	Superior gluteal	Not routine; test only in foot drop. To test, lie patient on his/her side and ask him/her to abduct the leg.

Table A2.4. Sensory test points, lower limb.

Location	Root	Nerve	Notes
Mid anterior thigh	L2	Femoral nerve	
Medial knee	L3	Femoral nerve	
Medial malleolus	L4	Saphenous nerve (from femoral nerve)	
Lateral malleolus	L5	Lateral cutaneous nerve of calf (from superficial peroneal nerve)	
Dorsum of foot, first webspace	L5	Deep peroneal nerve	
Lateral border of foot	S1	Tibial nerve	Or test sole of foot

Sensation

Spinothalamic tracts. The technique and instruction is similar to the upper limb examination. Standard dermatomal test points are listed in Table A2.4; again, if you suspect peripheral neuropathy, test from distal to proximal to elicit a glove and stocking pattern.

Dorsal columns. Test either proprioception or vibration sense, using the technique described in the upper limb examination. If you suspect that the dorsal columns will be abnormal (e.g., clear-cut glove and stocking numbness), vibration may be the better test because you can go proximally from the big toe → ankle joint → patella → anterior superior iliac spine relatively quickly, to identify the level of dorsal column loss.

Pitfall: Contradicting signs

> Do not be confused by apparently contradictory signs (e.g., hypertonia, hyporeflexia, upgoing plantars) or an inconsistent sensory examination. Real patients may not always follow 'textbook' scripts. Rely on the most concrete signs first (particularly tone, plantars, clonus, reflexes) and give less weight to more subjective signs (e.g., sensation). If signs are truly mixed, present what you have found and explain what you found to be inconsistent, rather than disregarding some signs or force-fitting it into a certain script.

Cerebellar

The heel-shin test can only be done if the patient has good vision and has power greater than grade 3. If cerebellar dysfunction is suspected, tandem gait is a helpful additional test, if time permits.

Neurology (Limbs)

Gait

Before proceeding, ask if the patient is able to walk, and ask the examiner if it is safe to do so. If there is a wheelchair at the bedside, verify that the patient requires a wheelchair to mobilise, instead of cheerfully asking the patient to walk — which betrays your failure of inspection. Common gaits include a spastic gait, high-stepping gait (foot drop), waddling gait (proximal weakness), Parkinsonian gait, and ataxic gait. Stress the gait if the abnormality is not obvious (e.g., tandem gait or stand on tiptoe). Consider doing Romberg's test if there is dorsal column loss.

Subsequent steps may further localise the pathology, and are described in specific clinical syndromes. Checking the back and neck for scars is particularly important in both spastic and flaccid diplegia.

Clinical Syndromes

Interpretation of the neurological examination is very logical. Principles of localisation and key differentials do not differ whether the stem is 'examine lower limb' or 'examine upper limb'. The two universal questions are:

1. **Where is the lesion?** First decide if the pathology is in the pyramidal tracts or extrapyramidal tracts (Parkinsonism and mimics), or if it is a cerebellar problem. If it is a pyramidal tract issue, distinguish between UMN and LMN lesions, then localise the lesion further along the neuroaxis. Figures A2.1 and A2.2 provide an overview of localisation. Table A2.5 provides a precis of localising LMN lesions.
2. **What is the lesion?** Each localisation comes with specific aetiologies to consider.

This is discussed in further detail in individual clinical syndromes.

Clinical syndrome	Key features
1. Bilateral UMN (UL or LL)	UMN signs in bilateral UL/LL
	± sensory, cerebellar dysfunction
2. Unilateral UMN (UL or LL)	UMN signs in left or right UL/LL
	± sensory, cerebellar dysfunction
3. Mixed UMN and LMN signs	UMN signs with wasting ± fasciculation, or bizarre distribution of UMN signs
4. LMN + normal sensation	Any distribution of weakness
	LMN signs
	Normal sensation
5. LMN + abnormal sensation	LMN signs
	Sensory loss ± Charcot foot

(Cont'd)

Clinical syndrome	Key features
6. Foot drop	Weak ankle dorsiflexion on screening
	High steppage/circumducting gait
7. Finger/wrist drop*	Weak wrist flexion on screening
8. Claw hand*	Unilateral weak/wasted/clawed hand
9. Cerebellar signs only	Stem: difficulty walking, falls rather than weakness
	Scanning speech, upward rebound in pronator drift
	Unilateral or bilateral cerebellar signs
	No weakness or sensory loss
10. Parkinsonism only*	Mask-like facies, hypophonic speech
	Pill-rolling rest tremor
	Cogwheel and leadpipe rigidity
	No weakness or sensory loss

*These syndromes tend to come with a 'examine the upper limbs' stem rather than a 'examine lower limbs' stem.

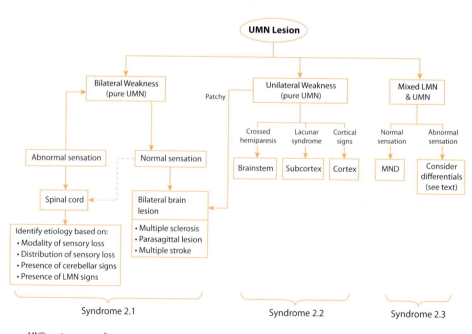

MND: motor neuron disease

Figure A2.1. Localisation overview for UMN lesions.

Neurology (Limbs)

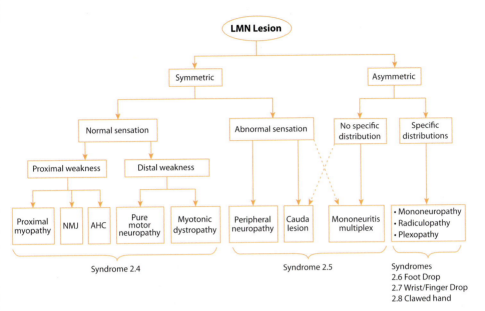

AHC: anterior horn cell; NMJ: neuromuscular junction

Figure A2.2. Localisation overview for LMN lesions.

Table A2.5. Precis of localisation in LMN lesions.

Lesion	Prototype	Distribution of weakness	Sensation	Distinguishing features
AHC	Motor neuron disease	Proximal or distal	Normal	Fasciculations. Mixed UMN signs in MND
Root and plexus	Radiculopathy	Myotomal	Dermatomal loss	Asymmetric
Peripheral nerve	Diabetic neuropathy	Distal	Symmetrical glove and stocking loss	
Mono-neuropathy	Carpel tunnel syndrome	In distribution of nerve	In distribution of nerve	Asymmetric
NMJ	Myasthenia gravis	Distal	Normal	Fatigability
Muscle	Dermatomyositis	Mostly proximal. Distal in myotonic dystrophy	Normal	Some myopathies have pathognomic features

Neurology (Limbs) – Clinical Syndromes

2.1 | Bilateral UMN Signs

Spastic paraparesis/quadriparesis usually localises to the spinal cord. Cord lesions often affect sensation, with each cord lesion leading to a unique pattern of sensory involvement. Certain entities (we think of them as "spastic paraparesis plus" syndromes) display additional features e.g., cerebellar dysfunction or peripheral neuropathy. For a brain lesion to cause hemiparesis, bilateral hemispheres must be involved (e.g., a parasagittal lesion, multifocal demyelination, or strokes). Sensation is typically normal unless the brainstem is involved or the brain lesion is large enough to affect both motor and sensory areas.

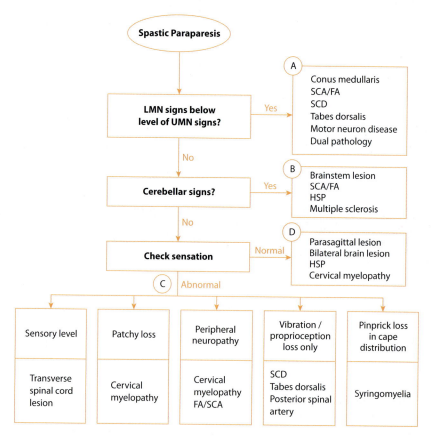

FA: Friedreich's ataxia; HSP: hereditary spastic paraparesis; SCA: spinocerebellar ataxia; SCD: subacute combined degeneration

Figure A2.3. Localisation of spastic paraparesis.

Where is the Lesion

The approach to spastic paraparesis begins with recognising bilateral UMN signs. Once you notice bilateral hypertonia, ankle clonus >3 beats, hyperreflexia, upgoing plantars, or an UMN pattern of weakness (flexors stronger than extensors in upper limbs, and/or extensors stronger than flexors in lower limbs), enter the algorithm for spastic paraparesis (Figure A2.3).

Conceptually it is important to distinguish between a *motor level* and the entity of *'mixed UMN and LMN signs'* (Table A2.6). In either entity, *both* UMN and LMN signs are observed, but the distribution differs.

Table A2.6. Motor level vs. Mixed UMN and LMN signs.

	Motor level	Mixed UMN and LMN signs
Pathology	Cord lesion at a specific level. This can be traumatic, degenerative, neoplastic, infective, or so on.	Pathology affecting both corticospinal tracts (hence UMN) and anterior horn cells or peripheral nerves (hence LMN). See below for examples.
Signs	LMN at level of lesion. UMN below level of lesion. Normal above level of lesion.	To be certain that the signs reflect a 'mixed' picture and not motor level, LMN signs must appear at or below the level of UMN signs.
Example	A C6 cord lesion leads to depressed biceps jerk (C5/6), brisk triceps jerk (C7), and UMN signs in the lower limbs.	Upgoing plantars and absent ankle jerks in a conus medullaris lesion.

Power testing confirms bilateral weakness and can help to localise the LMN level.

Cerebellar examination (including tandem gait in lower limb) is next (as long as power ≥3). Spine lesions alone do not cause cerebellar signs. Bilateral cerebellar signs with spastic paraparesis can be explained by a brainstem lesion, which affects both cerebellum and descending corticospinal tracts, or by a "spastic paraparesis plus" syndrome.

Sensation. Both pinprick (spinothalamic tract) and vibration/proprioception (dorsal columns) must be tested. If the lower limbs are affected but upper limbs are spared, check sensation going up the thoracic dermatomes to identify a sensory level at which sensation becomes normal again. Consider the modality and distribution of sensory loss:

- Clear sensory level (transverse cord lesion).
- Patchy distribution of sensory loss (cervical myelopathy).
- Peripheral neuropathy pattern (Friedreich's ataxia, spinocerebellar ataxia).

- Isolated loss of vibration/proprioception sense (posterior spinal cord lesion).
- Isolated loss of pinprick sensation in a 'cape-like' distribution over C5-8 dermatomes (syringomyelia).
- Completely normal sensation.

Scars. For spastic paraparesis cases, always examine the back and neck for a scar!

Localisation groups

Four localisation groups are discussed in the subsequent pages:

A. Spastic paraparesis with mixed LMN signs.
B. Spastic paraparesis with cerebellar signs.
C. Spastic paraparesis with sensory loss (normal cerebellar, no LMN signs).
D. Spastic paraparesis alone (normal sensation, normal cerebellar, no LMN signs).

What is the Lesion (A): Spastic Paraparesis + Mixed LMN Signs

This situation confuses many. It really isn't so complicated — all it means is that both spine and peripheral nerves are affected by the same or concomitant pathologies.

1. Sensation affected

Single pathology:

- **Conus medullaris lesion**: particularly if there is a history of back pain, a lower back scar, or early urinary dysfunction.
- **Spinocerebellar ataxia**[1], **Friedreich's ataxia**[2]: young patients with spastic paraparesis, cerebellar signs, ± peripheral neuropathy, often with signs of chronicity.
- **Subacute combined degeneration**: B12 deficiency affects the descending corticospinal tracts, dorsal columns, and peripheral nerves. Either dorsal column involvement or peripheral neuropathy may be more prominent.
- **Tabes dorsalis (syphilis)**: uncommon nowadays.

---

[1] Spinocerebellar ataxia/degeneration: A hereditary disorder with multiple subtypes and inheritance patterns. In addition to progressive corticospinal and cerebellar degeneration, additional features vary with the subtype and may include peripheral neuropathy, extrapyramidal and autonomic dysfunction, developmental delay, and cognitive impairment.

[2] Friedreich's ataxia: an autosomal recessive trinucleotide repeat disorder. Its onset is in the teenage years and patients are unable to walk by their 20s. Apart from upper motor neuron and cerebellar features, patients may have dorsal column loss, peripheral neuropathy, reduced vision and hearing, and bladder dysfunction. Associations include scoliosis, cognitive impairment, hypertrophic obstructive cardiomyopathy, and diabetes. There is no treatment. Mean life expectancy is 37 years.

Neurology (Limbs)

Dual pathology: many combinations of UMN disease + LMN disease are possible. Common examples include cervical myelopathy + diabetic polyneuropathy, and cervical myelopathy + lumbar radiculopathy.

2. Sensation normal

- **Motor neuron disease** (use the euphemism 'anterior horn cell disease'). Look for prominent fasciculations and wasting. This is discussed further in Syndrome 2.3.
- Any of the above causes (sensory involvement can be mild and undetectable).

What is the Lesion (B): Spastic Paraparesis + Cerebellar Signs

Spastic paraparesis and bilateral cerebellar signs localises to either:
- A brainstem lesion, which affects both cerebellum and descending corticospinal tracts (these are in close proximity and share the same vascular supply), or
- A "spastic paraparesis plus" syndrome.

1. **Brainstem lesions**: look closely for cranial nerve involvement (or offer to examine cranial nerves at the end)
    - Multiple sclerosis – can cause spastic paraparesis with cerebellar signs by either (i) brainstem lesion or (ii) lesions separated in space (spine + cerebellum).
    - Brainstem infarct.
    - Space-occupying lesion (e.g., tumour, abscess).

2. **Spastic paraparesis plus syndrome**:
    - **Spinocerebellar ataxia, Friedreich's ataxia**: young patients with spastic paraparesis, cerebellar signs, ± peripheral neuropathy, often with signs of chronicity.
    - **Hereditary spastic paraplegia**[3]: young to middle-aged patients, lower limbs more affected than upper limbs. Some variants have cerebellar signs. Sensation may be spared or mildly affected.

---

[3] Hereditary spastic paraplegia: a genetic syndrome with variable inheritance (most commonly autosomal dominant). It is characterised by length-dependent degeneration of corticospinal tracts (hence lower limbs are more affected than upper limbs). Some patients have cerebellar signs, while others may have mild sensory defects.

What is the Lesion (C): Spastic Paraparesis + Sensory Loss

The pattern and modality of sensory loss is diagnostically critical.

1. Clear sensory level

Key signs

- Bilateral sensory loss.
- Sensory level (e.g., ↓ up to T10/umbilicus, normal above).
- May have urinary disturbance (e.g., patient on urinary catheter)[4].
- ± Back scar.

This suggests a **transverse spinal cord lesion** which may be due to:

- Trauma.
- Neoplastic (metastases, lymphoma, meningioma).
- Infective (e.g., abscess).
- Inflammatory (transverse myelitis; e.g., multiple sclerosis, viral infection).
- Vascular (e.g., vasculitis, spinal artery thrombosis).
- Degenerative (very common in cervical and lumbar spine, unlikely in thoracic spine).

2. Patchy bilateral sensory loss

The key differential here is **cervical myelopathy**. This tends to cause a non-specific 'gloves and socks' distribution of sensory loss. However, it can be quite variable and patchy.

Additional signs that may be seen in cervical myelopathy include:

- Finger escape sign (deficient adduction of ulnar 2 fingers).
- Positive Hoffman's sign.
- Slow grip and release.
- Unsteady lower limb gait (sensory ataxia from dorsal column dysfunction).

---

[4] There are differences in the presentation of extramedullary (e.g., spondylosis, metastases) vs. intramedullary spinal lesions (e.g., syringomyelia). Making this distinction is generally not expected in PACES.

3. Peripheral neuropathy pattern

In distal > proximal sensory loss, consider:
- Patchy sensory loss as in cervical myelopathy.
- Friedreich's ataxia, spinocerebellar ataxia.
- Dual pathology (e.g., cervical myelopathy plus diabetic neuropathy).

4. Isolated loss of vibration and proprioception sense

This is a lesion that affects only the posterior spinal cord, i.e.:
- Subacute combined degeneration of the cord.
- Tabes dorsalis.
- Posterior spinal artery occlusion.
- Less likely: Multiple sclerosis.
  Cervical myelopathy.
  Friedreich's ataxia/spinocerebellar ataxia.

5. Isolated loss of pinprick sensation in a 'cape like' distribution (over C5-8 dermatomes)

This is pathognomic of **syringomyelia**, in which decussating spinothalamic tracts are affected by an enlarging syrinx, but sparing the dorsal columns. There may be asymmetry to the 'cape' distribution (i.e., one side more significantly affected than the other). The syrinx may extend into the lower brainstem causing Horner's syndrome, bulbar palsy, facial numbness, and ataxia.

What is the Lesion (D): Spastic Paraparesis Alone

With normal sensation, a cord lesion is less likely as it would be unusual to affect only descending motor tracts but not sensory tracts. Key differentials are:

Mainly lower limbs affected
- Parasagittal brain lesion (e.g., meningioma; recall that the lower limbs are in the parasagittal region of the motor homunculus).
- Hereditary spastic paraparesis (particularly if longstanding from young).

Affects both lower and upper limbs, or only lower limbs
- Bilateral cortical lesion (e.g., multifocal strokes or demyelination).
- Cerebral palsy.
- Cervical myelopathy remains a consideration as sensory involvement can be patchy.

The features of the causes of spastic paraparesis are summarised in Table A2.7.

Table A2.7. Spastic paraparesis: aetiologies and features.

Lesion		Sensory loss	LMN signs	Cerebellar signs
"Whole" cord lesion	Transverse cord lesion	All modalities below level		-
	Conus medullaris*	All modalities below level	At level of lesion	-
	Cervical myelopathy	Patchy sensory loss		-
	Multiple sclerosis with transverse myelitis	Below level of transverse myelitis		If brainstem involved
Focal cord lesion	Subacute combined degeneration	Dorsal column loss ± peripheral neuropathy	-	-
	Tabes dorsalis	Dorsal column loss	-	-
	Posterior spinal artery occlusion			
	Syringomyelia	Pinprick loss in cape-like distribution	At level of syrinx	-
"Spastic paraparesis plus" syndromes	Friedreich's ataxia	Peripheral neuropathy is prominent		Common
	Spinocerebellar ataxia	May have peripheral neuropathy		Common
	Hereditary spastic paraparesis*	Peripheral neuropathy/sensory findings usually absent or mild.		Some variants
Brain	Brainstem lesion	Variable	-	Common
	Parasagittal lesion*	-	-	-
	Bilateral cortical lesions	-	-	-
Others	Motor neuron disease	-	Diffuse	-

*Affects lower limbs only, upper limbs spared.

Look for Complications

Look for complications, particularly:
- Mobility – comment on the presence of any walking aid, motorised wheelchair, and fall risk.
- Urinary function – comment on the use of urinary catheters or diapers.

Neurology (Limbs)

Requests

Requests will depend on the clinical suspicion, for example:

- *Suspect multiple sclerosis*: examine cranial nerves for relative afferent pupillary defect, internuclear ophthalmoplegia, and fundoscopy for optic neuritis.
- *Suspect congenital cause*: take a family history or examine the patient's family members.
- *Suspect spinal cord lesion*: doing a per-rectal examination for saddle anaesthesia, examining the back for any scar (if not already done), and examining the upper limbs for a level (if not done).
- *Suspect subacute combined degeneration*: taking a nutritional history and checking the conjunctivae for pallor.
- *Suspect Friedreich's ataxia*: doing cardiovascular examination for hypertrophic cardiomyopathy, doing blood glucose for diabetes, and examining the spine for scoliosis.

Scripts

Spastic paraparesis plus syndrome

This young gentleman has spastic paraparesis. Both lower limbs are wasted with pes cavus deformity. There are upper motor neuron signs of hypertonia, clonus, brisk knee and ankle jerks, and upgoing plantars. Power is 3/5 proximally and distally. There is peripheral loss of pinprick sensation. He is unable to walk and has a wheelchair at the bedside. There is no urinary catheter and he is not on diapers. In summary, this young man has spastic paraparesis and peripheral neuropathy. Differentials include spinocerebellar ataxia and Friedreich's ataxia, and I will also like to rule out a conus medullaris lesion and subacute combined degeneration.

This patient is likely to also have cerebellar dysfunction, but you will not be able to do cerebellar testing in the lower limbs with a power of ≤ 3. Consider checking for cerebellar signs in the upper limbs. If sensory loss is very mild, hereditary spastic paraplegia is also a possible differential.

Transverse spinal cord lesion

This middle-aged lady has spastic paraparesis. She has bilateral upper motor neuron weakness with hypertonia, clonus, brisk knee and ankle reflexes, and upgoing plantars. There is a sensory level at the nipples and the upper limb reflexes are normal. Cerebellar examination is normal. She is able to walk with the aid of a quad-stick and does not have evidence of urinary dysfunction. The clinical localisation is a thoracic spinal cord lesion, probably at T4. There is no back scar to suggest prior trauma or instrumentation. Possible aetiologies include neoplastic lesions, abscess, transverse myelitis, or a vascular process.

A degenerative process is uncommon in the thoracic spine and should not be offered here.

Cervical myelopathy

This elderly gentleman has a depressed biceps reflex, brisk triceps reflex, and inverted supinator jerk. Upper limb power is 3/5 in shoulder abduction, elbow flexion, and wrist extension (C5/C6), and 4/5 in elbow extension, finger flexion, and abduction (C7 and below). There is minimal sensory loss. I also note a positive Hoffman sign and a surgical scar on the posterior neck. The clinical localisation is to the cervical spine at the C5/6 level. Differentials include cervical myelopathy, spinal trauma, neoplasm, abscess, transverse myelitis, and vascular lesions at that level, for which he has undergone surgery.

Neurology (Limbs)

Neurology (Limbs) – Clinical Syndromes

2.2 | Unilateral UMN Signs

Spastic hemiplegia localises to the contralateral brain or brainstem and is most commonly due to a cerebrovascular accident. This is usually considered too easy for PACES, but you still might get a case pulled from the ward and would be expected to perform to a high level.

Where is the Lesion

Recognise unilateral weakness with UMN signs. After completing the standard limb examination, proceed to screen the cranial nerves (e.g., check for facial droop, screen eye movements, and check speech — you will not be able to do a full cranial nerve examination) and for cortical signs (line bisection is a good quick screen.

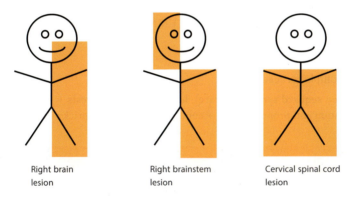

Figure A2.4. Conceptual distribution of weakness in UMN lesions.

You should be able to describe the syndrome (e.g., a lacunar syndrome, partial anterior circulation syndrome, focal cortical syndrome). Localisation hinges on the presence of:

- **Cerebellar signs**.
- **Cranial neuropathy**. Recall that cortical lesions lead to contralateral limb and cranial nerve deficits, while brainstem lesions lead to crossed hemiparesis (affects ipsilateral uncrossed cranial nerve nuclei, and descending corticospinal fibres that cross to supply the contralateral limbs) (Figure A2.4). Be able to distinguish between a UMN vs. LMN CN VII palsy (page 98).
- **Cortical signs** (e.g., hemineglect, gaze preference, abnormal line bisection).

	LEFT hemiparesis with...	Localisation
1. **Crossed hemiparesis**	RIGHT CN III palsy	RIGHT midbrain
	RIGHT CN VI or LMN VII palsy	RIGHT pons
	RIGHT CN XII palsy (tongue deviates to right)	RIGHT medulla
2. **Ipsilateral CN palsy**	LEFT UMN CN VII palsy	RIGHT subcortex/cortex
3. **Hemispheric syndrome**[5]	LEFT hemineglect	RIGHT cortex[6]
4. **Lacunar syndromes**[7]		
– ataxic hemiparesis	LEFT dysmetria	RIGHT subcortex
– sensorimotor	LEFT numbness	RIGHT subcortex
– pure motor	(nothing else)	RIGHT subcortex
5. **Focal cortical syndrome**	Focal left UMN weakness e.g., pure wrist weakness	RIGHT subcortex/cortex (classically embolic)

6. **Other considerations**

   - Patchy UMN weakness or multiple UMN deficits that do not fit into a single lesion:
     - Multiple sclerosis.
     - Multiple cortical strokes.
   - Brown sequard syndrome (rare): left spastic hemiparesis + ipsilateral loss of vibration and proprioception + contralateral loss of pinprick sensation.

What is the Lesion

Not every hemiparesis is a stroke! The key to identifying aetiology is the time course of symptoms, but this is something that you will not be able to elicit in a physical examination station. Consider:

1. **Differentials to a cerebrovascular accident**

   - Inflammatory (e.g., multiple sclerosis).
   - Neoplastic.
   - Infective (e.g., abscess).

---

[5] You are unlikely to get a total anterior circulation syndrome (i.e., dense middle cerebral artery infarct) as such patients cannot cooperate with clinical examination.

[6] The lower limbs may be relatively spared in a cortical lesion, as the lower limb homunculus lies in the anterior cerebral artery territory.

[7] The naming convention is confusing. Hemispheric syndromes are named according to the side of the infarct (right hemispheric syndrome = right middle cerebral artery infarct with left-sided weakness), but lacunar syndromes are named according to the side of deficit (left ataxic hemiparesis = right brain lacunar stroke with left-sided weakness).

Neurology (Limbs)

2. **Mechanism of cerebrovascular infarct**
   - Haemorrhagic
   - Ischaemic
     - Cardioembolic — irregularly irregular pulse
     - Artery-to-artery embolism — carotid bruit
     - Large vessel disease
     - Small vessel disease — capillary glucose marks, request blood pressure
       — proxy markers for cardiovascular disease (e.g., sternotomy scar, lower limb amputations)

Look for Complications

Consider patient's function in terms of:
- Fine motor tasks (e.g., whether patient is able to button shirt or use a handphone).
- Mobility — use of walking aid or wheelchair.
- Swallowing — use of nasogastric tube.
- Urinary function — requirement for urinary catheter or diapers.

Sample Scripts

Ataxic hemiparesis

This elderly gentleman has left-sided weakness with left-sided hypertonia, brisk reflexes, and dysmetria. He ambulates with a walking stick and a spastic gait. Sensation is normal. There are no cortical signs. This is a left ataxic hemiparesis syndrome which localises to the right subcortical region, although right brainstem is also possible. Possible aetiologies include infarct, haemorrhage, demyelination, neoplasm, or abscess. I note he is in atrial fibrillation, which may be the underlying mechanism of stroke. I will like to complete my examination by checking blood pressure, urine dipstick for glycosuria, and examining the cardiovascular system.

Crossed hemiparesis

This middle-aged lady has left-sided weakness, left-sided hypertonia, brisk reflexes, and loss of pinprick sensation. She also has a right lower motor neuron CN VII palsy affecting the upper and lower face. There are no cerebellar signs or cortical signs. This is a crossed hemiparesis syndrome and the localisation is to the right pons. Possible aetiologies of the lesion include infarct, haemorrhage, demyelination, neoplasm, or abscess. Incidentally I note a saphenous vein graft scar, which is suggestive of cardiovascular disease. I would like to complete my examination by checking the rest of the cranial nerves and examining the pulse for atrial fibrillation.

Neurology (Limbs) – Clinical Syndromes

2.3 | Mixed UMN and LMN Signs

This is case is confusing to the uninitiated, but easy once you know what to look for. Be sure to distinguish 'mixed UMN and LMN signs' from a UMN level (Table A2.6).

Where is the Lesion

There are two distinct syndromes with true mixed UMN and LMN signs — (1) a pathology that affects both spine and peripheral nerves, and (2) motor neuron disease. Sensation is the key to distinguish between the two.

Sensation abnormal

These conditions tend to present as spastic paraparesis plus features of peripheral neuropathy (depressed ankle jerks, distal sensory loss) and are discussed further on page 32. A brief list includes:

- Conus medullaris lesion.
- Subacute combined degeneration.
- Tabes dorsalis (syphilis).
- Spinocerebellar ataxia, Friedreich's ataxia.
- Dual pathology (e.g., cervical myelopathy with diabetic neuropathy).

Sensation normal

This is suggestive of motor neuron disease. The classic picture of amyotrophic lateral sclerosis (ALS), one of the more commonly encountered types of motor neuron disease, is:

- Mixed UMN and LMN signs *in the same segment* (e.g., wasting and brisk reflexes in the same limb). Note that there are pure UMN and pure LMN variants of ALS[8].
- Distribution is often asymmetrical, and may not resemble spastic paraparesis.
- Prominent fasciculations in the limbs and tongue (remember to look in the mouth).
- Absolutely normal sensation.

---

[8] Variants of ALS:
– Pure UMN variant – primary lateral sclerosis
– Pure LMN variant – progressive muscular atrophy
– Cranial nerve dominant variant – progressive bulbar palsy

Neurology (Limbs)

What is the Lesion

Motor neuron disease is a diagnosis of exclusion. Differentials must be considered — especially in cases with predominant LMN or UMN signs.

Differentials to motor neuron disease with a predominantly lower motor neuron picture: (these differentials do not strictly have mixed UMN and LMN signs)

- **Multifocal motor neuropathy**: patchy, asymmetrical LMN weakness; does not always obey the distal > proximal pattern of a neuropathy.
- **Neuralgic amyotrophy** (Parsonage-Turner syndrome, Brachial neuritis): acute-onset of pain and patchy weakness of the upper and/or middle brachial plexus, with or without sensory involvement.
- **Spinobulbar muscular atrophy** (Kennedy's disease): gradual progression, without UMN signs, associated with endocrinopathies and gynaecomastia.
- **Monomyelic amyotrophy** (Hirayama disease): localised anterior horn cell disease; usually a young Asian male with wasting and LMN weakness limited to a single limb, which develops over 5 years and then plateaus.

Differentials to motor neuron disease with a predominantly upper motor neuron picture: (these differentials do not strictly have mixed UMN and LMN signs)

Differentials: predominant UMN

- **Hereditary spastic paraparesis**: spastic paraparesis ± urinary dysfunction.
- **Multiple sclerosis**: check for unilateral cranial nerve and cerebellar signs, which are less likely in ALS.

Look for Complications

Consider patient's function in terms of:
- Fine motor tasks (e.g., whether patient is able to button shirt or use a handphone).
- Mobility – use of walking aid or wheelchair.
- Swallowing – use of nasogastric tube, gastrostomy tube.
- Urinary function – requirement for urinary catheter or diapers.

Sample Scripts

Motor neuron disease

This middle-aged gentleman has mixed upper and lower motor neuron signs. His left lower limb and right upper limb are wasted and fasciculating, yet showing UMN signs of hypertonia, brisk reflexes, and upgoing plantars. Power is 2/5 in the left lower limb and 3/5 in the right upper limb. The tongue is fasciculating at rest. Sensation is normal. I was unable to examine the cerebellar system due to weakness. The diagnosis is anterior horn cell disease. Functionally, he is still able to use a handphone with his left hand, which is his dominant hand, and he ambulates with a motorised wheelchair. There is no evidence of a nasogastric or gastrostomy tube.

Use 'anterior horn cell disease' as a euphemism in front of the patient.

Neurology (Limbs) – Clinical Syndromes

2.4 | LMN Signs + Normal Sensation

This case requires the candidate to go beyond the standard upper or lower limb examination routine to look for additional features suggestive of specific conditions (Figure A2.5). It can be very easy (e.g., if one screens for grip myotonia in all upper limb cases and clinches the diagnosis right at the start) or very difficult (e.g., if one forgets to test fatigability and completely misses a case of myasthenia). A few tips are all it takes to make 80% of these cases 'very easy'!

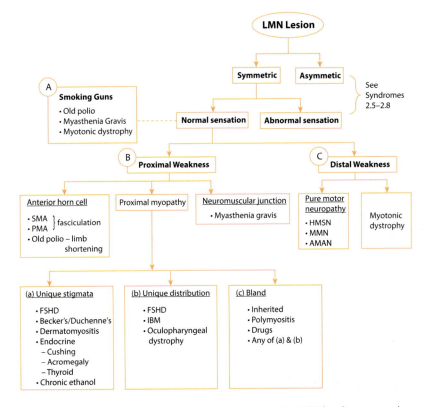

AMAN: acute motor axonal neuropathy; FSHD: facio-scapulo-humeral dystrophy; HMSN: hereditary motor and sensory neuropathy; IBM: inclusion body myositis; MMN: multifocal motor neuropathy; PMA: progressive muscular atrophy; SMA: spinal muscular atrophy

Figure A2.5. Localisation of LMN signs with normal sensation.

Where is the Lesion

LMN weakness with absolutely normal sensation localises to the neuromuscular junction, muscle, anterior horn cell, and occasionally a pure motor neuropathy.

Tip: Relatively preserved reflexes

> Reflexes may seem relatively 'normal' in some of these cases. Tendon reflexes are usually depressed in demyelinating neuropathies (which tend to be diffuse), but proximal reflexes may be relatively spared in axonal neuropathies (which are length dependant). Reflexes may also be preserved in myopathies and neuromuscular junction lesions.

'Smoking gun' quick screen routine

We suggest this quick screen for old polio, myasthenia gravis, and myotonic dystrophy in all cases of LMN weakness with normal sensation. These signs are quick to elicit, lead to one clear diagnosis, and are common in PACES.

- **Inspect the limb** for a shortened, wasted limb (old polio).
- **Inspect the face** for bilateral ptosis (myasthenia or myotonic dystrophy), facial diplegia (myotonic dystrophy), and frontal balding (myotonic dystrophy).
- **Check for fatigability** (myasthenia gravis):
  - Eyes: use prolonged upward or lateral gaze (>20 seconds); if the eyes are beginning to droop but very slowly, hold up one eyelid with a finger (this counters frontalis activity and leads to the contralateral eye drooping more rapidly).
  - Limbs: test bilateral shoulder abduction power, which should be symmetrical. Have the patient rapidly adduct and abduct one shoulder 20 times, then retest shoulder abduction, comparing the power of the fatigued and non-fatigued side.
- **Check for myotonia** (myotonic dystrophy):
  - Grip myotonia (if not previously done): have the patient make a tight fist, and then release quickly. Difficulty unclenching the fist suggests grip myotonia (myotonic dystrophy).
  - Percussion myotonia: percuss the thenar eminence over a finger, then quickly remove the finger (continuing to applying pressure on the thenar eminence may prevent visualisation of percussion myotonia).

'Smoking gun' negative

After excluding these obvious diagnoses, consider if weakness is proximal or distal:
- Symmetrical proximal weakness, after ruling out old polio and myasthenia gravis, localises to anterior horn cell disease or myopathies.
- Symmetrical distal weakness suggests a distal myopathy, pure motor neuropathy, or anterior horn cell disease.

What is the Lesion (A): Smoking Guns

1. Old poliomyelitis

Key features are:
- Stem may be suggestive of a childhood or longstanding illness.
- Limb shortening and wasting.
- May have contractures or other signs of chronicity.
- Fasciculations are not commonly seen.
- LMN signs.
- Normal sensation.

2. Myotonic dystrophy

The critical step is to test for grip and percussion myotonia. Key features (not all may be present) include:
- **Distal** weakness (in Type 1[9]) with normal tone and normal/reduced reflexes.
- Myopathic facies: frontal balding, bilateral ptosis, bilateral facial droop, temporalis and masseter wasting.
- Myotonia: ocular (difficulty opening eyes after firm closure), grip, and percussion.
- Normal sensation and cerebellar function.

3. Myasthenia gravis

Key features may include:
- Proximal > distal weakness with normal tone and normal/reduced reflexes.
- Bilateral ptosis.
- Fatigability of eyes, limbs, and speech.
- Normal sensation and cerebellar function.

What is the Lesion (B): Proximal Weakness

Having ruled out polio and myasthenia gravis, symmetric proximal LMN weakness with normal sensation generally localises to:
- Anterior horn cell: spinomuscular atrophy, progressive muscular atrophy, and differentials.
- Myopathies: congenital, inflammatory, endocrine, and drug-induced.

---

[9] Weakness may be proximal in Type 2 myotonic dystrophy, which is less common.

The strategy to distinguish between specific aetiologies is to:

- Look for unique peripheral stigmata — mainly through careful inspection of the face, neck/chest, and hands.
- Pay attention to distinctive patterns of weakness.
- Then consider the remaining causes that present relatively 'bland' with no unique peripheral stigmata or distribution of weakness.

1. Unique peripheral stigmata

These conditions present with LMN proximal weakness, normal sensation, and unique peripheral stigmata. In addition to proximal weakness with normal sensation, distinguishing features include:

Anterior horn cell disease including (see Syndrome 2.3)
- Progressive muscular atrophy
- Spinal muscular atrophy
- Monomyelic amyotrophy
- Spinobulbar muscular atrophy

- Prominent fasciculations of limbs and tongue.

Myopathies

(a) **Facio-scapulo-humeral dystrophy (FSHD)**
- Overriding scapula (viewed from front) with polyhill sign (selective wasting of biceps and trapezius, preservation of deltoids).
- Winging of scapula (viewed from back).
- Facial weakness without ptosis.
- ± Bilateral foot drop (weakness is distal in lower limbs, but proximal in upper limbs).

(b) **Dermatomyositis**
- Rashes: heliotrope, photosensitive rash in shawl distribution.
- Hands: Gottron's papules, mechanics hands.

(c) **Endocrine causes**
- Cushing's syndrome with steroid myopathy – central obesity, skin thinning, supraclavicular adiposity, abdominal striae.
- Hyper/hypothyroidism – goitre, tremor.
- Acromegaly – spade-like hands, coarse facial features.

(d) **Chronic ethanol use**
- Unique stigmata: dupuytren's contracture, parotidomegaly.
- Other features of chronic liver disease.

(e) **Becker's/Duchenne's muscular dystrophy**
- Calf hypertrophy (unlikely in PACES).

2. Distinctive patterns of weakness

Most of these causes lead to proximal upper and lower limb weakness with none or mild facial involvement.

There are however some with distinctive patterns of weakness:

Differential

(a) Upper limbs: Proximal weakness
 Lower limbs: Distal weakness (often with foot drop)

FSHD

(b) Upper limbs: Distal weakness (forearm flexors)
 Lower limbs: Proximal weakness (thigh extensors)

Inclusion body myositis

(c) Prominent ocular/facial weakness

Occulopharyngeal dystrophy
FSHD
Anterior horn cell disease

3. Bland aetiologies

Aetiologies that present relatively 'bland' with no unique peripheral stigmata and proximal weakness in both upper/lower limbs include:

- Inherited: limb girdle muscular dystrophy, mitochondrial myopathies.
- Inflammatory: Polymyositis.
- Metabolic/drugs: Drug-induced myopathy (e.g., steroids, statins, colchicine, chloroquine, cyclosporine).
- Any of the previous causes, as unique stigmata may not be obvious.

What is the Lesion (C): Distal Weakness

Symmetric distal LMN weakness with normal sensation generally localises to a pure motor neuropathy, distal myopathy, or anterior horn cell disease.

(a) **Pure motor neuropathy**
 - Hereditary motor sensory neuropathy (one variant of Charcot-Marie-Tooth disease): prominent features of chronicity (e.g., inverted champagne bottle appearance (distal wasting) with pes cavus, clawing of toes, and achilles tendon contracture).
 - Multifocal motor neuropathy: often a patchy distribution.
 - Acute motor axonal neuropathy (AMAN): a pure motor variant of Guillain-Barré syndrome which presents acutely.

(b) **Distal myopathy**   i.e., myotonic dystrophy — look again for it!

(c) **Anterior horn cell disease**   can also lead to distal weakness

Look for Complications

Finish off by looking for complications.

1. **Comment on patient's function, for example**:
   - Mobility – use of walking aid or wheelchair.
   - Fine motor tasks (especially in distal weakness).
   - Swallowing – use of nasogastric tube, gastrostomy tube.
2. **Comment on respiratory muscle function**
   - Respiratory muscle weakness, especially in myasthenia gravis and myopathies
     > Consider checking neck flexion and counting from 1 to 20

     Obviously a patient with impending respiratory failure will not be in PACES.
3. **Look for extra-neurological complications**

   For example, in myotonic dystrophy, look for:
   - Cataracts — visual problems, previous cataract surgery
   - Cardiomyopathy — implantable cardiac device
   - Hypogonadism — gynaecomastia and testicular atrophy
   - Endocrinopathy — smooth diffuse goitre, glucose check marks

Sample Scripts

Myotonic dystrophy

This middle-aged gentleman has myotonic dystrophy. There is myotonic facies with frontal balding, facial diplegia, and bilateral ptosis. The limb examination is significant for distal weakness, as well as grip and percussion myotonia. Sensation and cerebellar function is normal. Functionally he is ambulant with a stick and has an endoscopic gastrostomy tube. In terms of extra-neurological manifestations, I notice an implantable cardiac device and a small goitre. I will like to complete my examination by asking for a family history and examining the cardiovascular system.

Comment: Grip and percussion myotonia are signs specific to myotonic dystrophy. If these were clear cut, you may wish to state the diagnosis upfront.

Myasthenia gravis

This young lady has myasthenia gravis. She has bilateral, fatigable proximal weakness in the upper limbs with normal sensation. I also note bilateral fatigable ptosis with non-conforming ophthalmoplegia (see Syndrome 3.1) and a midline sternotomy scar suggesting previous thymectomy. Functionally she is able to walk without aid. There is no weakness of neck flexion or inability to count to 20, which would have made me concerned about respiratory muscle weakness.

Myopathy, no clear specific aetiology

This middle-aged gentleman has symmetrical proximal weakness in the upper limbs, with reduced tone, reflexes, and intact sensation. Cerebellar function is normal. The clinical localisation is to the muscle. There is no fatigability to suggest neuromuscular junction disease. There are no fasciculations to suggest anterior horn cell disease. Multifocal motor neuropathy is less likely as the weakness is very symmetrical.

In terms of aetiology of muscle disease, there is no overriding scapula to suggest facioscapulohumeral dystrophy, no rash or Gottron's papules to suggest dermatomyositis, and no obvious endocrinopathy such as Cushing's syndrome. Possible aetiologies include inherited muscular dystrophies such as limb girdle muscular dystrophy or inflammatory conditions (e.g., polymyositis, drug-induced). I will like to take a history for drugs and ethanol use, as well as ask about any family history of muscle problems. Functionally he is able to walk without aid.

Neurology (Limbs) – Clinical Syndromes

2.5 | LMN Signs + Distal Numbness

The patient with symmetrical LMN distal weakness with distal numbness almost always has peripheral neuropathy (Figure A2.6). This is usually an easy case, but occasionally candidates will be fooled by a mimic — a mononeuropathy, root, plexus, or cauda equina lesion.

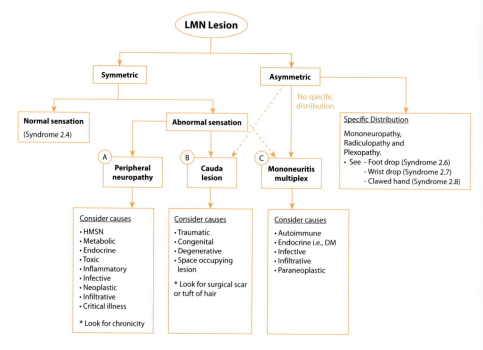

HMSN: hereditary motor and sensory neuropathy

Figure A2.6. Localisation of LMN lesion with distal numbness.

Where is the Lesion

Having detected distal weakness with LMN signs, consider if signs are consistent with peripheral neuropathy, or if there are any inconsistent features suggestive of a mimic.

Is this a peripheral neuropathy?

Key features of peripheral neuropathy
- Symmetrical distal > proximal weakness (which may include distal wasting, bilateral foot drop, and high steppage gait).

Neurology (Limbs)

- Glove-and-stocking pattern[10] of distal > proximal sensory loss (typically in all sensory modalities, although the different modalities may not be equally affected).
- May have predominant sensory involvement, predominant motor involvement, or both.

Features inconsistent with peripheral neuropathy
- Lower back scar or tuft of hair (low spinal cord lesion).
- Use of urinary catheter/intermittent catheterisation (may occur for example in diabetic autonomic neuropathy, but look hard for a spinal cord lesion).
- Signs are not symmetrical and bilateral (i.e., they are asymmetric, patchy, or localised to one/several myotomes or dermatomes).

Other differentials and key distinguishing points

1. **Cauda equina lesion (in lower limb weakness)**
   - Weakness follows a myotomal pattern (e.g., L4 and below) rather than distal > proximal. In practice this resembles the distal weakness of peripheral neuropathy and is not easy to tell apart, particularly if many myotomes are affected.
   - Early sphincter (bladder/bowel) involvement (urinary/bowel).
   - ± Sacral numbness.
   - Lower back scar or tuft of hair.
2. **Mononeuropathy, root, or plexus lesion**
   - Unilateral LMN weakness and/or numbness in the distribution of one peripheral nerve, or one or several adjacent nerve roots.
   - Unilateral LMN foot drop, wrist drop, or claw hand (see Syndromes 2.6–2.8).
3. **Mononeuritis multiplex**
   - Patchy, asymmetric weakness + numbness in the distribution of multiple peripheral nerves.

What is the Lesion (A): Peripheral Neuropathy

Look for stigmata to suggest a specific cause of peripheral neuropathy (Table A2.8). It would be embarrassing to miss clear-cut features of chronicity suggesting hereditary motor sensory neuropathy, or an obvious Charcot foot or lower limb amputation stump to suggest diabetes.

There are differences in the extent of sensory vs. motor deficit in each of these causes, but remembering these nuances would ordinarily not be expected in PACES.

---

[10] Caveat: The glove and stocking pattern may not be present in predominantly demyelinating processes such as chronic inflammatory demyelinating polyneuropathy (CIDP).

Table A2.8. Common causes of peripheral neuropathy.

	Cause	Peripheral stigmata
Congenital	HMSN (Charcot-Marie-Tooth)	Chronicity: distal wasting, pes cavus, clawed toes, contractures Thickened nerves
Metabolic/endocrine	Diabetes mellitus	Insulin injection/glucose check marks Coronary bypass, peripheral vascular disease Diabetic dermopathy
	B12 deficiency	Glossitis, anaemia
	Hypo/hyperthyroidism	Goitre, signs of hyper/hypothyroidism
	Uraemia	
	Acromegaly	Spade-like hands, coarse facial features
Toxic	Alcohol	Parotidomegaly, Dupuytren's contracture
	Drugs: isoniazid, phenytoin, cisplatin, vincristine	Central line/port-a-cath in situ
	Metals: lead, mercury, arsenic	Lead lines in gums
Inflammatory	GBS, CIDP	
	Sjogren's syndrome*	
Infective	Leprosy	Thickened nerves
	HIV	
Neoplastic	Paraneoplastic (anti-Hu)	Cachexia
Infiltrative	Amyloidosis	
	Sarcoidosis	
Other	Critical illness	Tracheostomy scar

CIDP: chronic inflammatory demyelinating polyneuropathy; GBS: Guillain-Barré syndrome; HMSN: Hereditary motor sensory neuropathy

*Other rheumatologic diseases (e.g., rheumatoid arthritis, systemic lupus erythematosus, ANCA vasculitis) can present with peripheral neuropathy, although mononeuritis multiplex is more common.

What is the Lesion (B): Cauda Equina Lesion

The causes of a cauda equina lesion include:
- Traumatic.
- Congenital – spina bifida.
- Degenerative (i.e., low intervertebral disc prolapse).
- Space-occupying lesion – neoplasm, abscess.

Look for a lower back scar (spinal surgery) or tuft of hair (spinal bifida). Always request for a rectal examination.

What is the Lesion (C): Mononeuritis Multiplex

Mononeuritis multiplex appears daunting, but in reality there are only a short list of causes — i.e., a systemic process that affects peripheral nerves at random, and not all of them equally.

Common causes of mononeuritis multiplex:

- Autoimmune: Vasculitis (ANCA vasculitis, rheumatoid arthritis, lupus, Sjogren's)
- Endocrine: Diabetes mellitus
- Infective: Lyme disease, HIV, Leprosy
- Infiltrative: Amyloidosis, Sarcoidosis
- Paraneoplastic

Look for Complications

Look for complications in terms of:

- Function – mobility, use of walking aids.
- Continence – use of diapers, urinary catheter (especially cauda equina lesions).
- Complications of peripheral sensory loss (e.g., foot ulcers, amputations).

Sample Scripts

Hereditary motor sensory neuropathy

This young man has peripheral neuropathy as evidenced by symmetrical distal weakness with reduced tone and depressed reflexes, as well as a glove and stocking pattern of sensory loss. His feet have an inverted champagne bottle appearance with pes cavus, clawing of toes, and achilles tendon contractures. Examination of the back did not reveal any scar or cutaneous signs of spina bifida. The likely diagnosis is hereditary motor sensory neuropathy (Charcot-Marie-Tooth disease), although differentials include diabetes, chronic inflammatory demyelinating polyneuropathy, and drugs and toxins. In terms of function, he is ambulant with a high steppage gait. I am concerned about his fall risk. I will like to complete my examination by asking for a family history, checking capillary glucose, and examining his upper limbs.

Spina bifida

This young lady has bilateral weakness in ankle dorsiflexion, plantarflexion, and hip abduction accompanied by lower motor neuron signs of decreased tone, absent ankle jerks, and downgoing plantars. There is also numbness over the dorsum and sole of the foot. I notice a tuft of hair over the lower back with no overlying scar. The localisation is to the cauda equina and the likely diagnosis is spina bifida, although differentials include trauma and space-occupying lesions such as an abscess, neoplasm, or hematoma. Functionally, she uses a motorised wheelchair and has a urinary catheter. I will like to complete my examination with a rectal examination for anal tone, and examining the upper limbs.

Neurology (Limbs) – Clinical Syndromes

2.6 | Foot Drop

Foot drop follows a simple and logical algorithm, but is often poorly done. We recommend checking ankle dorsiflexion as an early screen, while inspecting the patient from the foot of the bed. This will allow you to identify unilateral foot drop early and incorporate additional steps (e.g., hip abduction) that are not a routine part of the lower limb examination.

Where is the Lesion

Foot drop can be due to a bilateral UMN disorder, a generalised LMN process, sciatic plexus, L5 root, sciatic nerve, or peroneal nerve lesion. Localisation follows a simple algorithm (Figure A2.7).

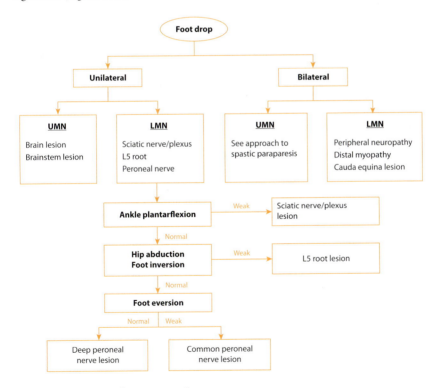

HMSN: hereditary motor and sensory neuropathy

Figure A2.7. Localisation of foot drop.

1. **Exclude bilateral foot drop**
   - Bilateral LMN foot drop: peripheral neuropathy (Syndrome 2.5) or distal myopathy (myotonic dystrophy, facioscapulohumeral dystrophy, etc.; Syndrome 2.4).
   - Bilateral UMN foot drop: usually a spinal cord lesion (Syndrome 2.1).
2. **Exclude UMN foot drop**
   - Look for UMN features including hypertonia, clonus, hyperreflexia, upgoing plantars, or UMN pattern of weakness.
   - The causes of unilateral UMN weakness are discussed in Syndrome 2.2 and include brain and brainstem lesions.
3. **Consider sciatic nerve or plexus lesions**
   - A sciatic nerve lesion affects many more muscles, causing weak ankle plantarflexion, a depressed ankle jerk, and a larger area of numbness.
   - A plexus lesion may affect certain nerve roots but not others, resulting in a myotomal pattern.
4. **Distinguish peroneal nerve vs. L5 root lesion**
   - The critical test is hip abduction and foot inversion — these are weak in a L5 lesion, but normal in a peroneal nerve lesion.
   - Sensory loss is over the lateral leg in an L5 lesion, but over the 1st webspace or dorsum of foot in a peroneal nerve lesion.
5. **If peroneal nerve, distinguish deep vs. common peroneal nerve lesion**
   - A common peroneal nerve lesion also affects the superficial peroneal nerve, causing weak foot eversion and a larger patch of numbness over the dorsum of the foot.

Table A2.9 summarises the key differences between each cause of LMN foot drop.

Table A2.9. Localisation of LMN foot drop.

Action	Root and nerve		L5 root	Peroneal nerve Deep	Peroneal nerve Common	Sciatic nerve	Sacral plexus
Ankle dorsiflexion	L5	Deep peroneal	Weak	Weak	Weak	Weak	Weak
Ankle plantarflexion	S1	Tibial	Strong	Strong	Strong	**Weak**	**Weak**
Hip abduction	L5	Superior gluteal	**Weak**	Strong	Strong	Strong	Weak
Foot inversion	L4-5	Tibial	**Weak**	Strong	Strong	Weak	Weak
Foot eversion	L5	Superficial peroneal	Weak	Strong	**Weak**	Weak	Weak
Sensory loss			Lateral leg	Only 1st webspace	Dorsum of foot	Extensive	

What is the Lesion (A): Peroneal Nerve Lesion

Causes of a peroneal nerve lesion:
- Most common: compressive neuropathy at the fibular head (common peroneal nerve lesion) due to prolonged bed rest or trauma.
- Trauma and Iatrogenic – look for a scar at the fibula head (fracture, surgery).
- Causes of mononeuropathy (e.g., diabetes mellitus).
- As part of a mononeuritis multiplex (diabetes, vasculitis, etc.; see page 55).

What is the Lesion (B): L5 Root, Sciatic Nerve, and Plexus Lesions

The causes here overlap. The more common causes may include:

	L5 root	Sacral nerve	Sacral plexus
(a) Compressive /traumatic	Prolapsed disk	Post op (hip) Prolonged sitting Postpartum	Postpartum
	Hematoma Neoplasm	Hematoma Neoplasm	Hematoma, retroperitoneal Neoplasm
(b) Vasculitis	Possible	Possible	–
(c) Inflammatory			Radiation
(d) Metabolic			Diabetic amyotrophy

Look for Complications

Look for patient's function and mobility. Pay attention to the patient's footwear and use of any aids (e.g., an ankle foot orthosis).

Sample Scripts

Common peroneal nerve lesion

This middle-aged gentleman has left-sided foot drop, weak ankle dorsiflexion, and foot eversion. Ankle plantarflexion, foot inversion, and hip abduction are normal. Tone and reflexes are normal, and plantars are downgoing. There is sensory loss over the dorsum of the foot. The lesion localises to the common peroneal nerve. I note a surgical scar over the fibula head, suggesting that past trauma may be the cause of this lesion. Functionally, he walks with a high steppage gait on the left and does not use any orthosis. I am concerned about his fall risk as he appears to be tripping over often.

L5 nerve root

This middle-aged gentleman has a left foot drop with weak ankle dorsiflexion, weak hip abduction, and weak foot inversion. Ankle plantarflexion is normal. Tone and reflexes are normal. There is a patch of sensory loss over the lateral leg. The lesion is in the L5 nerve root. Possible causes include degenerative lumbar spine disease, trauma, compression by a space-occupying lesion, as well as causes of a mononeuritis multiplex. He appears to be comfortable, although I will like to take a history for back pain or trauma. Functionally he is ambulant with a stick. I will like to complete my examination by checking anal tone and doing a straight leg raise.

Neurology (Limbs) – Clinical Syndromes

2.7 | Finger/Wrist Drop

We recommend screening wrist dorsiflexion (asking the patient to cock the wrists up as in checking for asterixes) at the start of the upper limb examination, along with pronator drift. This will allow early identification of finger or wrist drop and facilitate smooth performance of additional steps (particularly brachioradialis testing) which is not routine.

Where is the Lesion

Isolated LMN finger or wrist drop is most likely a radial or C7 root lesion. The localisation algorithm is simple:

1. **Ensure isolated unilateral LMN wrist drop; exclude more complex disorders**
   - Rule out an **UMN disorder** – this can present as wrist drop as upper limb UMN disorders cause greater weakness of extensors than flexors in the upper limb.
   - Rule out **generalised distal weakness** (e.g., bilateral wrist drop) – consider a peripheral neuropathy or distal myopathy (Syndromes 2.4, 2.5).
   - Rule out concomitant **ulnar or median nerve palsies**. Test finger abduction and grip strength in slight wrist extension (slight extension of wrist flexors allows optimal action of dorsal interossei). Testing these actions in wrist flexion will lead to spurious weakness.
   - Consider **cortical wrist drop** if there is no sensory involvement. This is a small cortical stroke (classically embolic) affecting only a small region of the motor homunculus. There may not be UMN signs if the area of infarct is small. The presence of sensory involvement makes cortical wrist drop unlikely, as this small lesion will not affect the sensory gyrus.

2. **Differentiate radial nerve vs. C7 root lesion**
   - **Motor**: The key test is the **brachioradialis muscle** (supplied from C6 root via the radial nerve), which is weak in a radial nerve lesion at the spiral groove of humerus or above, but unexpectedly strong in a C7 lesion. To test the brachioradialis, check elbow flexion in forearm mid-pronation, or forearm supination in full elbow extension (the biceps is responsible for forearm supination in 90 degrees elbow flexion, as well as elbow flexion in forearm supination).
   - **Sensory**: Test pinprick sensation at the **palmar aspect of the middle finger** (supplied from C7 root via median nerve). This is affected in a C7 lesion, but spared in a radial nerve lesion.

3. **In a radial nerve lesion, find the level of the lesion** — at the posterior interosseous nerve (PIN), spiral groove, or axilla. The higher the lesion, the more extensive the weakness.

Lesion at...	Motor weakness in...	Numbness over...
Forearm or elbow (PIN)	Finger extension Wrist extension – slightly weak[11]	Nil or 1st dorsal webspace only
Spiral groove of humerus	Finger and wrist extension Brachioradialis, ↓ supinator jerk	Extensor aspect of forearm
Axilla	Finger and wrist extension Brachioradialis, ↓ supinator jerk Triceps, ↓ triceps jerk	Extensor aspect of arm and forearm

What is the Lesion (A): Radial Nerve

Look closely for deformities and scars. Consider both local causes as well as causes of a mononeuropathy in general. This will include:

- Trauma – e.g., humeral fracture (radial nerve lesion at the spiral groove — there may be a scar as humeral fractures with nerve injury are likely to be operated on).
- Compressive neuropathy – e.g., Saturday night palsy (radial nerve lesion at the spiral groove), crutch palsy (radial nerve lesion at the axilla).
- Part of a mononeuritis multiplex – e.g., diabetes, vasculitis.
- Inflammatory mononeuropathy – e.g., multifocal motor neuropathy.

What is the Lesion (B): C7 Root

The lesion here is of the cervical spine or brachial plexus. Look for neck scars.
    Aetiologies may include:

- Degenerative – cervical disc prolapse (most common).
- Traumatic.
- Space-occupying lesion (e.g., neoplasm, abscess, hematoma).

Look for Complications

Assess patient's function, for example, test his/her ability to write or button a shirt.
    Look for the presence of aids (e.g., a wrist splint).

---

[11] Fine print: the extensor carpi ulnaris, but not the extensor carpi radialis, is affected in a PIN lesion. Therefore in a PIN lesion, there may be slight weakness of wrist extension with radial deviation of the wrist.

Sample Scripts

Radial nerve lesion at the spiral groove

This gentleman has a right wrist drop. There is weakness of finger and wrist extension, weakness of the brachioradialis muscle, and diminished supinator jerk. However, triceps jerk and elbow extension is preserved. He has loss of pinprick sensation over the dorsal aspect of the forearm. There is also a surgical scar over the right upper arm. This localises to a right radial nerve lesion at the level of the spiral groove. (It is not a C7 root lesion because the brachioradialis is weak, and sensation over the palmar aspect over the middle finger is normal.) The likely aetiology is traumatic humeral fracture, which is consistent with the scar. Functionally he is able to write with a wrist splint. I will like to complete my examination by examining the lower limbs and cranial nerves for any other nerve lesions that would suggest mononeuritis multiplex.

C7 Root lesion

This patient has weak elbow extension, depressed triceps jerk (radial/C7), and weakness of wrist and finger extensors (radial/C7). However, brachioradialis power and supinator jerk is preserved (radial/C6). There is sensory loss including over the palmar aspect of the middle finger. The localisation is to the C7 nerve root. In terms of aetiology, there are no neck scars to suggest cervical spine instrumentation. Possible causes include a cervical disc prolapse, cervical spine or brachial plexus trauma, or a space-occupying lesion such as a neoplasm or abscess. Functionally he is able to write and open a bottle cap unaided.

Neurology (Limbs) – Clinical Syndromes

2.8 | Unilateral Weak/Wasted/Claw Hand

It is easy to miss an upper limb mononeuropathy because fine hand movements are not a routine part of the upper limb examination. Have a high index of suspicion for an upper limb mononeuropathy if there is asymmetric distal upper limb weakness. Better yet — identify a mononeuropathy during inspection by noticing wasting of thenar or hypothenar eminences, clawing of the hand, or abnormal grip and release screen.

Where is the Lesion

You will need to distinguish between a medial nerve, ulnar nerve, T1 root, and more complex lesion.

1. **Ensure isolated wasted/claw hand; rule out more complex disorders**
   - Rule out an UMN disorder.
   - Rule out a bilateral disorder which will require consideration of a peripheral neuropathy, distal myopathy (Syndrome 2.5), or syringomyelia (Syndrome 2.1).
   - Beware of a mixed median + ulnar or T1 root lesion.
2. **Distinguish between a median nerve, ulnar nerve, and T1 root lesion.** The key rules are:
   - **Motor**: The ulnar nerve supplies all intrinsic hand muscles except the 'LOAF' muscles (lateral two lumbricals, opponens pollicis, abductor pollicis brevis, and flexor pollicis brevis), which are supplied by the median nerve. The key tests are thumb abduction, little finger abduction, and Froment's sign.
   - **Sensory**: In the palmar aspect, the lateral 3.5 digits are supplied by the median nerve, and the medial 1.5 digits are supplied by the ulnar nerve.
   - Beware the T1 root lesion, which causes motor weakness in both ulnar and medial nerve distributions, but leads to numbness over the medial (inner) arm instead.

	Ulnar nerve lesion	Median nerve lesion	T1 root lesion
Inspection	Clawed ring and little finger	Thumb externally rotated (simian hand)	
	Hypothenar wasting	Thenar wasting	Thenar + hypothenar wasting
	Wasted small muscles (dorsal guttering)		Wasted small muscles (dorsal guttering)

(Cont'd)

Neurology (Limbs)

	Ulnar nerve lesion	**Median nerve lesion**	**T1 root lesion**
Motor	Weak little finger abduction	Weak thumb abduction	All finger abduction weak
	Weak 1st dorsal interossei (Froment's sign)		Weak 1st dorsal interossei
Sensory	Numb ulnar 1.5 fingers	Numb median 3.5 fingers	Numb medial arm

3. **In a median or ulnar nerve lesion, distinguish between high or low lesion**
   - The key muscle is the flexor digitorum profundus (FDP), which receives its nerve supply in the forearm and is therefore spared in a low lesion. Test the FDP of the radial two fingers (index and middle) in a median nerve lesion, or of the ulnar two fingers (ring and little) in an ulnar nerve lesion; to test the FDP, immobilise the middle phalanx and ask the patient to flex the distal interphalangeal joint.

	High lesion (above wrist)	**Low lesion** (wrist or below wrist)
Inspection		Pronounced claw hand (ulnar nerve – the ulnar paradox)
Motor	Flexor digitorum profundus weak	Flexor digitorum profundus spared
Sensory	Hypothenar numbness (ulnar) Thenar numbness (median)	Hypothenar/thenar eminence sensation normal

What is the Lesion (A): Ulnar and Median Nerve

Important causes include:

	Ulnar nerve lesion	**Median nerve lesion**
• Trauma	Elbow fracture	Cubital fossa injury (e.g., surgical, fracture)
	Tardy ulnar nerve palsy in cubitus valgus	
• Compressive	Cubital tunnel compression	Carpal tunnel syndrome

- Part of a mononeuritis multiplex (e.g., diabetes, vasculitis).
- Inflammatory mononeuropathy (e.g., multifocal motor neuropathy).

Look closely for deformities and scars.

Carpal tunnel syndrome

This is most common median nerve lesion. Look carefully for scars over the carpal tunnel suggesting previous release surgery. Attempt provocative tests, such as:

- Tinel's sign: percuss over the carpal tunnel; a positive test is if this leads to shooting parasthesias in the median nerve distribution.

- Phalen's manoeuvre: have the patient flex both wrists by placing the backs of the hands against each other. Pain and paraesthesia in the median nerve distribution within 1 minute of wrist flexion is a positive test.

Look for secondary causes of the carpal tunnel syndrome:

- Rheumatological – rheumatoid arthritis, other connective tissue diseases.
- Endocrine – diabetes, hypothyroidism, acromegaly.
- Oestrogen-related – contraceptive pill use, pregnancy.
- Other – renal impairment (dialysis-related amyloidosis).
- Occupational/recreational – repetitive strain, vibrating tool use.

What is the Lesion (B): T1 Root

The causes of a T1 root lesion include:

- Cervical spine lesion – trauma, disc prolapse, myelopathy, space-occupying lesion.
- Lower brachial plexus lesion – brachial neuritis, Klumpke's palsy, trauma.
- Apical lung lesion – classically a pancoast tumour involving the T1 nerve root.

Look for Complications

Consider the patient's function, particularly fine motor tasks (e.g., writing, buttoning shirt).

Sample Scripts

Carpal tunnel syndrome

My patient is a middle-aged lady with a left carpal tunnel syndrome. She has thenar wasting and weakness of thumb abduction, with numbness in the lateral 3.5 digits. This is a low median nerve lesion as evidenced by preserved power of distal phalanx flexion in the index and middle finger, as well as the absence of thenar eminence numbness. There is a scar over the volar aspect of the wrist, suggesting previous carpal tunnel release surgery. Functionally she is able to use a handphone and button her shirt. To identify underlying risk factors for carpal tunnel syndrome, I would like to examine her hands, thyroid system, and visual fields, and ask for an occupational history.

Neurology (Limbs) — Clinical Syndromes

2.9 | Cerebellar Signs Only

Be alert to a stem of 'difficulty walking' or 'falls' rather than weakness, the presence of scanning speech when greeting the patient, or upward rebound when doing pronator drift. The examination would be otherwise normal until cerebellar function is tested — which can make you quite anxious.

Demonstrate Cerebellar Signs

After completing the examination of the upper/lower limbs, also examine the cranial nerves to complete the cerebellar examination[12].

Limbs

a. Dysmetria.
b. Dysdiadochokinesia.
c. Dyssynergia on heel-shin test.
d. Truncal ataxia (e.g., a patient who is unable to maintain balance sitting upright. Such severe cerebellar disease is unlikely in PACES).
e. Ataxic/broad-based gait – if not obvious, stress gait by doing tandem gait.

Cranial nerves

f. Multidirectional or vertical nystagmus – be able to distinguish the unidirectional, horizontal or rotational nystagmus of a peripheral vestibular lesion from the multidirectional or vertical nystagmus of cerebellar disease.
g. Jerky pursuit – test smooth pursuit by asking the patient to follow an object with his/her eyes as you move it across the visual field slowly. The patient with cerebellar disease is unable to do so.
h. Hypermetric saccades – ask the patient to look alternately between a finger and a pen. The gaze overshoots in cerebellar disease.
i. Scanning speech – the classic test phrase is "British Constitution".

The rest of the neurological examination should be unremarkable without weakness, sensory deficit, or extrapyramidal features.

What is the Lesion

The first step is to ascertain that the patient indeed has isolated cerebellar signs (1, 2). Having done so, the key distinction is between unilateral (3) and bilateral (4) cerebellar signs.

---

[12] (Not required in PACES) The lesion can be further localised to specific parts of the cerebellum — the flocculonodulus (f-i), vermis (d, e), or cortices (a-c, e).

1. Non-isolated cerebellar signs

Be alert to several patterns of cerebellar signs in combination with other pyramidal or extrapyramidal signs:

- Unilateral UMN + ipsilateral cerebellar signs: suggests the lacunar syndrome of ataxic hemiparesis or a brainstem lesion.
- Bilateral UMN + cerebellar signs: brainstem lesion or the 'spastic paraparesis plus' syndromes (Friedreich's ataxia, spinocerebellar ataxia, hereditary spastic paraparesis; see Syndrome 2.1).
- Scattered UMN + cerebellar signs: consider demyelinating lesions separated in space (i.e., multiple sclerosis).
- Cerebellar + extrapyramidal signs: consider multiple system atrophy.
- Cerebellar + cranial nerve signs: brainstem lesion.

2. Ataxia alone

Be cautious of patients with ataxia alone and no other cerebellar signs. Differentials to cerebellar disease in this situation include:

- Sensory ataxia – dorsal column dysfunction (subacute combined degeneration, posterior spinal artery infarct, tabes dorsalis).
- Cortical ataxia – normal pressure hydrocephalus. These patients would have predominant findings of gait instability and broad-based gait; dysmetria and ocular signs are usually absent.

3. Unilateral cerebellar signs

This is suspicious for a focal lesion:

- Vascular: infarct, haemorrhage.
- Inflammatory: multiple sclerosis.
- Space-occupying lesion: cerebellopontine angle tumour, abscess, hematoma – examine cranial nerves (especially hearing) and look for a post-auricular scar.

Note: Patients with unilateral cerebellar disease may not have the cranial nerve signs of cerebellar dysfunction.

4. Bilateral cerebellar signs

This is more likely a systemic cause:

- Toxic/metabolic: excessive alcohol ingestion, hyperglycaemia, Wilson's disease (copper), Wernicke encephalopathy (thiamine deficiency).
- Drugs: antiepileptic drugs (especially phenytoin), chemotherapy (e.g., cytarabine).
- Infective (e.g., viral cerebriitis).

Neurology (Limbs)

- Paraneoplastic.
- Inflammatory: Miller-Fisher syndrome, multiple sclerosis.
- Degenerative: multiple system atrophy.
- Hereditary: neurodegenerative ataxias (e.g., spinocerebellar ataxia, Friedreich's ataxia, ataxia telangiectasia).

This is not a hard and fast rule; a unilateral cerebellar hemisphere lesion can cause bilateral (although asymmetric) cerebellar signs, as cerebellar tracts are partly crossed.

Look for Complications

Check patient's gait, use of walking aids, and comment on complications such as falls or old fractures.

Sample Scripts

Unilateral cerebellar signs

My patient has left-sided cerebellar signs as evidenced by left dysmetria, dysdiadochokinesia, and an ataxic gait. I note the presence of a left post auricular scar suggesting that she may have had a previous cerebellopontine angle lesion which was excised, although her hearing is normal at present. There is otherwise no weakness and no cranial nerve deficits. In summary she likely has an old left cerebellopontine angle lesion post excision, with residual cerebellar signs. Functionally she walks independently without aid.

Bilateral cerebellar signs

This middle-aged gentleman has bilateral cerebellar signs with ataxia, dysmetria, dysdiadochokinesia, multidirectional nystagmus, and jerky pursuit. There is no weakness or sensory loss, no extrapyramidal features, and no cranial nerve signs. I will like to take a drug history, alcohol use history, family history for neurodegenerative ataxias and Wilson's disease, and ask him about recent infections or weight loss. I will like to complete my examination by checking the fundi for optic neuritis, and doing a capillary glucose.

Neurology (Limbs) – Clinical Syndromes

2.10 | Parkinsonism

Parkinsonism is generally an easy case (in fact, some exam centres consider it 'too easy'), but catastrophic if missed. Patients may not have an obvious rest tremor — subtle cases can be missed if tone is not carefully examined. You will need to complete the standard upper/lower limb examination quickly then perform additional steps to demonstrate features of Parkinsonism (e.g., bradykinesia), as well as look for differentials to idiopathic Parkinson's disease.

Demonstrate Parkinsonism

Inspection: the diagnosis of Parkinsonism should really be suspected on inspection for:

- Mask-like facies.
- Hypophonic speech.
- Pill-rolling tremor at rest.

Examination features: additional steps must be performed to demonstrate the core features of Parkinsonism:

- Tone: cogwheel rigidity, leadpipe rigidity (note how to distinguish this from spasticity, page 19).
- Bradykinesia – demonstrate slow grip release or slow pronation/supination movements.
- Gait – difficulty initiation, shuffling gait with festination, stooped posture, reduced arm swing.
- Check handwriting – micrographia.

Look for Differentials to Idiopathic Parkinson's Disease

The majority of cases will be idiopathic Parkinson's disease (PD). Features consistent with idiopathic PD include asymmetric extrapyramidal signs, normal eye movements, normal cerebellar function, and postural or cognitive difficulty developing only late in the disease course.

Important differentials that appear in PACES include:

- Parkinsons-plus syndromes
    - Multiple system atrophy (MSA).
    - Progressive supranuclear palsy (PSP).

- Corticobasal degeneration (CBD).
- Dementia with Lewy bodies (DLB) – *unlikely in PACES*.
• Secondary Parkinsonism
- Vascular Parkinsonism.
- Drug-induced, particularly from antipsychotics.
- Wilson's Disease.
• Mimics
- Normal pressure hydrocephalus (NPH).

Suggested routine:	**Significance**
– Ensure signs are asymmetric	Symmetrical signs is not consistent with idiopathic PD
– Check cerebellar signs	Bilateral cerebellar signs – suspect MSA
– Check vertical gaze	Vertical gaze palsy, can be overcome with Doll's reflex[13] – suspect PSP
– Look for dystonia, alien limb	Suggest CBD
– Ask patient to 'show me how you brush your teeth'	Tests ideomotor apraxia (*unable to perform action that relies on semantic memory*) – suspect CBD
– Inspect for signs of vascular disease	In vasculopaths (e.g., coronary bypass scars, foot amputations), consider vascular Parkinsonism.
– Look for urinary catheter	Autonomic dysfunction occurs late in idiopathic PD – consider NPH, MSA
– Caution in a young patient	Less likely idiopathic PD, consider Parkinsons-plus, drug-induced, and Wilson's disease

Offer at end of exam:

– Postural blood pressure	Consider MSA
– Drug history	Possibility of drug-induced Parkinsonism
– Mini-mental state exam	Normal until late stage in idiopathic PD; suspect DLB

---

[13] The Doll's reflex distinguishes between a supranuclear and nuclear (i.e., midbrain) vertical gaze palsy. The Doll's reflex bypasses the supranuclear centres responsible for vertical gaze; therefore, in a supranuclear disorder, performing vertical Doll's reflex (i.e., moving the head up and down) elicits normal vertical eye movements. Conversely, vertical eye movements remain abnormal in a midbrain (nuclear) lesion.

Look for Complications

Look for:

- Functional status – mobility, activities of daily living.
- Dyskinesias from levodopa therapy – pay attention to dyskinesias including choreiform thrusting hip movements and lip smacking movements; do not confuse this with tremors.

Sample Scripts

Idiopathic PD

This elderly gentleman has features of Parkinsonism consistent with idiopathic Parkinson's disease. On inspection, he has mask-like facies, hypophonic speech, and a pill-rolling tremor most prominent in the left upper limb. There is cogwheel rigidity and bradykinesia, worse on the left. There is a festinating gait. There is no vertical gaze palsy to suggest progressive supranuclear palsy, no cerebellar signs to suggest multiple system atrophy, and no dystonia to suggest corticobasal degeneration. These features are consistent with idiopathic Parkinson's disease. He appears to be early in the course and is functionally mobile without aid. I will like to complete my examination by taking a drug history, conducting a mini mental state examination, checking his postural blood pressure and urinary function, and asking about previous strokes.

Inconsistent with idiopathic PD

This middle-aged lady has features of Parkinsonism that are inconsistent with idiopathic Parkinson's disease. On inspection, she has mask-like facies and hypophonic speech. There is bilateral cogwheel rigidity and bilateral bradykinesia. There are also bilateral cerebellar signs and a urinary catheter suggesting autonomic dysfunction. There is no vertical gaze palsy or dystonia. Features inconsistent with idiopathic Parkinson's disease include symmetrical signs, cerebellar dysfunction, and early autonomic dysfunction. I suspect multiple system atrophy.

Neurology (Limbs)

2.11 | Discussion Framework

Most examiners evaluate the candidate's clinical judgement by asking questions about investigations and management. This section provides a general framework to answer these questions, focusing on how to structure a sound answer, and principles that apply across all cases in this system. It must be tailored and prioritised to your list of differentials.

How Would You Investigate?

"I will like to confirm my diagnosis, identify the aetiology, and look for complications."

I. Discuss any potential emergency

Take myasthenia gravis or Guillain-Barré syndrome, for instance — offer to check a bedside negative inspiratory force or forced viral capacity to rule out impending respiratory failure.

II. Confirm diagnosis and investigate for aetiology

Go directly for investigations that will confirm the suspected diagnosis. Your choice of investigation reflects your understanding of neurological localisation — for example, asking for an MRI brain in a peripheral neuropathy betrays a lack of understanding.

Be aware that a number of neurological conditions are clinical diagnoses. For instance, in a case of suspected Parkinson's disease, you could say, *"The diagnosis of Parkinson's disease is clinical; however, investigations are useful to rule out Parkinsons-plus syndromes and differentials, especially if the presentation is atypical or the patient does not respond as well as expected to levodopa."*

1. **More history/examination**
   - Time course of neurological deficit is always helpful. For instance, vascular lesions develop acutely (in minutes), inflammatory lesions are subacute (hours to days), while neoplastic or degenerative lesions take much longer to develop.
   - Specific features that will distinguish between differentials.
   - Family history in heritable conditions.
2. **MRI brain/spine is useful in...**
   - UMN disorder: MRI the part (brain/spine) where the lesion localises to. Contrast is necessary if looking for infective, inflammatory, or mitotic lesions.
   - Suspected multiple sclerosis: MRI both brain and spine with contrast to look for dissemination in space and dissemination in time (e.g., both contrast enhancing and non-enhancing lesions).

- Parkinsonism: useful to look for differentials (normal pressure hydrocephalus), evidence of vascular Parkinsonism, and Parkinson's plus features (hummingbird sign in progressive supranuclear palsy, hot cross bun sign in multiple system atrophy).
- Suspected radiculopathy, plexus or cauda equina lesion: MRI lumbar spine and plexus.
- Little role in other LMN disorders.

3. **Neurodiagnostic tests are useful in LMN disorders**

    (a) **Nerve conduction study** – for anterior horn cell and nerve disorders:
    - Identifies pattern of sensory and motor involvement.
    - Distinguishes between demyelination (decreased conduction velocity) or axonopathy (reduced amplitude potentials), which is of diagnostic significance (details not required for PACES).

    (b) **Electromyography** – helpful for most LMN lesions:
    - Neuropathy or anterior horn cell disorders: large complexes, indicative of denervation.
    - Myopathy: small, polyphasic complexes.

4. **Lumbar puncture** is helpful in…
    - Guillain-Barré syndrome: looking for albuminocytologic dissociation.
    - Multiple sclerosis: looking for oligoclonal bands.
    - Other spinal lesions: for cytology, microbiology.

5. **Blood and other tests, for example:**
    - Peripheral neuropathy – look for systemic disorders that will cause a neuropathy (e.g., screen diabetes, B12, folate).
    - Stroke – stroke work-up including cardiovascular risk factor screen (fasting glucose, lipids), ECG, echocardiogram, Holter monitor, and carotid doppler.
    - Myasthenia gravis – acetylcholinesterase receptor antibodies (anti-AChR) and muscle specific kinase (anti-MUSK) antibodies, CT thorax for a thymoma.

III. Look for complications

- Urinary evaluation (e.g., post-void residual urine, ultrasound kidneys for hydronephrosis) for urinary complications in many neurologic disorders (particularly spinal cord disease).
- Swallowing assessment if lower cranial nerves are involved.
- Investigations for extra-neurological complications (e.g., in myotonic dystrophy) – ECG and 24 h holter monitoring, echocardiogram, bloods for glucose, thyroid status, slit lamp exam for cataracts.

How Would You Manage?

"Patient requires multidisciplinary management including specific treatment of the underlying disease, management of complications, and supportive management to maximise function." Conversely, many neurological diseases do not have specific treatment to reverse the underlying cause. *"Management of X is mainly supportive with multidisciplinary interventions to manage complications and maximise function."*

1. **Management of an emergency** *(very unlikely)*
   - Neurosurgical referral for trauma/cauda equina syndrome.
2. **Specific treatment** (if any)
   (a) **Neurological disease with secondary causes**
   - Stop causative drug/toxin.
   - Treat underlying cause (e.g., control diabetes, replace vitamin B12).
   - Treat underlying risk factors (e.g., anticoagulation of atrial fibrillation (stroke)).
   - Immunosuppression of rheumatologic disease (e.g., dermatomyositis).
   - Treat infection (e.g., HIV).

   (b) **Structural causes**
   - Surgical decompression in compressive neuropathy, cervical myelopathy.
   - Surgical resection of a space-occupying lesion.

   (c) **Primary neurological diseases**
   - Levodopa/dopamine agonist in Parkinson's disease.
   - Acetylcholinesterase inhibitors (pyridostigmine) and thymectomy in myasthenia gravis.
   - Immunosuppression.
     - Guillain-Barré syndrome – IVIg or plasma exchange.
     - Myasthenia gravis – IVIg or plasma exchange acutely, long-term maintenance immunosuppression.
     - Chronic inflammatory demyelinating polyneuropathy – steroids.
   - Disease-modifying therapy in multiple sclerosis (plus steroids for flares).
   - Riluzole to delay the onset of ventilator dependence in motor neuron disease.

Pitfall: Not everything is treated with steroids

> Steroids have little role in the acute treatment of Guillain-Barré syndrome or myasthenia flare. The correct treatment is IVIg or plasma exchange.

3. **Management of complications**
   - Neurological complications (e.g., urinary retention (catheterisation), dysphagia (gastrostomy tube)).
   - Management of other organ involvement (e.g., cataracts, endocrine, cardiac complications in myotonic dystrophy).
   - Psychosocial complications (e.g., depression).
4. **Supportive management and maximisation of function**
   - Patient education.
   - Physiotherapy, occupational therapy to maximise function.
   - Assistive devices (e.g., splints, ankle-foot orthosis, mobility devices).
   - Home modification.
   - Vaccination.
   - Genetic counselling and screening of family members (in genetic diseases).

Sample Scripts

Facioscapulohumeral Dystrophy

I will like to investigate to confirm my diagnosis, search for aetiology, and look for complications.

- I will confirm my diagnosis by doing nerve conduction study and electromyography looking for normal nerve conduction but myopathic (small) complexes.
- I will like to look for aetiologies by taking a family history, taking a history for steroid use, joint pains, and rashes, checking thyroid panel, and offering a gene test for facioscapulohumeral dystrophy.
- I will like to look for complications by referring for swallowing assessment.

Management is supportive as there is no disease-modifying therapy available. The patient will benefit from physiotherapy, assistive devices such as an ankle-foot orthosis as he has foot drop, and vaccination. I will also like to offer genetic counselling and screening of family members (autosomal dominant inheritance pattern).

Physical Examination

3 | Neurology (Cranial Nerves)

Additional resources and examination videos available at:
www.nigelfong.net/paces-resources.html

The cranial nerve examination is intellectually interesting and fluid, without a fixed order of examination. Some candidates struggle due to unfamiliarity with cranial nerve localisation, but this actually follows a set of straightforward, logical rules. Signs are generally obvious, but one must know what to look for and use correct technique to accurately pick them up.

Walk-Through and Tips

Initial Approach

Look at the stem, which usually gives the patient's presenting complaint (e.g., diplopia, difficulty seeing, slurred speech).

Approach the patient with a warm greeting, make eye contact, smile, and give a handshake — this initial screen can reveal obvious dysarthria, facial droop, or ptosis. Be attuned to the presence of any bilateral deficit (bilateral facial droop, bilateral ptosis), which can be more subtle. Look at the blinking of the eyes — one eye that does not blink is the first indication of a LMN CN VII palsy. Have a look at the bedside for prism glasses, eye patches, etc.

Position yourself. Have the patient sit at the edge of the bed or on a chair. Sit yourself one arm length's distance opposite the patient, with your face at the same height as that of the patient's (raise or lower the bed as necessary). This is critical particularly for testing of eye movements and visual fields.

Decide on the order of examination based on the stem and this screen. Go for the highest yield examination first.
- Ptosis, obvious extraocular eye movement palsy → Examine eyes first, then other cranial nerves.
- Facial droop → Examine CN V, VII, VIII first, then the eyes, followed by the lower cranial nerves and limbs.
- Dysarthria, dysphasia → Examine lower cranial nerves first.
- Examining CN II to CN XII in order is a fall-back only if nothing is detected on screening and no helpful clue is given in the stem.

Eyes (CN II, III, IV, VI)

Ptosis. Look for ptosis; if present, check for fatigability on prolonged upward gaze (myasthenia). If ptosis is subtle or equivocal, it can be made more prominent by lifting one eyelid and watching for worsening ptosis of the contralateral eyelid (lifting one eyelid removes the ability of the frontalis muscle to compensate for ptosis). If ptosis obscures your view of the pupil, ask the patient to elevate one eyelid with his/her fingers as you examine the eyes, or seek permission to do so on behalf of the patient.

Pupil size. Ask the examiner to turn off the room lights. Illuminating the eyes dimly with a pen-torch held away from the patient, ask the patient to look into the distance and observe for anisocoria in the dark (Horner's syndrome). Turn the lights back on and observe for anisocoria in the light (CN III palsy). It is important to examine for Horner's syndrome with the lights off because the pathology here is *failure to dilate* rather than *failure to constrict* — this can be subtle in the light and easy to miss. If the examiner instructs that there is no need to turn the lights off, there is probably no anisocoria; he/she is helping you to save time.

Pupillary reflexes. Check for a direct pupillary reflex by bringing the pen-torch in from the side and observing for constriction (illuminating from the side is preferable so as not to induce photophobia). Use the swinging torchlight test to check for relative afferent pupillary defect (RAPD) — do not do it too quickly, but spend at least 3 seconds on each eye. The eye with a CN II (i.e., *afferent*) problem will dilate when the light is swung onto it. Remember that in bilateral symmetrical CN II defects, there will be no *relative* defect and therefore no RAPD. Testing accommodation is not routine but should be done if the pupils are not reactive (Argyll-Robertson pupil).

Check visual acuity. If required, allow the patient to don his/her spectacles for this step. Ask the patient to cover one eye while you test visual acuity in the other, with some reading material or a pocket-sized Snellen chart. If unable to read, try (in order) counting fingers, hand movement, then light perception.

Eye movements. Observe the eyes in the primary position (are they down and out?). Whip out your red hat pin and ask the patient if he/she sees double in the primary position. Instruct the patient to keep his/her head still, follow your red hat pin with his/her eyes, and inform you if he/she sees double. Check eye movements in all 9 positions, being sure to go to the extremes of abduction and adduction. If there is diplopia, ask the patient to cover one eye and report whether the inner or outer image disappears (covering the abnormal eye results in the outer image disappearing). Monocular diplopia is unlikely in the neurology station. Look also for nystagmus. If it is present, characterise the nystagmus (see footnote 14 on next page), check saccades (hold up a finger and a pen some distance apart and ask the patient to look at the finger, then quickly at the pen, again at the finger, and so on) and slow pursuit (ask the patient to follow your finger as you slowly and smoothly move it left to right). Dysmetric saccades and jerky pursuit suggest cerebellar disease.

Confrontational visual field testing should be done if the complaint/stem relates to the eyes. It may be omitted if there are other clear lesions and you are running out of time. Both patient and examiner should cover one eye (e.g., patient covers the left eye, you cover the right eye). Ask the patient to fix his gaze on your nose and tell you once he can see a red pin being brought in from the side. Holding the red hat pin equidistant between yourself and the patient, bring the red hat pin in gradually from each of the 4 quadrants (top right, bottom right, top left, bottom left). Report any hemianopia or quadrantanopia.

Pitfall: Examining the eyes

> Many cranial nerve stations involve an abnormality in the eyes, and careful eye examination is critical. Common mistakes include:
> 1. Missing Horner's syndrome due to failure to notice subtle ptosis, or neglecting to dim the room lights.
> 2. Relying solely on the patient's reporting of diplopia during eye movement testing, rather than objective determination of abduction/adduction deficit. The former is often unreliable, so do look carefully for asymmetrical or incomplete (not just absent) eye movements. The exception is in complex ophthalmoplegia (as in myasthenia gravis), where the patient may report diplopia in multiple positions even with only subtle ophthalmoplegia.
> 3. Failure to 'stress' the eye movements (i.e., not testing extreme right/left gaze). It is important to have the patient look far to the left and right as a subtle CN VI palsy can be otherwise missed.
> 4. 'Unfair' positioning of the patient, examiner, or pin during confrontational visual field testing. Remember that the basis of this test is the comparison of the patient's and candidate's visual fields.
>   - Candidate's face must be positioned directly opposite the patient's. Asymmetric positioning, or examining the patient lying down, will lead to inaccuracies.
>   - Pin must be held equidistant between the patient and the examiner.
>   - Pin must not cross vertical or horizontal meridian.

---

[14] **Interpretation of Nystagmus**: pendular nystagmus is always central, while jerk nystagmus can be central or peripheral. Specific patterns may suggest particular localisations:
- **Peripheral vestibular lesion**: Horizontal uni-directional nystagmus, fast phase away from side of lesion, suppressed with visual fixation and fatigable with continued gaze.
- **Central vestibular lesion**: Horizontal, vertical or multi-directional nystagmus, fast phase toward side of lesion. Visual fixation and continued gaze has no effect.
- **Cerebellar lesion**: Multidirectional gaze evoked nystagmus, jerky pursuit, hypermetric saccades (overshoot when trying to alternate between two objects).
- **Visual deprivation pendular nystagmus**: multidirectional nystagmus with oscillations of equal amplitude and velocity (no fast or slow component), in a blind patient.
- **Foramen magnum lesion**: downbeat nystagmus.
- **Medulla lesion**: upbeat nystagmus.

Face (CN V, VII, VIII)

CN VII. Test the facial nerve in its branches — ask the patient to look up and observe for forehead furrowing (temporal), close their eyes tight and bury the eyelashes completely (zygomatic), smile (buccal), and puff out cheeks (marginal mandibular). If a facial droop is seen, verify whether the CN VII palsy is of a lower motor neuron (affects whole face) or upper motor neuron (spares frontalis and orbicularis occuli) pattern.

CN V. Check sensation in CN V_1, V_2, and V_3 using cotton wool (please do not use your fingers). Appropriate test points are on (1) the forehead above the pupil, (2) the cheek below the pupil, and (3) lower jaw below the second test point. Do not test too laterally as there is overlap with C2/3 territory laterally. A single sensory modality is adequate; unlike in the limbs, separate testing of spinothalamic and dorsal column tracts provides no additional information. Finally, ask the patient to open his jaw against resistance (motor of CN V).

CN VIII. Check hearing using a 512 Hz tuning fork (do not use 128 Hz). If (and only if) this is abnormal, proceed with the Rinne and Weber's test. Rinne's test is performed by placing a vibrating tuning fork on the mastoid bone (bone conduction). When the patient can no longer hear the vibration, move the same tuning fork to the external auditory meatus (air conduction) and ask if the vibration is now audible; this should normally be audible as air conduction is physiologically superior to bone conduction. Weber's test is performed by placing a vibrating tuning fork on the middle of the forehead and asking whether it is heard equally in both ears or louder in one ear. The interpretation of Rinne's and Weber's tests are given in Table A3.1.

Table A3.1. Interpretation of Rinne's and Weber's tests.

	Conductive hearing loss	Sensorineural hearing loss	Normal
Rinne	Bone conduction better than air conduction	Air conduction better than bone conduction	Air conduction better than bone conduction
Weber	Central or lateralise to bad ear	Lateralises to good ear	Central

Lower cranial nerves (CN IX, X, XI, XII)

CN IX, X, XII. Ask the patient to open his/her mouth and observe the tongue at rest in the mouth (fasciculations, wasting). Then ask the patient to say 'Ahhhh' and look for palatal elevation — the side of a CN X palsy fails to elevate normally, and the uvula deviates to the contralateral side. Ask the patient to protrude his tongue (tongue deviates to the side of the CN XII palsy). Speech is not routinely checked unless there is a lower cranial nerve palsy or the stem suggests so (see Syndrome 3.5).

CN XI. Ask the patient to turn his/her head to the left and right against resistance, and to shrug his/her shoulders. Pay attention not just to the strength of movement, but also the sternocleidomastoid bulk.

Putting it together

By this time, you should be able to decide if there is a single or multiple cranial nerve palsy. Always look carefully for head and neck **scars** (note that trans-sphenoidal surgery leaves no scar).

Pitfall: Missing scars

> Missing a scar in the cranial nerve examination (or any PACES station, for that matter) is a cardinal sin. Understand why this might happen and therefore how to avoid this pitfall:
> 1. Not knowing where to look – examine the entire cranium and bilateral neck, but pay special attention to the post-auricular space.
> 2. Scars hidden by hair – ask the patient to lift up long hair so that you can look behind the ear for a post-auricular scar (helpful patients may show you the scar or inform you that there are none).
> 3. Failure to localise the lesion – if one does not recognise that a CN VIII + CN V lesion localises to the cerebellopontine angle, one might not search for the post-auricular scar.

Additional tests are performed to localise the defect further, based on what has been found. For example:

- Most cranial nerve palsies → check upper limb for pronator drift and cerebellar signs.
- If speech is abnormal → test speech (see Syndrome 3.5).
- If there is ptosis → check fatigability; and if there is suspicion for Horner's syndrome, check T1 dermatomal wasting/weakness and examine neck for cervical lymph nodes or masses or scars.
- If there is a RAPD or multiple sclerosis is a possibility, fundoscopy may be offered.

Many cranial mononeuropathies (CN III, VI, internuclear ophthalmoplegia, Bell's palsy) recover within 4–6 weeks and are therefore rarely listed for exams, although occasionally you may get a case pulled from the wards. Therefore cases with some degree of chronicity (e.g., resected cerebellopontine angle tumours, myasthenia gravis, base of skull lesions) are more likely to feature.

Clinical Syndromes

The four rules of cranial nerves (Table A3.2) are always helpful.

Table A3.2. Prof Loong's four rules of cranial nerves[15].

	Rule	Implication
1	Cranial nerves come from the brainstem	Always consider a brainstem lesion in contiguous cranial nerve involvement (e.g., V/VI/VII/VIII), and check the limbs for pronator drift and cerebellar signs.
2	Cranial nerves pass through the base of skull	A base of skull lesion (e.g., meningitis, tumour) can affect any cranial nerve in any combination.
3	Cranial nerves travel in clubs	Specific combinations of cranial nerve palsies localise to specific locations in which they are found together (e.g., III, IV, VI, V_1 = superior orbital fissure).
4	Cranial nerves are peripheral nerves	Cranial nerves are affected by anterior horn cell, peripheral nerve, neuromuscular junction, and muscle disease.

The main clinical syndromes present for the cranial nerve examination are as follows:

Clinical syndrome	Key features
1. Multiple CN palsy	Multiple CN impairment (conforming or nonconforming) ± long tract signs
2. Ophthalmoplegia	Impaired extraocular eye movements ± diplopia May have ptosis and/or abnormal pupils
3. Ptosis	Unilateral or bilateral ptosis May have abnormal pupils
4. Facial droop	Facial droop on inspection Reduced blinking
5. Speech abnormality	Abnormal speech Lower cranial nerve palsy

Other syndromes include visual loss, optic neuropathy (RAPD), and hemianopia: these lend themselves nicely to a consultation station and are covered in the consultation section.

---

[15] Credits: These 4 rules were developed by the late Prof Loong Si Chin (National Neuroscience Institute, Singapore), a respected neurologist and tutor whom many of us learnt from.

Neurology (Cranial Nerves) – Clinical Syndromes

3.1 | Multiple Cranial Nerve Palsy

Multiple cranial nerve palsies are usually good fun and not difficult to localise once you are familiar with this approach. Remember not to miss scars!

Where is the Lesion

The localisation of a multiple cranial nerve palsy is given in Figure A3.1. The key steps are:

A. Does it conform to a known cranial nerve 'club'?
B. Does it correspond to a part of the brainstem?
C. If no, consider:
   o Base of skull disease.
   o Myasthenia gravis.
   o Peripheral nerve.
   o Muscle disease.
   o Anterior horn cell disease.

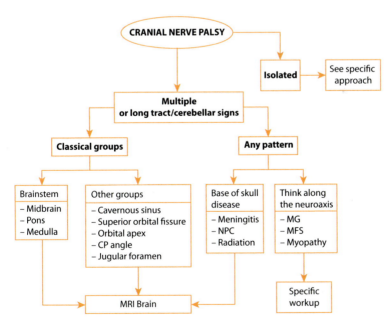

CP angle: cerebellopontine angle; MFS: Miller-Fisher syndrome; MG: myasthenia gravis; NPC: nasopharyngeal carcinoma

Figure A3.1. General approach to cranial nerve palsy.

A. Cranial Nerve Clubs

The cranial nerve 'clubs' are groups of cranial nerves that pass through the same space and therefore may be affected by a lesion at that space. Note that the clubs are sometimes incomplete with only some cranial nerves in each syndrome affected.

Syndrome	CN palsies	Possible aetiologies
1. **Orbital apex**	CN II (relative afferent pupillary defect) CN III, IV, VI, V_1 ± Proptosis	• Thyroid eye disease • Tumour (pituitary adenoma, meningioma, cranio-pharyngioma) • Vascular: cavernous sinus thrombosis, aneurysm • Infective (e.g., abscess)
2. **Superior orbital fossa**	CN III, IV, VI, V_1	
3. **Cavernous sinus**	CN III, IV, VI, V_1-V_2	
4. **Cerebellopontine angle lesion**	CN VIII ± CN VII ± CN V ± ipsilateral cerebellar	• Tumour (e.g., acoustic neuroma) – look for scar, cervical lymph nodes, and stigmata of neurofibromatosis
5. **Jugular foramen**	CN IX, X, XI	• Tumour • Trauma

Further distinction between possible aetiologies may not be possible on physical examination alone. History — in particular time course — is key; for instance an acute lesion is likely vascular or traumatic, while a chronic progressive lesion may be neoplastic.

B. Brainstem Lesions

Recall that CN III-IV arises in the midbrain, CN V-VII in the pons, and CN IX-XII in the medulla; a lesion of these parts of the brainstem may affect the corresponding cranial nerves. Brainstem lesions are more likely if there are long tract or cerebellar signs, especially crossed signs (e.g., left face + right body) or bilateral signs.

1. **Brainstem lesions**

    a) **Midbrain** – CN III, IV palsy ± long tract signs ± cerebellar signs
    b) **Pons** – CN V-VIII palsy ± long tract signs ± cerebellar signs
    c) **Medulla** – CN IX-XII palsies ± long tract signs ± cerebellar signs

The lesion may be vascular (infarct, haemorrhage), demyelinating, or a space-occupying lesion (neoplasm, abscess, etc.).

2. **Lateral medullary syndrome**
   - Crossed sensory loss in the ipsilateral face (S4*) and contralateral limbs (S1*).
   - Ipsilateral Horner's syndrome – ptosis, miosis, anhidrosis (S3*).
   - Ipsilateral palatal paralysis, hoarseness of voice (motor nuclei of CN IX*).
   - Ipsilateral cerebellar signs (S2*) without limb weakness.

*This unique pattern of involvement arises because of the anatomical location of specific tracts and cranial nerve nuclei in the lateral medulla (Table A3.3). *Note that CN XII nuclei, descending corticospinal tracts, and dorsal columns are located in the medial medulla and are therefore unaffected in a lateral medullary syndrome.*

Lateral medullary syndrome is classically a focal infarct affecting the posterior inferior cerebellar artery, although it can happen with focal demyelination.
   - Proceed to examine pulse for atrial fibrillation and look for stigmata of diabetes.

3. **Medial medullary syndrome**
   - Ipsilateral CN XII lesion (i.e., wasted tongue and tongue deviation to abnormal side) (M4).
   - Crossed hemiparesis with contralateral limb weakness (M1).
   - Contralateral loss of vibration and proprioception sense (M2).
   - Ipsilateral internuclear ophthalmoplegia (M3).

This is classically a focal infarct of the lower basilar artery/medial branches of vertebral artery, although it can well happen with focal demyelination.
   - Proceed to examine pulse for atrial fibrillation and look for stigmata of diabetes.

Table A3.3. Lateral organisation of the brainstem.

4 Medial structures (and deficit if lost) *Medial structures start with 'M'*	4 Lateral structures (and deficit if lost) *Side structures start with 'S'*
M1. Motor pathways/corticospinal tract (contralateral weakness)	S1. Spinothalamic pathway (contralateral loss of pain and temperature)
M2. Medial lemniscus (contralateral loss of proprioception and vibration)	S2. Spinocerebellar pathway (ipsilateral cerebellar signs)
M3. Medial longitudinal fasciculus (ipsilateral internuclear ophthalmoplegia)	S3. Sympathetic tract (ipsilateral Horner's syndrome)
M4. Motor cranial nerve nuclei of CN III, IV, VI, and XII (those that are factors of 12)	S4. Sensory nucleus of V (loss of ipsilateral facial sensation)
	Additionally, the motor nuclei of cranial nerves V, VII, IX, and XI are in the lateral brainstem.

C. Non-conforming Multiple CN Palsy

The key is to consider a base of skull process, and remember that cranial nerves are also peripheral nerves.

1. **Motor ± sensory involvement**
   (a) **Base of skull lesion** – can affect any cranial nerve at random. Possible causes:
   - Neoplasm (particularly nasopharyngeal carcinoma in Chinese) – look for cervical lymphadenopathy.
   - Basal meningitis – particularly tuberculous.
   - Fibrosis from prior radiation therapy.
   - Trauma.

   (b) **Peripheral nerve process**
   - Miller-Fisher syndrome – classic triad of ataxia, ophthalmoplegia, and areflexia.
   - Mononeuritis multiplex (page 55).

2. **Only motor involvement**
   (c) **Myasthenia gravis**
   - Variable complex ophthalmoplegia.
   - Look for fatigability on prolonged upgaze and counting from 1 to 20.
   - May also affect limbs – test repeated shoulder abduction.

   (d) **Myopathy** (see Syndrome 2.4). The myopathies have characteristic patterns of cranial nerve involvement. For instance, prominent ocular involvement is seen in occulopharyngeal muscular dystrophy and mitochondrial myopathies, while facioscapulohumeral dystrophy spares the eyes[16].

   (e) **Motor neuron disease (progressive bulbar palsy)**
   - Look for fasciculations.
   - Does not usually affect eye movements.

Look for Complications

- Check speech.
- Check swallowing – consider offering a bedside swallowing test and formal speech therapy assessment.
- If patient is unable to fully close eyes, express your concern for exposure keratitis.

---

[16] Further reading: Barohn RJ, Dimachkie MM, Jackson CE. A pattern recognition approach to patients with a suspected myopathy. *Neurol Clin* 2014 32(3):569–93.

Sample Scripts

Myasthenia gravis

This young lady has multiple cranial nerve palsies with variable complex ophthalmoplegia, fatigable ptosis, dysphonia, and fatigable speech. There is also fatigable proximal weakness in the upper limbs. Sensation and cerebellar function is normal. The likely diagnosis is myasthenia gravis. I am concerned about her respiratory status as her neck flexion is weak, and will like to do a bedside negative inspiratory force.

Cerebellopontine angle lesion

This middle-aged gentleman has right-sided sensorineural hearing loss as evidenced by decreased hearing on the right, air conduction better than bone conduction on Rinne's test, and Weber's test lateralising to the left. He also has right-sided lower motor neuron facial droop which does not spare the frontalis muscle. There is a right post-auricular scar. I suspect that he has had a previous cerebellopontine angle lesion, such as a cerebellopontine angle tumour, which has since been resected.

Neurology (Cranial Nerves) – Clinical Syndromes

3.2 | Ophthalmoplegia

Ophthalmoplegia is reasonably straightforward. Very often the syndrome is given away by a stem of 'difficulty seeing', 'double vision', or if you note an eye patch or prism glasses by the bedside. Be sure to observe the eyes in the primary position and 'stress' extreme right/left gaze so as to identify a subtle CN VI palsy.

Approach

Determine if a single cranial nerve palsy can explain the pattern of ophthalmoplegia:

A. CN III
B. CN VI   } See subsequent sections
C. CN IV
D. Internuclear ophthalmoplegia, one and a half syndrome

Important negatives that must be fulfilled before calling it a single cranial nerve palsy are:

- No other cranial nerve deficit.
- No cerebellar signs (brainstem lesion).
- No long tract signs, particularly no crossed hemiparesis (brainstem lesion).
- No fatigability (myasthenia gravis).
- No thyroid eye signs.

If the pattern of ophthalmoplegia does not fit any of the above, consider:

- Cranial nerves 'clubs' (Syndrome 3.1).
- A brainstem lesion, particularly if there are long tract signs (Syndrome 3.1).
- Complex ophthalmoplegia (i.e., does not conform to any known pattern) which gives differentials of:
  - Myasthenia gravis.
  - Thyroid eye disease.
  - Miller-Fisher syndrome.
  - Chronic progressive external ophthalmoplegia (CPEO).
  - Causes of a mononeuritis multiplex.

A. Isolated CN III Palsy

Features

- Complete/partial ptosis of the affected eye.
- In primary position: divergent strabismus with affected eye 'down and out' (may not always be obvious).
- Impairment of all extraocular eye movements except abduction (CN VI) and depression (CN IV).

Checking CN IV in the presence of a CN III lesion

> Brownie points for ruling out a concomitant CN IV palsy in a CN III palsy. Remember that CN IV is responsible for depression in an adducted position, as well as intorsion. The former cannot be tested in a 'down and out' eye, but intorsion can. Have the patient attempt down gaze and discern whether the eye intorts by looking at a conjunctival vessel.

Further localisation: Distinguish between pupil-sparing and pupil-involved third nerve palsy. Recall that the parasympathetic fibres of CN III are on the outside of the nerve, so they may be affected in a compressive lesion but spared in a microvascular lesion, which preferentially affects the inner fibres.

	Pupil Sparing (isolated CN III)	**Pupil Involved** (isolated CN III)
Signs	Pupil not dilated, reacts to light 'Medical' third nerve palsy	Pupil dilated, unreactive to light 'Surgical' third nerve palsy
Aetiology	– Microvascular disease (i.e., diabetes, hypertension, vasculitis) – Trauma – Consider compressive lesion if incomplete ptosis[17] or fail to recover – Idiopathic	– Concern of compressive lesion (i.e., posterior communicating artery aneurysm) – Idiopathic

Fine print: the presence of contralateral ptosis suggests a III nerve nuclear lesion[18].

---

[17] The thought process here is: if the microvascular lesion is severe enough to cause complete ptosis and yet the pupils are spared, then a compressive lesion is unlikely. However, if there is incomplete ptosis, we are much less confident that we have ruled out a compressive lesion.

[18] A central midbrain nucleus supplies bilateral levator palpebrae superioris; a nuclear 3rd nerve palsy therefore results in bilateral ptosis.

B. Isolated CN VI Palsy

Features

- In primary position: convergent strabismus.
- Abduction failure/incomplete abduction in affected eye.
- Patient complains of horizontal diplopia on abduction of affected eye.

Common causes

- Microvascular disease (diabetes, hypertension, hyperlipidemia, vasculitis).
- Idiopathic.
- Trauma.
- False localising CN IV from raised intracranial pressure (unlikely in a well patient).

C. Isolated CN IV Palsy

CN IV palsies are rarely listed for PACES as they are subtle and may be identified only with cover-uncover testing and the Parks-Bielschowsky 3-step test (not expected in PACES).

Features

- In primary position: hyperopia of affected side (failure of depression) and head tilt away from affected side (due to failure of intorsion).
- Impaired depression of affected eye, worst in adducted position (inferior rectus depresses the eye in primary or abducted position, while superior oblique is the main muscle responsible for depression in the adducted position).
- Patient complains of vertical diplopia that is worst on looking down and away from the affected side.

Common causes

- Idiopathic.
- Trauma (due to long intracranial course).
- Microvascular disease (diabetes, hypertension, hyperlipidemia).
- Congenital.

D. Internuclear Ophthalmoplegia

These are rare syndromes with specific localisation value.

Features

(a) **Internuclear ophthalmoplegia (INO)**
  - In primary position: eyes central.
  - On lateral gaze, the affected eye fails to adduct and the contralateral eye abducts with nystagmus.

(b) **One and a half syndrome**
- In primary position: eyes central.
- Complete gaze palsy on affected side (neither abducts nor adducts).
- Internuclear ophthalmoplegia in contralateral eye (fails to adduct on contralateral gaze).

Localisation
- Unilateral INO
  - Normal convergence – pons (medial longitudinal fasciculus) on side of eye that does not adduct.
  - Abnormal convergence – dorsal midbrain (version centre) on side of eye that does not adduct.
- Bilateral INO – bilateral pons/midbrain.
- One and a half syndrome – midbrain lesion on side of complete gaze palsy, affecting the parapontine reticular formation (the 'one' — both eyes unable to look to the affected side) and median longitudinal fasciculus (the 'half' — INO looking to the opposite side).
- One and a half syndrome may be combined with a LMN CN VII palsy on the side of complete gaze palsy. This is the 'eight and a half syndrome', similarly caused by a slightly larger lesion on the side of the eye with complete gaze palsy, affecting the parapontine reticular formation (the 'one'), the medial longitudinal fasciculus (the 'half'), and the facial nerve nucleus causing an LMN CN VII palsy (the 'seven').

Aetiology – essentially the causes of a brainstem lesion:
- Small infarct, classically microvascular disease (most common).
- Focal demyelination (i.e., multiple sclerosis) – strongly suspect in bilateral INO.
- Focal haemorrhage.
- Small mass lesion (e.g., neoplasm).

Look for Complications

This will essentially be assessing the patient's functional vision and complications of poor vision (e.g., falls).

Sample Scripts

Third nerve palsy

This is an elderly gentleman with a right third nerve palsy. There is complete ptosis of the right eye, which is 'down and out' at rest. All extraocular movements are impaired except depression and abduction. There is pupil sparing. There are no other cranial neuropathies, no fatigability, no long tract signs, and no cerebellar signs. The likely cause of the third nerve palsy is microvascular disease, and I note capillary glucose check marks and evidence of peripheral vascular disease. Differentials include trauma and idiopathic causes. A compressive lesion, such as a posterior communicating artery aneurysm, is less likely with pupil sparing in complete ptosis, but must still be considered if he fails to improve. Functionally I note that he has an eye patch and is still able to read newspapers. I will like to complete my examination by checking the blood pressure and capillary glucose, and performing fundoscopy for diabetic and hypertensive changes.

Neurology (Cranial Nerves) – Clinical Syndromes

3.3 | Ptosis

The eyes have to be examined very carefully in a ptosis case. Examine for anisocoria in the dark so as not to miss Horner's syndrome. Ophthalmoplegia and fatigability may be subtle; a cursory 10-second upgaze will not do. Bilateral ptosis is subtle and easily missed. Comment on frontalis overactivity (wrinkles on the forehead) if present.

Approach

Ptosis arises from weakness of the levator palpebrae superioris, which is supplied by both CN III as well as ascending sympathetic fibres. Keeping the eyes open also requires normal peripheral nerve, neuromuscular junction, and muscle function (Table A3.4). Anterior horn cell disease tends not to affect the eyes prominently.

Table A3.4. Key causes of ptosis.

	Unilateral	Bilateral
CN III	Isolated CN III palsy CN III in club or brainstem lesion	Nuclear CN III[19]
Sympathetic fibres	Horner's syndrome	
Peripheral nerve		Miller-Fisher syndrome
Neuromuscular junction	Myasthenia gravis	Myasthenia gravis
Muscle		Myopathy
Other causes	Aponeurotic ptosis (or senile ptosis), congenital ptosis	

Key questions to answer are:

1. Is this an isolated ptosis, or are there other cranial nerve palsies, long tract, or cerebellar signs? In particular, consider:
   - Cranial nerve clubs (Syndrome 3.1).
   - Brainstem lesion, with long tract signs or contiguous CN palsies (Syndrome 3.1).
   - Myopathy (lower cranial nerves, proximal limb muscles affected).
   - Miller-Fisher syndrome (areflexia, ataxia).

---

[19] A central midbrain nucleus supplies bilateral levator palpebrae superioris; a nuclear 3rd nerve palsy therefore results in bilateral ptosis.

2. Is ptosis unilateral or bilateral?
   - Look for any blepharoplasty scar (eyelid lift surgery). Unilateral ptosis + a contralateral blepharoplasty scar = bilateral ptosis!
3. In the eyes, look out for:
   - Miosis – Horner's syndrome.
   - Ophthalmoplegia – CN III.
   - Dilated pupil – CN III.
   - Fatigability – Myasthenia gravis.
4. If all else is not found, consider 'local causes' (e.g., senile ptosis) or a loose aponeurotic fold (unlikely in PACES).

A. Unilateral Ptosis

Isolated unilateral ptosis, having ruled out multiple cranial nerve palsy or a brainstem lesion, gives the following key differentials:

- CN III palsy (see Syndrome 3.2).
- Horner's syndrome.
- Myasthenia gravis – can affect both eyes asymmetrically.
- Local causes.

Horner's syndrome

Key features

- Ipsilateral partial non-fatigable ptosis.
- Miosis.
- ± Anhidrosis (in a first- and second-order Horner's syndrome).

Localisation. Horner's syndrome can arise from a disruption anywhere along the sympathetic supply. Recall that:

- The first order sympathetic neuron descends from the hypothalamus through the brainstem into the cervical spinal cord.
- The second-order sympathetic neuron in the cervical spinal cord travels through the brachial plexus over the lung apex and ascends to the superior cervical ganglion, which is in close proximity to the common carotid artery bifurcation.
- The third-order neuron ascends with the internal carotid artery through the skull base into the cavernous sinus, joining CN V_1 into the eye.

The causes of Horner's syndrome are given in Table A3.5. In practice, having ruled out other cranial nerve palsies, long tract, or cerebellar signs, the remaining steps in the examination routine will be to:

- Test for anhidrosis by feeling the facial skin. Normal facial skin feels slightly oily, while an anhidrotic face feels gritty. Anhidrosis is present in a 1st and 2nd order Horner's syndrome.
- Examine the upper limbs, particularly paying attention to intrinsic muscle wasting (T1 root) and pinprick loss in a shawl-like distribution (syringomyelia).
- Examine the neck, particularly looking for scars, examining for cervical lymph nodes, and auscultating for a carotid bruit.
- Offer to auscultate the lungs.

Table A3.5. Localisation and important causes of Horner's syndrome.

Order	Localisation	Features	Important causes
1st	Brainstem	Long tract, cerebellar signs Lateral medullary syndrome (page 85)	Infarct, demyelination, space-occupying lesion
	Cervical spine	UMN signs below level	Syringomyelia (page 35) Degenerative, trauma, etc.
2nd	Brachial plexus	C5-T1 root weakness	Trauma, iatrogenic (e.g., central line insertion)
	Lung apex	T1 root wasting and weakness	Pancoast tumour
3rd	Cervical ganglion	Neck pain, carotid bruit Cervical lymph nodes	Carotid dissection, thrombosis Tumour, infiltration, trauma
	Skull base	Non-conforming CN palsy	Tumour, basal meningitis, old radiation therapy
	Cavernous sinus	CN III, IV, VI, V_1-V_2 palsy	Tumour (e.g., pituitary adenoma) Cavernous sinus thrombosis, aneurysm
	Superior orbital fissure	CN III, IV, VI, V_1 palsy	Infective (e.g., abscess)

B. Bilateral Ptosis

The key differentials, having ruled out multiple cranial nerve palsy or a brainstem lesion, are:
- Myasthenia gravis.
- Myopathy.
- Miller-Fisher syndrome.
- Nuclear CN III palsy.

Because myasthenia is so common in PACES, the first step is to test for fatigability.

1. **Fatigable bilateral ptosis**

Fatigability is the hallmark of myasthenia gravis. This will be accompanied by other features of myasthenia, such as proximal weakness and ophthalmoplegia. Frontalis overactivity, which is not usually present in a myopathy, may be the first clue to suspect myasthenia.

2. **Non-fatigable bilateral ptosis**

Rule out

- Fatigability (myasthenia gravis).
- Miosis (Horner's syndrome).
- 'Down and out eye' (CN III palsy).

Look for features to suggest a cause

- **Myotonic dystrophy**: frontal balding, facial diplegia, distal wasting and weakness of hands, percussion and grip myotonia.
- **Other myopathies**: LMN proximal weakness with normal sensation (Syndrome 2.4).
- **Mitochondrial disorders** (e.g., chronic progressive externalophthalmoplegia (CPEO)): multidirectional ophthalmoplegia (often severe), ptosis, orbicularis oculi weakness.
- **Miller-Fisher syndrome**: Complex ophthalmoplegia, ataxia, areflexia.

Sample Scripts

Horner's syndrome

My patient is an elderly lady with a left-sided Horner's syndrome as evidenced by partial ptosis, miosis, and anhidrosis of the left face. The eye movements are normal and there are no other cranial neuropathies. However she is clubbed and has wasting of the intrinsic muscles of the left hand, associated with weakness of finger abduction. This is worrisome for a neoplasm in the lung apex. There are no cervical lymph nodes or neck scars. I will like to complete my examination by performing a respiratory examination and taking a smoking history.

Myasthenia gravis

This young gentleman has bilateral fatigable ptosis with compensatory frontalis hyperactivity, variable complex ophthalmoplegia, and a nasal voice which gets softer counting to 20. The rest of the cranial nerves are normal; in particular, there are no CN III, IV, or V palsies to suggest superior orbital fissure or cavernous sinus syndrome. There is no limb weakness. The diagnosis is ocular myasthenia gravis. I note a midline sternotomy suggesting a prior thymectomy. I will like to complete my examination by checking negative inspiratory force and forced vital capacity, as well as asking for a drug history.

Neurology (Cranial Nerves) – Clinical Syndromes

3.4 | Facial Droop

Gross facial asymmetry is obvious on inspection. More subtle facial nerve lesions may appear as:
- One eye does not blink, or blinks less/incompletely.
- Nasolabial fold is less marked on one side.
- Bilateral facial droop

This is generally an easy case.

Approach

Step 1: Is this an isolated unilateral facial droop?
- If there are cranial nerve palsies (particularly CN V and VIII) – approach as for multiple cranial nerve palsy (Syndrome 3.1).
- In bilateral facial droop – consider a more generalised cause. Applying the four rules of cranial nerves (Table A3.2) readily results in a list of differentials and suggestions on what to examine next (Table A3.6).

Table A3.6. Causes of bilateral facial droop

	Cranial Nerve Rule	Differential of bilateral facial droop	Also examine...
1.	Cranial nerves come from the brainstem	Pons lesion (infarct, haemorrhage, neoplasm, demyelination) – can affect both facial nerves if large enough.	Long tract signs Other cranial nerves
2.	Cranial nerves pass through the base of the skull	Basal meningitis (e.g., tuberculous) Base of skull neoplasm (nasopharyngeal carcinoma)	Cervical lymph node
3.	Cranial nerves travel in clubs	(Not applicable)	
4.	Cranial nerves are peripheral nerves	Guillain-Barré/Miller-Fisher syndrome Bilateral parotid lesion (e.g., mumps, Sjogren's syndrome) Bilateral Bell's palsy NMJ – myasthenia gravis Myopathy – myotonic dystrophy, facio-scapulohumeral dystrophy, etc.	Ataxia, areflexia Parotidomegaly Fatigability Myotonia, winging of scapulae

Step 2: Is this UMN or LMN facial nerve palsy?

- Examine both the upper and lower face carefully. A sample routine could include:
  - Furrowing of forehead on upward gaze (frontalis – temporal branch).
  - Forceful eye closure/ability to completely bury eyelashes (orbicularis occuli – zygomatic branch).
  - Smile (multiple muscles – buccal branch).
  - Puff out cheeks (buccinator – buccal branch).
- UMN facial nerve palsy spares the upper face (frontalis and orbicularis occuli) which receive bilateral innervation.
- Facial synkinesis (e.g., corner of mouth twitches when patient blinks), reflecting aberrant regeneration, occurs in LMN facial nerve palsy. It *does not occur in UMN disease.*

A. UMN CN VII Palsy

Key features

- Facial droop/loss of nasolabial fold.
- Sparing of the frontalis and orbicularis occuli.

The next step is to look for ipsilateral UMN signs (e.g., spastic hemiparesis). This is discussed in Syndrome 2.2.

B. LMN CN VII Palsy

Consider aetiologies by thinking along the course of the facial nerve (the 5 Ps):

Location	Lesion	Other signs
Pons	Infarct, demyelination	Crossed hemiparesis, cerebellar
Posterior fossa	Cerebellopontine angle lesion	CN VIII ± CN V palsy
		Post auricular scar
		Cutaneous neurofibroma
	Base of skull lesion	Non-conforming CN palsy
		Bloody rhinorrhoea
Petrous part of temporal bone	Ramsay Hunt syndrome	Vesicles on otoscopy
	Cholesteatoma	Hearing loss
	Complicated otitis media	Otitis media on otoscopy
Parotid	Infiltrative parotid tumour	Parotid lump/scar
		Cervical lymphadenopathy
Peripheries	Mononeuritis multiplex	Other neuropathies
	Bell's Palsy	

Practically, after ruling out other CN palsies, long tract signs, and cerebellar signs, a possible routine would be to:

- Inspect for parotid and post-auricular scars carefully – ask for permission to lift the patient's hair (some patients may even point out their scar to you).
- Palpate the parotid and for cervical lymph nodes.
- Offer otoscopy (for vesicles, cholesteatoma) and formal hearing assessment.

In the absence of a secondary cause, the most likely diagnosis is Bell's palsy.

Look for Complications

A number of important complications arise in facial nerve palsy:

- Exposure keratitis due to inability to close eyes completely.
- Impact on speech.

Suggested Scripts

Bell's palsy

This middle-aged gentleman has a right lower motor neuron facial nerve palsy as evidenced by a right-sided facial droop with frontalis weakness and inability to bury the eyelashes. His hearing and other cranial nerves are normal. There are no long tract or cerebellar signs. There is no scar and no palpable parotidomegaly or cervical lymphadenopathy. The likely diagnosis is Bell's palsy. I will like to check the corneal reflex and perform otoscopy to look for vesicles, otitis media, or cholesteatoma. I note that he is using an eye patch; he may have had exposure keratitis.

Tip: Do all Bell's palsies warrant an MRI scan?

> **Honest answer**: it depends on local practice norms, resource availability (whether the patient presents to a tertiary centre or primary care), the medicolegal environment, and often the clinician's comfort level.
>
> **Exam answer**: Bell's palsy is a clinical diagnosis, but imaging is warranted if:
> - The history or physical signs are atypical.
> - It continues to worsen after 3 weeks.
> - It fails to improve within 4 months.

Neurology (Cranial Nerves) – Clinical Syndromes

3.5 | Speech Abnormality

This is a difficult case. Speech examination itself is challenging, but there will usually be other signs (cranial nerves and limbs) that you can go by.

Approach

Examination Routine

A suggested routine for the 'patient has speech difficulty' stem may include:

- Greeting the patient and engaging in small talk → assess for dysphonia or hypophonia (Parkinsonism).
- Inspecting and screening pronator drift. Look for any hemiparesis (cortical – dysphasia), ataxia (cerebellar), or tremor (Parkinson's disease).
- Saying "British constitution" or counting to 20 → assess for cerebellar dysarthria.
- Saying "ba ba ba" → tests lips (VII nerve).
- Saying "la la la" → tests tongue (XII nerve).
- Saying "ka ka ka" → tests palate (X nerve).
- Asking the patient to name his/her favourite colour, what he/she had for breakfast → check for expressive dysphasia (Broca's area, frontal lobe).
- Asking the patient to follow instructions (e.g., close eye) → check for receptive dysphasia (Wernicke's area, temporal lobe).
- Asking the patient to repeat "no ifs, ands, or buts" → check for conductive dysphasia (Arcuate fasciculus).
- Asking the patient to name objects (e.g., watch, pen) → check for nominal dysphasia (Angular gyrus, temporal-parietal lobe).
- Examining the rest of the cranial nerves in the usual way.
- Checking for cortical signs (e.g., line bisection), visual fields, and long tracts.

Interpretation

Begin by distinguishing:

- Dysphonia – cannot produce sound.
- Dysarthria – can produce sound, but unclear.
- Dysphasia – can produce clear sound, but difficulty saying meaningful words.

1. **Dysphonia**
   - Commonly hypophonia in Parkinson's disease (see Syndrome 2.10).
   - Local (e.g., vocal cord) lesions, unlikely in PACES.
2. **Dysarthria**
   - Cerebellar dysarthria.
   - Flaccid dysarthria – Bulbar palsy (LMN palsy of cranial nerves IX, X, XI, or XII).
   - Spastic dysarthria – Pseudobulbar palsy (UMN palsy of cranial nerves IX, X, XI, or XII).
3. **Dysphasia**
   - First, distinguish receptive vs. expressive vs. other dysphasias.
   - Next, localise to the appropriate cortical region and do other tests for that cortical region (e.g., 2 point discrimination in a parietal lobe lesion).
   - This is usually considered unfair for PACES and will not be covered in further detail here.

Tips: On diagnosing the cause of dysarthria

> 1. The distinction between flaccid and spastic dysarthria is challenging. Few non-neurologists are confident in calling speech spastic vs. flaccid, so it is best to look for other clues of UMN vs. LMN disease (e.g., fasciculations, limb signs, jaw jerk).
> 2. To cause spastic dysarthria, a bilateral UMN lesion is necessary. Unilateral stroke will not cause pseudobulbar palsy because cranial nerve nuclei (except CN VII and XII) receive bilateral cortical innervation. Therefore, unilateral brain lesions tend not to cause cranial nerve deficits apart from UMN facial droop and possibly an UMN XII lesion.
> 3. Do not be confused by a mix of UMN and LMN signs — this suggests motor neuron disease.

A. Flaccid Dysarthria – Bulbar Palsy

Key signs

- Wasted ± fasciculating tongue.
- Absent palatal movement *(not discriminatory)*.
- Nasal speech, a weak and soft voice with slurring of labial ("Ba") and lingual ("La") consonants.
- Drooling.
- Dysphagia ± nasogastric tube.
- Depressed or normal jaw jerk.

Localisation	Aetiology	Signs
Brainstem	Infarct, demyelination	Long tract signs, cerebellar signs
	Syringobulbia	Pinprick loss in shawl-like distribution
		Horner's syndrome, UMN signs in lower limb
Anterior horn cell	Motor neuron disease	Prominent fasciculations
		Hypertonia and brisk reflexes in wasted limb
Peripheral nerve	Guillain-Barré	Symmetric LMN weakness, areflexia
	Base of skull disease	Non-conforming cranial nerve palsy
Neuromuscular junction	Myasthenia gravis	Fatigable speech
		Fatigable ptosis, ophthalmoplegia

Practically, after ruling out other cranial nerve palsies, long tract, and cerebellar signs, a possible routine will be to:

- Inspect the tongue carefully for fasciculation.
- Test fatigability of speech (count 1 to 20).
- Look carefully for scars and radiotherapy marks.
- Examine upper limbs carefully (or offer to, if you do not have time).

B. Spastic Dysarthria – Pseudobulbar Palsy

Key signs

- Sluggish palatal movement (not discriminatory).
- Small, stiff, spastic tongue (cannot say "la la la").
- High pitched and slow speech, imprecise articulation, and a strained quality ('Donald Duck' speech).
- Brisk jaw jerk.
- Emotional lability (also known as pseudobulbar affect).
- UMN signs in limb.

Localisation: A bilateral UMN lesion is required — consider:

- Multiple sclerosis.
- Motor neuron disease – look for mixed UMN and LMN signs (e.g., brisk reflexes in a wasted limb), prominent fasciculations.
- Bilateral stroke.

C. Cerebellar (Ataxic) Dysarthria

Key signs

- Irregular speech with a variable rate and intonation pattern. This may be jerky and explosive, or slow and scanning.
- Other cerebellar signs (e.g., multi directional gaze-evoked nystagmus, jerky pursuit, bilateral dysmetria).

This is discussed further in Syndrome 2.9.

Look for Complications

Important complications to consider in a lower cranial nerve case include:

- Functional speech impairment.
- Swallowing dysfunction and aspiration risk – use of nasogastric tube, percutaneous gastrostomy tubes.

Sample Scripts

Base of skull disease

This middle-aged lady has multiple lower cranial nerve palsies including left-sided reduced palatal elevation, left-sided tongue wasting, and deviation to the left on tongue protrusion. Her speech is nasal and soft, with slurring of labial consonants ("ba ba ba") and lingual consonants ("la la la"). She also has dysphagia requiring the use of a nasogastric tube. There are skin changes consistent with chronic radiation dermatitis in the left neck. The clinical localisation is to the base of the skull, such as post-radiotherapy neuropathy or leptomeningeal processes like carcinomatosis or tuberculous meningitis. Differentials include mononeuritis multiplex and anterior horn cell disease. There are no long tract or cerebellar signs to suggest a brainstem lesion, and no fatigability to suggest myasthenia*. I will like to complete my examination by checking the gag reflex, examining the limbs, and doing a bedside swallowing test.

*Additionally, myasthenia tends not to cause wasting.

Bulbar palsy

This patient has multiple lower cranial nerve palsies. He has dysarthria with a weak and soft voice, reduced bilateral palatal movement, and bilateral facial droop. In the limbs there is proximal weakness in both upper limbs with intact sensation. Additionally there are fasciculations of the tongue and limb. There is no fatigability. The likely diagnosis is anterior horn cell disease, although my differentials include myasthenia gravis and myopathies. I will like to complete my examination by checking the gag reflex, examining the limbs, and doing a bedside swallow test.

Neurology (Cranial Nerves)

3.6 | Discussion Framework

As with the neurology (limbs) chapter, this section provides a general framework to answer examiners' questions, focusing on how to structure a sound answer, and principles that apply across all cases in this system. It must be tailored and prioritised to your list of differentials.

How Would You Investigate?

"I will like to confirm my diagnosis, identify the aetiology, and look for complications."

I. Rule out any potential emergency

For example:
- In a pupil-involved CN III palsy – offer urgent MRI brain and neurosurgical consult.
- In myasthenia gravis – offer to check negative inspiratory force (should be more negative than −30 cm H_2O) and forced vital capacity (ensure >20 mL/kg)

II. Confirm diagnosis and investigate for aetiology

Go directly for investigations that will confirm the suspected diagnosis.

1. **More history/examination**
   - Time course of neurological deficit is always helpful – vascular lesions develop acutely (in minutes), inflammatory lesions are subacute (hours to days), while neoplastic or degenerative lesions take much longer to develop.
   - Specific features that will distinguish between differentials.
   - Family history in heritable conditions.
2. **MRI**
   - MRI Brain if localisation is to the brain or brainstem.
   - MRI specific parts (e.g., orbits, facial nerve) for more specific attention.
   - In suspected multiple sclerosis, do MRI brain + spine looking for dissemination in space and dissemination in time.
3. **Neurodiagnostic tests are useful in LMN disorders**
   - Myasthenia gravis: Repetitive nerve stimulation, single fibre electromyogram.
   - Nerve conduction study and electromyography – see discussion in Chapter 2.10.
4. **Investigation of systemic disease**
   - CT neck/thorax in Horner's syndrome.

- Refer ENT for nasoendoscopy if concerned about nasopharyngeal cancer (especially in southern Chinese populations).
- Bloods (e.g., screen cardiovascular risk factors, autoantibodies in myasthenia gravis).

III. Look for complications

- Swallowing assessment if lower cranial nerves are involved.
- Ophthalmological assessment for exposure keratitis in a Bell's palsy.

How Would You Manage?

"Patient requires multidisciplinary management including specific treatment of the underlying disease, management of complications, and supportive management to maximise function."

If there are no specific treatment, *"Management of X is mainly supportive with multi-disciplinary interventions to manage complications and maximise function."*

1. **Management of an emergency**
   - Neurosurgical referral for surgical 3rd nerve palsy.
   - Intubation for myasthenia with respiratory compromise.
2. **Specific treatment** (if any)
   - Surgical treatment for a structural lesion/tumour.
   - Immunosuppression (e.g., steroids in Bell's palsy, IVIg/plasma exchange in myasthenia flare).
   - Acetylcholinesterase inhibitors (e.g., pyridostigmine) in myasthenia.
   - Treat metabolic cause (e.g., control diabetes, treat thyroid disorder).
3. **Management of complications**
   - For example, exposure keratitis in Bell's palsy – lubricant eye drop, eye patch, referral for tarsorraphy if severe.
   - Modified diet consistency, nasogastric or gastrotomy tubes in swallowing dysfunction.
4. **Supportive management to maximise function**
   - Patient education.
   - Speech therapy.
   - Optical correction (e.g., prism glasses for diplopia).
   - Hearing aids.
   - Vaccination.
   - Genetic counselling and screening of family members (in genetic diseases).

Sample Scripts

Post-radiotherapy lower cranial nerve dysfunction

Investigations: I will like to confirm my diagnosis and look for complications. First I will like to take a history of past head and neck cancer and prior radiotherapy. I will like to do an MRI brain and neck looking for leptomeningeal neoplasm or tuberculosis. I may consider lumbar puncture, sending CSF for cytology and acid-fast bacilli, smear and culture. I will send the patient for swallowing assessment.

Management: Although the underlying cause of radiation cannot be reversed, my patient will benefit from multidisciplinary management to mitigate complications and maximise function. This includes speech therapy consult for recommendations on diet consistency and minimising aspiration risk, vaccinations, patient education, and management of comorbid conditions.

Physical Examination

4 | Cardiology

Additional resources and examination videos available at: www.nigelfong.net/paces-resources.html

The cardiology station has a reputation for being unpredictable. Most candidates score well in cases of prosthetic valves or classical aortic stenosis, while a barely audible mitral stenosis or congenital heart disorder will prove tricky even for the best of candidates. While much is at the mercy of the exam centre (and examiner), the candidate's best bet is to have experienced as many cases as possible and learn some tricks to maximise one's yield even in difficult cases, which this chapter seeks to help with.

Acronyms used in this section:

AS	Aortic stenosis	HCM	Hypertrophic cardiomyopathy
AR	Aortic regurgitation	PDA	Patent ductus arteriosus
MS	Mitral stenosis	VSD	Ventricular septal defect
MR	Mitral regurgitation	ASD	Atrial septal defect
TR	Tricuspid regurgitation	AF	Atrial fibrillation
PS	Pulmonary stenosis	LLSE	Lower left sternal edge
PR	Pulmonary regurgitation		

Walk-Through and Tips

Listen to the stem

This tends to be less informative than in the other systems but listen to the presenting symptom, for example, palpitations (look for AF and its potential aetiologies such as MS), syncope (HCM? AS?), or breathlessness (non-specific but already an indication for valve replacement).

General inspection

Size up the patient's age; in a younger patient, be particularly alert for congenital conditions such as VSD, HCM, and cyanotic diseases. Two critical questions that must be answered on general inspection are:

(1) **Is there cyanosis and/or clubbing?** If so, suspect congenital cyanotic heart disease or endocarditis. It is exceedingly difficult to accurately interpret the many murmurs of congenital heart disease without first suspecting congenital disease.

109

(2) **Is this a prosthetic valve case?** Look for scars — if there is a sternotomy or mitral valvotomy scar, listen very hard for prosthetic clicks and check for a saphenous vein graft scar. Note that a sternotomy + saphenous vein graft scar does not always imply coronary artery bypass (CABG) alone as there can be a concomitant prosthetic valve, while the absence of a saphenous vein graft scar does not exclude CABG as the internal mammary artery alone can be used. If prosthetic clicks are heard, determine whether there are one or two clicks, and time it against the carotid pulse.

It is also helpful to pay close attention to the neck. Prominent pulsations in the neck suggest either Corrigan's sign (AR, which prompts a careful examination for a collapsing pulse) or giant c-v waves (TR). Other clues which may be identified here include marfanoid habitus (?AR) or dysmorphic facies (congenital heart disease?), respiratory distress, bedside apparatus (e.g., left ventricular assist device), or a malar flush (rare).

Peripheries

Begin with the hands. Inspect for clubbing and peripheral stigmata of infective endocarditis. Check the right radial pulse rate and rhythm, timing it over at least 10–15 seconds so as not to miss any atrial fibrillation. Simultaneously palpate the left radial pulse to elicit radial-radial delay. Radiofemoral delay is not routinely performed, but must be done later if there is a unexplained systolic murmur or audible PDA. Remember that the character of the pulse is best assessed at the carotid, although a difficult-to-palpate radial pulse may be the first clue of AS.

Collapsing pulse is an important sign because the early diastolic murmur of AR can be difficult to hear without prior clinical suspicion. It is a reliable sign provided that good technique is employed. Place your right hand *over* the patient's wrist and locate the radial pulse with your fingertips. Shift your fingers to position your middle phalanges over the radial pulse; as the middle phalanges are less sensitive, the pulse should be barely palpable now. Ask the patient if he/she has any shoulder pain and warn that you will raise his/her arm. Placing your left hand below the patient's elbow as a support, lift the patient's arm gradually. If doing so makes the radial pulse strongly palpable even with your insensitive middle phalanges, you can be confident that there is a collapsing pulse; prime yourself to listen very carefully for AR or a PDA later. If you are unsure, lower the arm gradually — the collapsing pulse is often still felt as little as 20–30 degrees above the horizontal meridian, then disappears. Raise the arm again slightly and the collapsing pulse reappears. Some examiners may give you a blood pressure should you ask for one — look out for a wide pulse pressure (AR) or narrow pulse pressure (AS).

Pitfall: The collapsing pulse

> The collapsing pulse is a reliable sign but tends to be poorly performed. Some common errors:
> - Do not lift with the palpating hand. This leads to inconsistent pressure application and under- or over-diagnosis of a collapsing pulse. Place your right hand above — not under — the wrist to avoid lifting with the palpating hand.
> - Do not lift the arm exceedingly rapidly. It is gravity — not the rate of elevation — that makes the pulse collapse. Doing so demonstrates a poor understanding of the collapsing pulse and can cause patient discomfort.
> - Do not palpate both the brachial and radial pulse simultaneously or seek to elicit a brachial-radial delay. This false teaching has been propagated but is simply baseless.

Move on to the face, looking in the eyes for conjunctival pallor and scleral icterus. Warn the patient before checking for conjunctival pallor — do not simply pull down the eyelid without permission. Look in the mouth for a high arched palate and dental hygiene (brownie points in a prosthetic valve case).

The neck is critical. Clearly distinguish a JVP from the carotid pulse — the JVP is occludable, not palpable, has two waveforms, and rises with right hypochondrial pressure. Prominent pulsations in the neck might be Corrigan's sign (AR) or giant c-v waves (TR). TR is a diagnosis best made in the neck — on auscultation, TR can be tricky to distinguish from VSD and MR. If no prominent pulsations are seen, inspect for the level of the JVP (elevated in congestive heart failure). If the JVP is not obvious, look at the neck from different angles — its pulsations are often more apparent from the side-view than looking straight-on.

Precordium

Inspect the chest carefully, paying attention to all scars — look out for a mitral scar hidden below the breast, the double scar of a re-do sternotomy, or more than 3 subcostal drain site scars (a sternotomy usually comes with 3 drain scars — if there are 6, look for two sternotomies). Look out for an implantable cardiac device (suspect HCM in a young patient with an implantable cardiac device) and see if the apex beat is visible.

Palpate for the apex beat. This can be challenging especially in a patient of larger body habitus. If the apex is not palpable, turn the patient left lateral to repalpate, and also check the right side for dextrocardia. Determine the location of the apex beat — the most lateral and inferior point at which it is still palpable, counting from the sternal angle — as well as its character. In AR/MR, the apex is displaced and diffuse over a large area (volume overload/thrusting). In AS, the apex is undisplaced and prolonged (pressure overload/heaving). In MS, the apex is undisplaced and tapping (a clear, non-prolonged 'tap' which represents the first heart sound).

Palpate for a parasternal heave (right ventricular hypertrophy) and thrills (VSD) at the lower left sternal edge. Palpate for a palpable pulmonary component of the second heart sound (pulmonary hypertension).

Pitfall: Beware of breasts

> Particularly for male candidates — practice handling large breasts sensitively and smoothly. Two slick methods are to (a) use the dorsum of your contralateral hand to gently lift the breast from below, or (b) use fingertips of your contralateral hand to exert an upward pressure on the upper breast, which will elevate the nipple complex and allow you to palpate below it. At all costs do not appear to grope or caress the breast!

Before picking up your stethoscope, by this stage you should be primed as to what to expect on auscultation (Table A4.1):

Table A4.1. Critical findings in common valvular lesions.

	AS	AR	MS	MR	VSD	TR
Before auscultation						
Pulse	Slow-rising	Collapsing	AF*	AF*		
Neck		Corrigan's				Giant c-v
Apex /LLSE	Undisplaced heaving	Displaced thrusting	Undisplaced tapping	Displaced thrusting	Parasternal thrill (often)	Parasternal heave (often)
Auscultation						
S1			Loud	Soft		
S2	Soft					
Murmur	ESM at aortic radiating to carotid	EDM at LLSE	MDM at mitral	PSM at mitral radiating to axilla	PSM at LLSE, very harsh	PSM at LLSE, soft, louder in inspiration

*Nonspecific, but most classically associated with MS.

Auscultation

This is the crux of the cardiovascular examination and is often harder than it looks. The first step to success is using the correct landmarks — directly over the apex beat (mitral), left sternal border in the 4th intercostal space (tricuspid), and left and right sternal border at the 3rd intercostal space (pulmonary and aortic). Do not stay in one spot but inch the stethoscope around (particularly in thin patients for whom protruding ribs may lead to poor contact between stethoscope and chest) — a soft murmur may only be audible at one spot.

Have the discipline to listen to each component of the cardiac cycle in turn — this is especially helpful in tricky cases with subtle signs or confounding sounds (breath or gastric sounds). First listen to the first and second heart sounds, paying attention to their sound (prosthetic?), volume (loud S1 – MS, soft S2 – AS, loud P2 – pulmonary hypertension), any split S2 (physiologic in inspiration, fixed split in ASD), and for any additional heart sounds (S3, S4). Next, listen for murmurs, with your finger on the carotid (not radial) pulse for timing. For each murmur, determine its timing, character, and location in which it is loudest. Elicit change with respiration by asking the patient to breathe in and out slowly, which changes intrathoracic pressure (note that 'breathe in and hold'/'breathe out and hold' does not lead to the desired changes in intrathoracic pressure during the 'hold' phase and can cause discordant findings).

Decide on how you would describe a murmur before moving to a new auscultation location, but be prepared to revise your description if the murmur is better heard elsewhere.

Check for radiation to the axilla and carotid (using the bell directly over the carotid pulse). Radiation means not only that the murmur is audible in these regions (a loud murmur may be audible across the entire precordium), but also that the murmur is at least as loud and of the same character as in the primary location.

Dynamic manoeuvres are next. First, turn the patient left lateral, repalpate the apex beat, and auscultate the apex with the bell for the soft mid-diastolic murmur of MS. If no clear murmurs have been heard thus far (or if there is MR), this is your second chance to listen for MS (or at least the loud S1 that would make you suspect MS). Next, sit the patient up and ask him/her to lean forward in full expiration. Auscultate for AR over a band from the lower left sternal edge to the aortic region (not just over the lower left sternal edge). Do Valsalva if you suspect HCM.

Pitfall: Help! I can't hear the murmur

> This is a common struggle with the cardiology station. Ideally only patients with clear, indisputable signs are listed, but this is unfortunately not always the case. Tips:
> 1. Auscultate well
>   - Ensure that auscultation begins in correct landmarks — e.g., some candidates auscultate the aortic and pulmonary areas too high, in the 1st intercostal space.
>   - Inch the stethoscope around and don't stay in one spot.
> 2. Don't just rely on the murmur
>   - AR (collapsing pulse) and TR (giant c-v waves) are diagnosed in the periphery.
>   - MS is notoriously soft. If the patient is in AF, has an undisplaced apex beat, and has a loud S1 and no other murmur, the diagnosis is likely MS even if you do not hear a mid-diastolic murmur. In this situation, you may wish to present the pertinent findings and state that you suspect MS but was unable to appreciate the expected mid-diastolic murmur. If you are very confident that the diagnosis is MS, you may take the calculated gamble of saying that you heard a mid-diastolic murmur (pays off if you are right, but disastrous if you are wrong).
> 3. Always listen to the entire cardiac cycle — are there two prosthetic valves instead of one? Is there mixed mitral valve disease instead of just MR?

Complete the examination by auscultating the lung bases for fluid overload and palpating for pedal oedema. If suspecting coarctation of the aorta or a PDA, auscultate between the scapulae and do radiofemoral delay. Palpate for a pulsatile liver if you suspect TR. Thank the patient and cover up.

Typical requests at the end of the cardiac examination are:
- Measuring the blood pressure.
- Looking for stigmata of endocarditis: fundoscopy looking for Roth spots and urine dipstick for microscopic haematuria.

Clinical Syndromes

The chapters ahead detail each of these clinical syndromes:

Clinical syndrome	Key features
1. Systolic murmur (one or multiple)	Systolic murmur May have large c-v wave, slow rising pulse
2. Diastolic murmur (one or multiple)	Obvious: diastolic murmur Not obvious: absence of silence in diastole ± AF, loud S1 (MS) ± Collapsing pulse (AR)
3. Systolic + diastolic murmur	Murmur in both systole and diastole Noisy precordium
4. Prosthetic valves	Sternotomy scar Metallic click
5. Cyanosis/clubbing	Clubbed, cyanotic ± Scars (sternotomy, lateral thoracotomy)
6. Dextrocardia	Absent apex beat – palpate contralateral side Right-sided pacemaker without explantation of left side

In each case, you will need to comment on:
- What is the valvular lesion(s)?
- What is the underlying aetiology?
- How severe is it?
- Are there any complications?

Cardiology – Clinical Syndromes

4.1 | Systolic Murmur

One hopes for an unmistakable aortic stenosis (AS) or mitral regurgitation (MR), and some candidates are indeed fortunate enough to get one. However, it is not uncommon to have a difficult or atypical systolic murmur. Look for a second murmur — listen carefully to all components of the cardiac cycle, particularly in diastole, and pay attention to whether the murmur sounds different in a different area.

Recognise the Murmur

Recognising the valvular lesion begins in the peripheries. Pay attention to the pulse, the presence of large c-v waves (TR), and any scars (thoracotomy scar – repaired congenital heart disease) or implantable cardiac devices (possible HCM).

On auscultation, pay attention to the timing of the murmur and where it is best heard (mitral: MR, left lower sternal edge: VSD or TR, pulmonary: PS, PDA, aortic: AS), changes with inspiration/expiration, and radiation.

Pitfall: The concomitant diastolic murmur

> Beware the concomitant diastolic murmur! Both mixed aortic and mitral disease are common, and in fact a systolic murmur is a common presentation of AR[20]. Tips:
> - After identifying the obvious systolic murmur, listen carefully to diastole.
> - In MR, ensure that S1 is not loud (a loud S1 would suggest concomittant MS).
> - Be suspicious if the apex beat is unexpected (i.e., if displaced in AS, or if undisplaced in MR).

The classic features of each valvular lesion are:

1. **Aortic stenosis**
   - Pulse: slow-rising.
   - Apex: undisplaced, heaving.
   - Heart sounds: soft S2.
   - Murmur: crescendo-decrescendo ejection systolic murmur best heard over the upper right sternal edge, radiating to the carotid. Note that 'ejection' more reliably describes the character of this murmur rather than its length.

---

[20] Heidenreich PA, Schnittger I, Hancock SL, Atwood JE. A systolic murmur is a common presentation of aortic regurgitation detected by echocardiography. *Clin Cardiol* 2004 27(9):502–6.

2. **Mitral regurgitation**
   - Pulse: may be in AF.
   - Apex: displaced, thrusting.
   - Murmur: pansystolic murmur best heard over the apex, radiating to the axilla. This murmur is not harsh (if harsh, think VSD) and constant in character and volume from start to finish.
   - Additional features in mitral valve prolapse: a mid-systolic click, murmur is harsher and begins later after S1.

Tip: Distinguishing AS vs. MR

> Distinguishing AS vs. MR is not always easy because:
> - The long ejection systolic murmur in severe AS, coupled with a soft S2, mimics the pansystolic murmur of MR.
> - The location in which the murmur is best heard is not always reliable (the gallavardin murmur in AS radiates to the apex, while posterior leaflet MR radiates to the upper right sternal edge).
>
> The following features may help in deciding between the two:
> - In severe AS, the pulse is slow-rising and often difficult to palpate. Despite being a reliable sign, it is often underappreciated.
> - Distinct S1 and S2 heart sounds (even if the ejection murmur is very long) favour AS, while the pansystolic murmur of MR tends to 'drown out' S1 and S2.
> - A blowing crescendo-decrescendo character ('woof woof') favours AS, while the MR murmur is constant in volume and character from start to finish. Appreciating this takes some experience.
> - The AS murmur is louder in the carotid than the mitral region, while the converse is true in MR.
> - Radiation to the axilla favours MR, while that to the carotid favours AS. A very loud murmur may be heard throughout the precordium.

3. **Ventricular septal defect**
   - Young patient (a helpful clue, but not always!)
   - Murmur: harsh pansystolic murmur best heard in the lower left sternal edge, with no change on inspiration. Does not radiate to the axilla but may radiate to the right lower sternal border.

Cardiology

Tip: Distinguishing VSD vs. MR

> The pansystolic murmur of VSD mimics MR. They can be differentiated based on the following:
> - VSD is often associated with a parasternal thrill. This is absent in MR.
> - Character: the VSD murmur is typically very harsh, loud, and higher pitched than the MR murmur.
> - VSD is louder in the lower left sternal edge than the apex, while MR is louder at the apex than at the sternal border. Loud VSDs and MRs may both be audible in the axilla, but the VSD will be softer in the axilla than at the lower left sternal edge.
> - Severe MR is likely associated with a displaced apex beat and atrial fibrillation.
>
> Not all VSDs are pansystolic. The murmur of a muscular VSD may be short and not pansystolic, thus resembling the ejection systolic murmur of AS. This is because ventricular contraction leads to occlusion of the VSD lumen. However, the VSD murmur will not radiate to the carotid.

4. **Tricuspid regurgitation**
   - JVP: giant c-v wave.
   - Murmur: pansystolic murmur best heard in the lower left sternal edge, louder in inspiration, not radiating to the axilla but may radiate to the right sternal edge or epigastrium. This murmur is typically not loud, as the pressures generated across the tricuspid valve are lower than in left-sided lesions (a very loud murmur is unlikely to be TR).
   - May also have pulsatile liver. You may request to examine for a liver.

TR may not be a lone lesion. It can be a complication of pulmonary hypertension due to another left-sided valvular lesion. Search for this left-sided lesion (e.g., MR/TR if there is a PSM radiating to axilla plus giant c-v wave)!

5. **Hypertrophic cardiomyopathy**
   - ± Implanted cardiac device (automated implantable cardioverter-defibrillator).
   - Pulse: jerky/bifid pulse.
   - Apex beat: double apical impulse (prominent presystolic pulse due to atrial contraction, if not in AF).
   - Heart sounds: S2 normal or reversed split in advanced disease[21].

---

[21] Reversed split = instead of inspiratory split S2, S2 is single in inspiration but split in expiration. This is due to delayed left ventricular emptying in left ventricle outflow obstruction, which becomes more prominent in expiration, increases intrathoracic pressure, and reduces venous return to the left heart.

- Classically *two* murmurs:
  - Pansystolic murmur best heard in the apex, radiating to the axilla (MR due to systolic anterior motion of anterior MV leaflet).
  - Ejection systolic murmur best heard in the lower left sternal edge, or along a band tracking from LLSE towards the aortic area, louder with Valsalva manoeuvre[22] (LV outflow tract obstruction murmur which mimics AS).

6. **Pulmonary area murmur**

This is unfamiliar territory for most. Consider where the murmur is best heard (infraclavicular = PDA, between scapulae = coarctation), whether the murmur is louder on inspiration (PS), associated with a collapsing pulse (PDA), radial-femoral delay (coarctation), or any other features of congenital heart disease.

a) **PS**: Ejection systolic murmur best heard in the upper left sternal edge which is louder on inspiration. May be associated with:
   i. Fixed split second heart sound = **ASD** with a pulmonary flow murmur
   ii. Midline sternotomy and lateral thoracotomy scars ± Blalock-Taussig shunts = repaired **tetralogy of Fallot**
   iii. None of the above = de novo **pulmonary stenosis**

b) **PDA**: Ejection systolic murmur best heard in the left infraclavicular region, associated with a collapsing pulse (Note: the diastolic component may be inaudible).

c) **Coarctation of the Aorta**: Systolic murmur best heard in the upper left sternal edge, radiating to the back between the scapulae, associated with radio-femoral delay.

There may be a thoracotomy scar in cases of repaired PDA/coarctation.

Tip: Dual systolic murmurs

> Situations in which dual systolic murmurs may arise include:
> (a) Ejection + pan systolic murmur
> - AS + MR dual pathology.
> - AS with gallavardin phenomenon.
> - Hypertrophic cardiomyopathy.
> (b) Dual pansystolic murmurs
> - MR complicated by pulmonary hypertension and TR. The only clue will be giant c-v waves.

---

[22] In hypertrophic cardiomyopathy, reduced preload (increased intrathoracic pressure from the strain phase of Valsalva, squatting to standing, beta blockers, dehydration) reduces left ventricle filling and increases left ventricular outflow tract obstruction. Therefore, these manoeuvres accentuate the outflow tract obstruction murmur of hypertrophic cardiomyopathy. Conversely, AS gets softer with Valsalva and squatting to standing.

Look for Complications

The complications in the cardiology station are quite standard and can be summarised using the acronym 'PACE':

- **P**ulmonary hypertension: palpable pulmonary component of second heart sound, parasternal heave.
- **A**trial fibrillation: if so, comment on the presence of ecchymoses that suggest over-anticoagulation.
- **C**ongestive cardiac failure: elevated jugular venous pressure, bibasal crepitations, and pedal oedema.
- **E**ndocarditis: Osler nodes, Janeway lesions, or splinter haemorrhages.

In addition, for the congenital lesions (ASD, VSD, PDA), comment on any evidence of Eisenmenger syndrome such as cyanosis or clubbing.

Describe Severity

In lieu of memorising severity classifications of each valvular lesion, this section presents a simplified approach. Any of the valvular lesions may be severe in the presence of:

(a) **Symptom**s – listen to the stem!

(b) **Haemodynamic consequences**
- Complications – congestive heart failure, pulmonary hypertension (left-sided lesions), AF (especially in MR), Eisenmenger syndrome (shunts).
- Effect on the pulse (small volume in severe AS, collapsing in haemodynamically significant PDA).
- Response of the left ventricle (dilated leading to displaced apex beat in severe MR).

(c) **Auscultation characteristics**
- Severe AS: long murmur, soft second heart sound.
- VSD: loud murmur likely suggests a small defect.

(d) **Echocardiographic features**
- Severe AS: valve area $< 1 \, cm^2$, transvalvular aortic velocity > 4 m/s, or transvalvular gradient > 40 mmHg (but consider the possibility of low-flow, low-gradient AS)
- Severe MR: regurgitant fraction $> 50\%$ or > 60 mL, etc.

Suggest Aetiology

Consider both primary valve disorders and secondary causes (annular dilation, iatrogenic, etc.). Prioritise your suggestions based on what is most likely in the patient (Table A4.2).

Table A4.2. Common causes of a systolic murmur.

	Primary valve disorder	Secondary causes
AS	Congenital bicuspid valve Calcific degeneration Rheumatic heart disease (unlikely lone AS) Infective endocarditis	
MR	Mitral valve prolapse (idiopathic, hereditary, connective tissue disease) Rheumatic heart disease (unlikely lone MR) Infective endocarditis	Papillary muscle rupture Annular dilation from - Ischaemic heart disease - Cardiomyopathy Previous mitral valvotomy
VSD	Congenital (idiopathic, syndromic)	Post myocardial infarct Iatrogenic (e.g., implantable cardiac device, mitral valvotomy)
TR	Congenital Carcinoid syndrome, drugs Rheumatic heart disease Infective endocarditis	Pulmonary hypertension – annular dilation Valve injury from pacemaker lead

Sample Scripts

Severe AS

This elderly lady who presents with syncope has a slow rising pulse, a heaving and undisplaced apex beat, and a grade 2/6 ejection systolic murmur best heard in the aortic region, radiating to the carotids. She is likely to have aortic stenosis which is severe as she is symptomatic with syncope. I did not note any evidence to suggest complications of heart failure, atrial fibrillation, pulmonary hypertension, or infective endocarditis. Possible aetiologies of aortic stenosis include congenital bicuspid valve and calcific degeneration.

Ischaemic MR

The positive physical signs are: a midline sternotomy scar* with saphenous vein graft scar, atrial fibrillation, a displaced apex beat, a grade 3/6 pansystolic murmur in the apex radiating to the axilla, and features of fluid overload including elevated jugular venous pressure, basal lung crepitations, and pedal oedema. Significant negatives are: no suggestions of infective endocarditis, and no parasternal heave or palpable pulmonary component of the second heart sound to suggest pulmonary hypertension. He is likely to have severe mitral regurgitation complicated by atrial fibrillation and heart failure. The aetiology of his mitral regurgitation may be mitral annular dilation from ischaemic cardiomyopathy. Other causes of mitral regurgitation include mitral valve prolapse, papillary muscle rupture due to ischaemia, infective endocarditis, and rheumatic heart disease.

If the scar were instead in the mitral position, consider mitral regurgitation as a consequence of prior mitral valvotomy for mitral stenosis.

Small VSD

This middle-aged gentleman has an undisplaced apex beat and a grade 4/6 harsh pansystolic murmur, best heard in the lower left sternal border and associated with a palpable thrill. This murmur does not radiate to the apex or carotid. He is likely to have a small ventricular septal defect. There is no clubbing or cyanosis to suggest Eisenmenger syndrome. There is no suggestion of congestive cardiac failure, pulmonary hypertension, or infective endocarditis.

Cardiology – Clinical Syndromes

4.2 | Diastolic Murmur

The key diastolic murmurs are AR and MS[23]. They are notoriously soft and barely audible.

Recognise the Murmur

1. **Aortic regurgitation**
   - Collapsing pulse (remember that the other cause of a collapsing pulse is a PDA).
   - Corrigan's sign.
   - Displaced thrusting apex beat.
   - Grade 2/6 decrescendo early diastolic murmur best heard in LLSE with patient sitting forward in full expiration. This murmur often has a blowing, cavernous, echoing sound.
   - There may also be a soft ejection systolic flow murmur.

2. **Mitral stenosis**
   - Malar flush.
   - (Often) atrial fibrillation.
   - Tapping, undisplaced apex beat.
   - Loud first heart sound.
   - Grade 2/6 rumbling mid-diastolic murmur best heard in the apex with the patient in the left lateral position.
   - ± Opening snap.

Look for Complications

These are the standard 'PACE' complications (see page 119 for details):

- **P**ulmonary hypertension.
- **A**trial fibrillation.
- **C**ongestive cardiac failure.
- **E**ndocarditis.

---

[23] The third diastolic murmur, not covered here, is pulmonary regurgitation. This is rare but may be seen in the setting of valvotomy for congenital pulmonary stenosis.

Tip: Improving your chances of picking up diastolic murmurs

> (1) Pay attention to the peripheries.
>   - AR should be suspected on the presence of prominent carotid pulsations (Corrigan's sign) and a collapsing pulse.
>   - AF with an undisplaced, unusually distinct ('tapping') apex beat should cause you to prick up your ears for an MS murmur.
>
> (2) Auscultate in the optimal locations. For MS, auscultate directly over the apex beat (remembering to repalpate for the apex beat after turning the patient left lateral) — as the MS murmur is soft, listening away from the optimum location may make it difficult to pick up. For AR, auscultate not just in the lower left sternal edge, but along a band tracking from the LLSE towards the aortic region.
>
> (3) Listen carefully and patiently. The mid-diastolic murmur of MS may be heard intermittently especially if the patient is in atrial fibrillation; you may not immediately notice an obvious murmur, only a loud first heart sound with the absence of silence in the diastole.

Describe Severity

AR/MS may be severe in the presence of:

(a) **Symptoms**

(b) **Haemodynamic consequences**
  - Complications – congestive heart failure, pulmonary hypertension, AF.
  - Effect on the pulse: wide pulse pressure (AR).
  - Response of the left ventricle: severely displaced apex beat (AR).
  - Response of the right heart: pulmonary hypertension, TR (MS).

(c) **Auscultation characteristics**
  - Severe AR: short murmur (rapid equalisation of aortic and left ventricular pressures) with soft second heart sound.
  - Severe MS: long murmur with an early opening snap. *(Note: Volume of murmur does not correlate with severity; in fact, severe MS is likely quite soft).*

(d) **Echocardiographic features**
  - Severe AR: regurgitant fraction > 50% or volume > 60 mL/beat, holodiastolic flow reversal in abdominal aorta, central jet width > 65% of left ventricular outflow tract, etc.
  - Severe MS: valve area < 1 cm^2, severe left atrial enlargement, elevated pulmonary artery systolic pressure.

Suggest Aetiology

Consider both primary valve disorders and secondary causes (Table A4.3); prioritise your suggestions based on what is most likely in the patient. Look hard for Marfan's syndrome in young patients with AR.

Table A4.3. Common causes of a diastolic murmur.

	Primary valve disorder	Secondary causes
AR	Congenital bileaflet valve Myxomatous/calcific degeneration Rheumatic heart disease Infective endocarditis	Annular dilation: - Connective tissue disease (e.g., Marfan's) - Inflammatory aortitis (e.g., ankylosing spondylitis) - Infective aortitis (e.g., syphilis) - Aortic dissection
MS	Rheumatic heart disease Calcific MS Infective endocarditis	Atrial myxoma

Sample Scripts

Aortic regurgitation

In the precordium, the apex is thrusting and displaced in the 6th intercostal space in the anterior axillary line. There is a grade 2/6 early diastolic murmur, best heard in the left lower sternal edge in full expiration. (There is also a soft ejection systolic murmur which does not radiate to the carotid; this may be a flow murmur). In the peripheries, there is a collapsing pulse. There are also features of arachnodactyly, positive thumb and ring sign, pectus excavatum, and a high arched palate. In terms of complications, there are no features of infective endocarditis, pulmonary hypertension, atrial fibrillation, or heart failure. In summary, this young gentleman has aortic regurgitation, which may be related to aortic root dilation from underlying Marfan's syndrome.

Mitral stenosis

This patient is in atrial fibrillation. There is an undisplaced, tapping apex beat. On auscultation, there is a loud first heart sound, followed by an opening snap and a rumbling grade 2/6 mid-diastolic murmur best heard at the apex. In the peripheries, I also notice extensive peripheral ecchymosis. Important negatives are the absence of features of pulmonary hypertension, infective endocarditis, or cardiac failure. In summary, this patient has mitral stenosis with atrial fibrillation. Causes of mitral stenosis include rheumatic heart disease and infective endocarditis.

Cardiology – Clinical Syndromes

4.3 | Systolic + Diastolic Murmur

This is a challenging case with two common pitfalls:

- The obvious (systolic) murmur is identified and the softer (diastolic) murmur is missed. This tends to occur because either peripheral clues are ignored (e.g., a collapsing pulse, or paradoxically undisplaced apex in a 'mitral regurgitation' case), or the candidate stops listening after picking up one murmur.
- It is difficult to characterise the murmurs in a noisy precordium. Try to isolate individual components of the cardiac cycle and listen to each in turn.

Recognise the Murmur

1. **Mixed aortic valve disease**
    - Findings of both AS and AR (i.e., ejection systolic murmur best heard at the aortic region, plus early diastolic murmur best heard in the lower left sternal edge).
    - Differential: AR with flow murmur (see note below).
2. **Mixed mitral valve disease**
    - Findings of both MS and MR (i.e., pansystolic murmur best heard in the apex, radiating to the axilla; with mid-diastolic murmur).
    - Differential: MR with flow murmur.
3. **Patent ductus arteriosus (PDA)**
    - ± Collapsing pulse (present only in a haemodynamically significant PDA).
    - Continuous machinery murmur best heard in the left infraclavicular area, radiating to the back. Note that the diastolic component may be soft and barely audible.

Identify the Dominant Lesion

The haemodynamic consequence of the valvular lesion on the left ventricle and pulse is the arbiter of which lesion is dominant.

Mixed aortic valve disease		Mixed mitral valve disease	
AS dominant	AR dominant	MS dominant	MR dominant
Undisplaced apex	Displaced apex	Undisplaced apex	Displaced apex
Small volume pulse	Collapsing pulse	Loud S1	Soft S1
Long systolic murmur	Short systolic murmur	Long diastolic murmur	Short diastolic murmur

Tip: AR or mixed aortic valve disease?

> As moderate-severe AR leads to increased flow across the aortic valve, many patients with AR have a soft ejection systolic murmur in the aortic position. This does not necessarily indicate mixed aortic valve disease, especially if the other features (displaced apex, collapsing pulse) point towards AR. For the purpose of PACES, we generally would advise offering the diagnosis of mixed aortic valve disease only if there is radiation of the systolic murmur to the carotid, or evidence of predominant AS.

Look for Complications

These are the standard 'PACE' complications (see page 119 for details):
- **P**ulmonary hypertension.
- **A**trial fibrillation.
- **C**ongestive cardiac failure.
- **E**ndocarditis.

Suggest Aetiology

Mixed aortic valve disease
- Congenital bicuspid valve.
- Rheumatic heart disease.
- Infective endocarditis.

Mixed mitral valve disease
- Rheumatic heart disease.
- Infective endocarditis.
- MS treated with valvotomy, then complicated by MR (in patients with a scar).

Sample Scripts

Mixed mitral valve disease

This middle aged lady has an irregularly irregular pulse, as well as a tapping and undisplaced apex beat. On auscultation, there is a loud first heart sound, a grade 2/6 mid-diastolic murmur best heard in the apex, and a grade 3/6 pansystolic murmur best heard at the apex, radiating to the axilla. She is likely to have mixed mitral valve disease. The dominant lesion is likely mitral stenosis as the apex is undisplaced and the first heart sound is loud. Possible causes include rheumatic heart disease and infective endocarditis. In terms of complications, there are peripheral ecchymosis, no suggestion of heart failure, no parasternal heave or palpable pulmonary component of the second heart sound to suggest pulmonary hypertension, and no stigmata of infective endocarditis.

Patent ductus arteriosus

This young man has a continuous murmur best heard in the left infraclavicular region. The apex is undisplaced. I looked for but did not find a collapsing pulse. The underlying diagnosis is likely a patent ductus arteriosus. There is no cyanosis or clubbing*, cardiac failure, pulmonary hypertension, or infective endocarditis.

*Cyanosis or clubbing would suggest shunt reversal (Eisenmenger syndrome), but in that case the murmur would no longer be loud (as shunt reversal obliterates the pressure gradient across the PDA that gives rise to the murmur).

Cardiology – Clinical Syndromes

4.4 | Prosthetic Valves

Prosthetic valves are probably the easiest cardiology case, but you will be expected to perform to a high standard. You must (a) recognise the case of prosthetic valves, (b) identify which valve is prosthetic, (c) state the likely underlying valve lesion, and (d) identify any complications. Some patients have a prosthetic valve plus a murmur.

Recognise the Prosthetic Valve

A case of prosthetic valves should be recognised on inspection. You will note:

- Midline sternotomy scar (without saphenous vein graft scar, unless concomitant coronary bypass has been done).
- Prosthetic clicks audible at the bedside.

Listen to the prosthetic click with your naked ear and time it against the carotid pulse. It is important to do so before auscultating as you may be confused if there are additional sounds or murmurs. The click audible to the naked ear always reflects valve closure; additional sounds such as opening clicks are usually not audible without a stethoscope. The timing of this click reliably indicates which valve is replaced:

- Single click before carotid pulse – mitral valve replacement.
- Single click after carotid pulse – aortic valve replacement.
- Two prosthetic clicks – dual valve replacement.

Auscultate the heart. There are some differences between tilting disc valves and ball and cage valves.

1. **Tilting disc valves** (e.g., St Jude, Bjork-Shiley)

These are straightforward and give a readily discernible prosthetic heart sound.

(a) Aortic	(b) Mitral	(c) Dual
– Midline sternotomy	– Midline sternotomy	– Midline sternotomy
– Click after carotid pulse	– Click before carotid pulse	– Dual prosthetic click
– Prosthetic S2	– Prosthetic S1	– Prosthetic S1 + S2

A soft flow murmur may be audible (systolic in an aortic valve replacement, diastolic in a mitral valve replacement).

2. **Ball and cage valves** (Starr-Edwards)

Ball and cage valves sound quite different. In addition to the prosthetic heart sound and metallic click, there will be an additional opening click (audible with the stethoscope but not the naked ear) and the rumble of turbulent bloodflow going past the ball in its cage. Therefore in a mitral ball and cage valve you will hear: prosthetic S1 –

native S2 – opening click – (flow murmur) – prosthetic S1. This flow murmur is diastolic and soft, if at all audible. In an aortic ball and cage valve you will hear S1 – opening click – (ejection murmur) – prosthetic S2.

The plethora of sounds can be confusing. It is critical to determine whether the ball and cage valve is in the mitral or aortic position. Timing is critical — identify the S1 sound as that which immediately precedes the carotid pulse and listen to whether this sound is native or prosthetic. If the S1 is prosthetic, then this is a mitral ball and cage valve. If the S1 is native, then this is an aortic ball and cage valve. If you are confused, put down the stethoscope and time the prosthetic click against the carotid pulse with your naked ears. If you hear a whole jumble of clicks, consider whether the patient has dual ball and cage valves.

3. **Bioprosthetic valves**

Bioprosthetic valves sound subtly different in quality from native valves, and there is no audible click. You will generally not be expected to distinguish between a native and bioprosthetic valve.

Look for Complications

Listen for any additional sounds and murmurs.

- Valvular thrombosis: are the valve sounds crisp?
- Valvular regurgitation: a regurgitant murmur is systolic in a mitral valve replacement but diastolic in an aortic valve replacement. A soft systolic flow murmur across an aortic prosthetic valve is normal.
- Patients can well have an unrelated murmur from their native valve.

Look for the standard 'PACE' complications (see Chapter 4.1):

- <u>P</u>ulmonary hypertension.
- <u>A</u>trial fibrillation.
- <u>C</u>ongestive cardiac failure.
- <u>E</u>ndocarditis.

Consider the effect of anticoagulation and haematological complications:

- Peripheral ecchymoses – anticoagulation use; if extensive, over-anticoagulation
- Anaemia and jaundice – suggests possible valve hemolysis.

Suggest Underlying Aetiology

The apex generally gives you the underlying aetiology:

- Undisplaced apex: stenotic lesion (i.e., AS/MS).
- Displaced apex: regurgitant lesion (i.e., AR/MR).
- Dual valve replacement: rheumatic heart disease, infective endocarditis.

Consider the underlying cause of AS/MS/AR/MR, for instance:
- Look for features of Marfan's syndrome or connective tissue disease.
- Saphenous vein graft scar suggests CABG, implying ischaemic heart disease.

Sample Scripts

Aortic valve replacement

This elderly lady has a midline sternotomy scar without saphenous vein graft scar, a metallic click that occurs after the carotid pulse, and a metallic second heart sound. The valve is well functioning with crisp sounds and a soft grade 2/6 systolic murmur, heard in the aortic region and not radiating to the carotid, which is likely a flow murmur. I note that she has a left hemiparesis, which makes me concerned about haemorrhagic stroke predisposed by anticoagulation or infective endocarditis with septic emboli, although I do not note any peripheral stigmata of endocarditis presently. There is no evidence of pulmonary hypertension or over-anticoagulation, and she is in sinus rhythm. In summary, my patient has an aortic valve replacement, and an old stroke. As her apex beat is undisplaced, the underlying disorder may be aortic stenosis.

Complex case

This young patient has a midline sternotomy without saphenous vein graft scar, along with multiple left and right inframammary scars. There is a prosthetic click audible to the naked ear. On examination of the precordium, the apex is displaced and there is a parasternal heave. The second heart sound is prosthetic. There are two murmurs — a harsh grade 3 ejection systolic murmur with no radiation and a grade 2 early diastolic murmur, both of which are best heard in the lower left sternal edge. In the peripheries, there is clubbing, a collapsing pulse, and a peripherally inserted central catheter. I looked for but did not find any cyanosis, Janeway lesions, or Osler nodes. There is no pedal oedema or elevated jugular venous pressure. Putting the signs together, this patient may have had complex congenital heart disease with an aortic valve replacement and likely a ventricular septal defect (differential: pulmonary stenosis), now complicated by aortic valvular regurgitation and infective endocarditis.

Cardiology - Clinical Syndromes

4.5 | Cyanosis/Clubbing

Congenital cyanotic heart disease cases are difficult. Be particularly alert if your cardiology patient is young — most of the other cardiac lesions except VSDs occur in middle-aged to older patients. The first step is to recognise that the patient is clubbed or cyanotic. This is critical — if missed, it becomes hard to put everything together later. Complex or multiple sternotomy and thoracotomy scars, or a syndromic-looking young patient, are also strong hints of congenital heart disease.

Recognise the Syndrome

The key differentiator is the presence of a PS murmur. As a general rule, if there is PS murmur or a Blalock-Taussig shunt, suspect tetralogy of Fallot. If there are prominent signs of pulmonary hypertension without a PS murmur, suspect Eisenmenger syndrome, which may in turn be due to a large VSD, PDA, or (less likely) ASD.

1. **Tetralogy of Fallot**
The signs in tetralogy of Fallot (TOF) are complex but can be worked through if one understands its anatomy and corrective procedures. The classic tetrad of TOF are a VSD, an overriding aorta, right ventricular hypertrophy, and pulmonary stenosis. This may be palliated initially with a Blalock-Taussig (B-T) shunt, a subclavian artery-pulmonary artery shunt that bypasses the pulmonary stenosis. The B-T shunt may be followed with definitive corrective surgery. Post correction, there is usually residual PS. There may also be residual VSD or PR due to abnormal valve anatomy post correction. There may also be secondary AR due to aortic valve deformity in abnormal outflow tract development and secondary MR due to cardiac dilation.

Therefore, signs that can appear in a patient with TOF include *(though not all will be present in a given patient)*:

- Cyanosis, clubbing, facial dysmorphisms (occasionally associated with TOF).
- Sternotomy: for subsequent corrective surgery.
- B-T shunt* (can be bilateral): thoracotomy scar, continuous murmur heard laterally, diminished ipsilateral radial pulse.
- Signs of pulmonary hypertension: parasternal heave, giant c-v waves, TR.
- Various murmurs – *the PS murmur is usually present, other murmurs may or may not occur*
    - PS* (ejection, pulmonary area, louder in inspiration) – residual post-correction.
    - VSD (pansystolic, lower left sternal edge) – residual post-correction.
    - MR (pansystolic, apex) – secondary to cardiac dilation.

- PR (early diastolic, pulmonary area, louder in inspiration) – post repair.
- AR (early diastolic, lower left sternal edge) – due to aortic valve deformity.
- Complications (e.g., AF, cardiac failure).

These signs are reasonably specific to TOF and distinguish it from an Eisenmenger syndrome case — note that B-T shunts are not performed for Eisenmenger syndrome.

Many murmurs are possible — at each auscultation location, listen carefully to each component of the cardiac cycle and pay particular attention to whether a given murmur is louder in inspiration or expiration.

2. Eisenmenger syndrome

Eisenmenger syndrome occurs due to reversal of a left to right shunt with the development of progressive pulmonary hypertension. Physical signs common to all cases of Eisenmenger syndrome are:

- Cyanosis, clubbing.
- Marked pulmonary hypertension – parasternal heave, loud P2 ± secondary TR.

While the common causes of Eisenmenger syndrome are a VSD or PDA (uncommon but possible in ASD), you are unlikely to encounter their pathognomic findings (i.e., murmurs, collapsing pulse). This is because shunt reversal has occurred in Eisenmenger syndrome; with equalisation of left- and right-sided ventricular pressures, there is little flow through a VSD or PDA. However, there may be additional murmurs present such as TR and PR secondary to the pulmonary hypertension.

Occasionally, some clues lead to an underlying diagnosis of PDA:

- Differential cyanosis and clubbing, more pronounced in the lower extremities ± left hand (the right innominate artery, being proximal to the PDA, does not receive any deoxygenated blood through the PDA).
- If there is concomitant coarctation of the aorta.
  - Radio-femoral delay.
  - Diminished left radial pulse, if coarctation occurs proximal to the origin of the left subclavian, or if the left subclavian has been used for repair.

3. Uncertain underlying diagnosis

Some patients do not fall neatly into either category — do not panic; focus on picking up all the signs and presenting what you find. In complex cases that do not fit neatly into one diagnosis, it may be wise to offer a diagnosis of 'complex cyanotic congenital heart disease' or 'pulmonary hypertension'.

Sample Scripts

Present what you find and do not try too hard to fit all the signs into one box. It may not always be possible!

Repaired tetralogy of Fallot

This young gentleman is clubbed, cyanotic, and has a midline sternotomy scar. He is in pulmonary hypertension with a palpable parasternal heave and a loud pulmonary component of the second heart sound. There is a grade 3/6 pansystolic murmur that is louder on inspiration and best heard over the left infraclavicular region. There is a grade 2/6 long diastolic murmur also best heard over the left infraclavicular region. He is in heart failure with a raised jugular venous pressure and bilateral pedal oedema. I suspect that he has repaired congenital cyanotic heart disease, which may be a tetralogy of Fallot, complicated with pulmonary hypertension and cardiac failure.

Eisenmenger syndrome

This young lady is clubbed and cyanotic. I note facial dysmorphism, such as hypertelorism and low-set ears. She has pulmonary hypertension with a palpable parasternal heave and a loud pulmonary component of the second heart sound. There is a soft pansystolic murmur best heard in the lower left sternal edge in inspiration, accompanied by giant c-v waves in the neck. I suspect she has congenital heart disease complicated by Eisenmenger syndrome. The murmur may be due to tricuspid regurgitation secondary to pulmonary hypertension; a differential will be ventricular septal defect.

PDA with coarctation of the aorta

My patient is a young gentleman who has differential clubbing of both feet and the left fingers but not the right hand. There is the presence of radial-radial and radio-femoral delay. On auscultation I note a continuous machinery murmur best heard over the left infraclavicular region, radiating to the back. He is in pulmonary hypertension with a parasternal heave and loud pulmonary component of the second heart sound. A possible unifying diagnosis is a patent ductus arteriosus with coarctation of the aorta, complicated by pulmonary hypertension and shunt reversal.

Cardiology – Clinical Syndromes
4.6 | Dextrocardia

Recognise the Pathology

Dextrocardia is actually is an easy case if you pick it up; most patients would have no other abnormality apart from dextrocardia. It can, however, easily become a complete disaster if missed. The key is to be sure about palpating the apex beat and not simply move on if the apex beat is not well-felt (in any case, it is important information for the other valvular lesions). If you are unable to palpate the apex beat, always check the right side and turn the patient left lateral. If, on inspection, you notice a right-sided pacemaker without a left-sided pacemaker scar (i.e., explanted left pacemaker), strongly suspect dextrocardia.

Look for Related Abnormalities

On examination, look for:
- Katargener's syndrome: coarse late inspiratory crepitations (bronchiectasis), sinusitis.
- Turner's syndrome (in a female): webbed neck, low set ears, dysmorphism.

Offer to complete the examination by examining the abdomen for a left-sided liver (situs inversus, which usually implies the absence of a significant cardiac malformation).

Cardiology

4.7 | Discussion Framework

This section provides a general framework to answer the examiner's questions, which must be tailored and prioritised to your list of differentials. The number of investigations and the management plan in cardiology are limited, so it becomes relatively easier to score in 'clinical judgement'.

How Would You Investigate?

"The definitive investigation to confirm my diagnosis is echocardiography. However, I will begin with simple investigations including an ECG and chest X-ray."

1. **ECG looking for...**
   - Left ventricular hypertrophy (in AS, AR).
   - Right ventricular hypertrophy (pulmonary hypertension).
   - P mitrale (MS).
   - Conduction abnormalities (calcification of conducting system in AS).
   - Atrial fibrillation (especially in mitral valve disease).
   - Signs of ischaemic heart disease (e.g., q waves, poor R wave progression in MR).

2. **Chest X-ray looking for...**
   - Signs of heart failure: cardiomegaly, pulmonary congestion.
   - Signs of LA enlargement (i.e., splaying of carina, double density sign/double right heart border in MS, MR).
   - Signs of congenital heart disease, such as boot-shape heart (tetralogy of Fallot), notching of ribs (coarctation of the aorta).

3. **2DE:**
   - Valve lesion: to confirm diagnosis, assess severity (Table A4.4), look for aetiology, and evaluate ejection fraction.
   - VSD, ASD: to examine the location, size of defect, direction of flow, and severity markers (e.g., LV dilation, pulmonary hypertension).

4. **Cardiac catherisation**: if planning for valve replacement, to assess if concomitant coronary artery bypass grafting is necessary.

5. **Blood tests**: standard blood tests will include:
   - For any patient with atrial fibrillation: PT/INR (if on warfarin), electrolytes, and thyroid function to look for secondary cause of atrial fibrillation.
   - For any prosthetic valve: PT/INR for warfarin.

Table A4.4. Simplified echocardiographic markers of severity in common valvular lesions.

AS	MS	AR	MR
• Valve area < 1 cm • Pressure gradient > 40 mmHg • Velocity > 4 m/s If ejection fraction is low, gradient may be low even in severe AS.	• Valve area < 1.5 cm^2 • Pulmonary hypertension	• Vena contracta width > 6 mm • Effective regurgitant orifice area > 0.3 cm^2 • Diastolic flow reversal in abdominal aorta	• Vena contracta width > 7 mm • Effective regurgitant orifice area > 0.4 cm^2 • Systolic flow reversal of pulmonary vein

How Would You Manage? (Valve Cases)

"My patient will benefit from a multidisciplinary team approach to management involving the cardiologist, cardiothoracic surgeon, dietitian, physiotherapist, and nurse counsellor, with the goal of treating the underlying cause, treating complications, and maximising function."

Surgery: In terms of treating the underlying cause, I would...

a) *If stem indicates that patient is symptomatic* → Offer valve replacement given that my patient is symptomatic, assuming that the breathlessness is due to valvular heart disease and I have ruled out other causes of shortness of breath.

b) Take a history for symptoms, assess ejection fraction on echocardiography, and offer valve replacement if there is an appropriate indication.
   - AS, AR, MS, MR: Indications are symptoms, decreased ejection fraction, haemodynamic complications, and concomitant cardiac surgery (Table A4.5).
   - VSD: small defects need not be closed; indications for closure are:
     – Infective endocarditis
     – Paradoxical embolism
     – Increasing pulmonary: systemic blood flow (Qp/Qs > 2)
     – Haemodynamic consequence (i.e., LV dilation or failure, pulmonary hypertension)
   - TR: treatment of heart failure, consideration of valve replacement.
   - Eisenmenger syndrome: surgery is contraindicated.

Medical therapy includes ... *(Tailor to what you find in the patient)*
- Management of underlying cause (e.g., treat ischaemic heart disease/infective endocarditis, aortic root screening in Marfan's syndrome).
- Management of heart failure (avoid diuretics in preload-dependant conditions; i.e., AS, HCM).

- Treat AF: rate or rhythm control plus anticoagulation (warfarin vs. direct oral anticoagulant, except in AF associated with MS or prosthetic valves whereby warfarin is the only option).
- Endocarditis prophylaxis in very limited cases (see below).

Supportive measures:
- Patient education.
- Smoking cessation.
- Influenza vaccination.
- Cardiac rehabilitation.
- Treatment of cardiovascular risk factors.

Table A4.5. Indications for surgery in common valvular lesions.

	AS	AR	MS	MR
Indications for surgery	Severe AS with - **Symptoms** - Decreased **EF < 50%** - Exercise hypotension - Decreased exercise tolerance Very severe AS (< 0.6 cm^2) alone Other cardiac surgery with moderate to severe AS	**Symptoms** EF < 50% LV dilation Repair of aortic root dilation Other cardiac surgery	**Symptoms** Pulmonary hypertension Other cardiac surgery	**Symptoms** EF < 60% LV dilation Other cardiac surgery
Surgical approach	AVR Transcatheter aortic valve intervention if high surgical risk Limited role for balloon valvuloplasty	AVR	Rheumatic MS: balloon valvuloplasty Calcific MS or not suitable: MVR	Repair if feasible if not, MVR

How Would You Manage? (Prosthetic Valve)

"My patient will benefit from a multidisciplinary team approach to management involving the cardiologist, cardiothoracic surgeon, dietitian, and nurse counsellor, with the goal of treating the underlying cause, treating complications, and maximising function."

- Regular follow up and echocardiographic assessment of valve function.
- Warfarin anticoagulation, targeting a typical INR of 2–3 for aortic valve replacement and 2.5–3.5 for mitral valve replacement (individualise based on risk profile).

- Dietician counselling on appropriate warfarin diet.
- Treatment of heart failure.
- Endocarditis prophylaxis.
- Other supportive measures.
  - Patient education.
  - Stop smoking.
  - Influenza vaccination.
  - Cardiac rehabilitation.
  - Treatment of cardiovascular risk factors.

Patient is Going For Procedure…

This question is a perennial favourite. Know the answer well and tailor it to your patient. Some examples are:

Patient with prosthetic valves, going for tooth extraction:
"My patient will require endocarditis prophylaxis with amoxicillin 2 g if there is no penicillin allergy. If bleeding risk is low, warfarin may be continued periprocedure. If the dentist prefers to stop warfarin, then bridging with low molecular weight heparin will be required."

Patient with prosthetic valves, going for knee replacement:
"My patient will not require endocarditis prophylaxis as this is not a highest-risk procedure. I will discuss perioperative management of anticoagulation with the surgeon. Patient will require bridging anticoagulation with low molecular weight heparin."

Patient with MS and AF, going for colonoscopy:
"My patient will not require endocarditis prophylaxis. I will discuss periprocedural management of anticoagulation with the endoscopist. If a biopsy is not planned, there may be the option of continuing anticoagulation. If a biopsy is planned, then the options are temporarily withholding anticoagulation or bridging with low molecular weight heparin."

Recommendation for endocarditis prophylaxis:
Endocarditis prophylaxis is indicated for the highest risk procedures in the highest risk patients (AHA 2007 guideline).

Highest risk procedures are:
1. Dental procedures including routine cleaning.
2. Incision or biopsy of respiratory mucosa.
3. Procedures on infected gastrointestinal, urinary, skin, or musculoskeletal tissue (not including routine endoscopies).
4. Surgery to place prosthetic valves or other prosthetic cardiac material.

Highest risk patients are:

1. Prosthetic intracardiac material – prosthetic valves or repair material (e.g., annuloplasty ring). Pacemaker leads do not count.
2. Previous infective endocarditis.
3. Cyanotic heart disease that is
   - unrepaired
   - repaired with residual shunt/regurgitation at or near to site of prosthetic patch/device
   - repaired within last 6 months
4. Heart transplant with valve regurgitation.

Regimen:

- PO amoxicillin 2 g if no penicillin allergy.
- Penicillin allergy: PO clindamycin 600 mg, clarithromycin 500 mg, or azithromycin 500 mg.

Physical Examination

5 | Abdomen

Additional resources and examination videos available at:
www.nigelfong.net/paces-resources.html

Aim to score in the abdominal station. The examination sequence can be completed ahead of time without rushing, key signs are clear and not difficult to elicit, there are only a few clinical syndromes, and interpretation is relatively straightforward.

Walk-Through and Tips

Listen to the stem

In a number of cases this is exceptionally helpful. For instance, "this patient presented with jaundice" immediately clues you in to likely hepatosplenomegaly rather than a renal case, even if jaundice is no longer present now that the patient has been treated. On the other hand, "this patient presented with abdominal pain" would mean that when discussing investigations and management you should consider causes of abdominal pain specific to your patient's context (e.g., ruptured/infected renal cyst in a patient with polycystic kidney disease, or spontaneous bacterial peritonitis in a patient with ascites). Some stems (e.g., "this patient had an abnormality detected on health screening") are less helpful, but at least they tell you that the patient is asymptomatic and the pathology is likely chronic.

Peripheries

Put the bed flat and expose the patient adequately. It is particularly critical to pull down the trousers to the inguinal creases, or you might miss a renal allograft scar.

Stand at the foot of the bed. An experienced clinician can often spot the renal patient at the foot of the bed — some clues include a sallow appearance, uremic pruritus, or obvious dialysis access. On the other hand, a liver patient may be deeply jaundiced. Look out also for cachexia or bronzing of skin (haemochromatosis). Abdominal scars, masses, or flank fullness may be visible from here. Bedside accessories are less common in the abdominal station, but should not be missed.

Hands and arms. Many important signs can be found here — particularly critical are dialysis fistulae and stigmata of chronic liver disease. Begin with both hands outstretched (for clubbing, leukonychia, and the fine tremor of calcinurin inhibitor use), wrists cocked upwards (for asterixes – unlikely in PACES), and hands flipped over to

141

inspect and feel the palms (for Dupuytren's contracture, palmar erythema). Work your way up the arms looking for dialysis fistulae and grafts — if any are present, identify:

- Their location and type – fistula (radiocephalic, brachiocephalic, or brachiobasilic) or graft.
- Whether they are working (i.e., there is an active thrill).
- Whether they are recently used (i.e., recent cannulation marks).

In the face, look for cushingoid features (steroid use), xanthelasma (primary biliary cirrhosis), frontal bossing and maxillary prominence (chronic haemolytic anaemia). Examination of the **eyes** for pallor and scleral icterus is critical to distinguish the causes of hepatosplenomegaly. Scleral icterus is sometimes confused with age-related dirty sclera — the former is uniformly yellow-tinged, while the latter tends to have patches of pigments. Look into the **oral cavity** (ulcers, gum hypertrophy from cyclosporine use, dental malocclusion in thalassaemia). Have a feel of the **parotids** for parotidomegaly (suggests potential alcohol-related liver disease).

Move downwards to the **neck** (parathyroidectomy scar, dialysis catheters, scars from previous tunnelled and non-tunnelled catheters), **axillae** (loss of axillary hair), and **chest** (spider naevi). Warn the patient that you will "feel around the nipple area for tissue growth" before palpating for gynaecomastia.

Some may prefer to sit the patient up to examine the cervical lymph nodes and back before moving on to the abdomen — this is a matter of preference. We prefer to go for the key signs in the abdomen first.

At the end of the peripheral examination you should have some idea of whether this is a renal, liver, or haematological case — but keep an open mind. Key peripheral signs are summarised in Table A5.1.

Abdomen

Inspect the abdomen. Look carefully for obvious masses, caput medusae, insulin or chelation injection marks, and scars. Critical scars include:

- Rutherford-Morrison scar (right or left iliac fossae) – renal allograft. Identify this early so as to be attuned to peripheral clues of the cause and complications of renal disease.
- Mercedes-Benz (rooftop) – liver transplant, pancreatectomy, or distal gastrectomy.
- Splenectomy (left hypochondrial) – trauma, transfusion-dependant haemolytic anaemia (to reduce transfusion requirements), severe immune thrombocytopenia.
- Laparotomy – multiple causes including bowel surgery, splenectomy, nephrectomy, transplant, and others. A laparotomy scar with a palpable renal allograft may be a simultaneous pancreas-renal transplant (the pancreas transplant may not be palpable) or a concomitant renal transplant and nephrectomy (e.g., in polycystic kidneys).
- Tenckhoff catheter or ex-tenckhoff sites (paraumbilical).

Table A5.1. Key peripheral signs in the abdominal examination.

	Renal	Liver	Haematological	Non-specific
Appearance	Sallow Uremic pruritus	Jaundiced^ Bronzed	Pale* ± Jaundiced^	Cachexia
Abdomen - inspection	Renal allograft Tenckhoff catheter	Ascitic drain Mercedes-Benz Caput medusae	Splenectomy Bone marrow aspirate	Laparotomy Chelation/ insulin marks
Hands and Arms	Dialysis fistulae	Clubbing Palmar erythema Dupuytren's	Central venous access lines/ports	Fingertip capillary glucose check marks Ecchymosis
Neck and Chest	Parathyroidectomy Dialysis catheters or old scars	Spider naevi Gynaecomastia Axillary hair loss	Hickmann line	
Face	Cushingoid facies Gum hypertrophy	Xanthelasma Parotidomegaly	Pallor* Dental malocclusion Frontal bossing	Scleral icterus^
Back	Nephrectomy		Bone marrow aspirate	

*Significant pallor is most likely haematologic disease, as liver patients with active or recent gastrointestinal bleeding are unlikely to be fit for PACES, and well-managed kidney patients are maintained at a haemoglobin of 10–11.5 g/dL.

^Jaundice and scleral icterus may be seen in both chronic haemolytic anaemias as well as chronic liver disease. Where severe, liver disease is more likely.

- Old ascitic drains (iliac fossa, usually left).
- Transcutaneous liver biopsy scars – may be difficult to spot.
- Nephrectomy scars are best seen at the back.

Bend down, make yourself comfortable, explain to the patient that you will now feel his/her tummy, and *before you even touch the abdomen* ask if there is any pain. Always keep an eye on the patient's face while palpating the abdomen.

General palpation. Superficial palpation can be done quickly, but deep palpation should be done systematically and carefully — most organomegaly can be identified, or at least suspected, at this step. This is particularly important in patients with isolated left lobe liver enlargement or a far lateral spleen, which can be missed with standard techniques of liver and spleen palpation. If you see any Rutherford-Morrison scar, palpate for a bean-shaped mass underlying it (i.e., a renal allograft).

Pitfall: The renal allograft

> This is usually a case to ace, but some stumble for the following reasons:
>
> 1. Missing a renal allograft. This usually occurs because of inadequate exposure such that the Rutherford-Morrison scar is not seen.
> 2. Making up signs of a transplant kidney, when one is not there.
>   - If a Rutherford-Morrison scar is seen but no allograft is felt beneath it, feel inferiorly and laterally as sometimes an old graft slides downwards.
>   - If none remain palpable, consider the following possibilities:
>   - Graft may be non-palpable due to large body habitus.
>   - Scar may have been for a hernia operation or appendectomy rather than a transplant – the hernia repair scar is typically at or inferior to the inguinal crease, while that of a renal allograft implantation is usually superior to the inguinal ligament.
>   - A graft nephrectomy may have been performed. Look for a second incision over the first scar.
> 3. Missing concomitant abdominal masses (e.g., renal transplant due to polycystic kidney disease). The usual trap is becoming too gleeful after identifying the transplant, and only performing cursory abdominal palpation thereafter. Do not let your guard down!

Liver. Begin palpation from the right iliac fossa, synchronising with the patient's breathing so as to feel the liver tip hitting your fingers as the patient inspires. If a liver is palpable, trace the entire liver outline, feel the liver surface, and check that you cannot get above it. Before you leave this space you must be able to describe the liver (pulsatile, nodular, smooth, craggy, firm, hard). If no liver is palpable, palpate leftwards along the costal margin so as not to miss an isolated left lobe liver enlargement. Percuss downwards in the mid-clavicular line to obtain the upper border of the liver, and upwards to confirm that the liver is dull. Using a ruler or tape measure, measure the liver span (>12 cm is enlarged). Measuring a liver span is superior to reporting the distance below the costal margin, as patients with pulmonary hyperinflation may have a pushed-down and palpable liver that is not actually enlarged.

Spleen. Remember again to begin palpation from the right iliac fossa. As you approach the spleen, place your left hand over the left lower ribs to 'splint' the spleen and make it easier to palpate. If no spleen is felt, palpate leftwards to avoid missing a lateral spleen, and turn the patient slightly right lateral to palpate a small spleen. The characteristics of the spleen is not diagnostically useful, unlike that of the liver. Percuss over any spleen and in the Traube's space (between the left 6th rib and costal margin in the mid-axillary line).

Pitfall: Missing a liver or spleen

> To avoid missing a liver or spleen:
> 1. Always start from the right iliac fossa, or a large liver/spleen may be missed.
> 2. After reaching the costal margin, always continue to palpate leftwards.
>   - Only the left lobe of the liver may be enlarged.
>   - Some spleens enlarge inferiorly rather than inferio-medially.
> 3. If the percussion note is dull but no liver or spleen is felt, try to re-examine.

Kidneys. The kidneys can be difficult to ballot. Do not ballot 'blind' but try to palpate for the kidneys first, so as to ballot precisely where a mass or fullness is felt — and certainly not too laterally (see pitfall). Warn the patient before proceeding to ballot. With the fingers of the balloting hand, make a firm upward thrust, while the palpating hand stays in the deep palpation position, ready to detect any upward bounce. If you do not feel anything, it is sensible to shift the balloting position slightly so as to increase your chance of pick up.

Pitfall: Missing a ballotable kidney

> To avoid missing a ballotable kidney:
> 1. Pay attention to peripheral clues. One's best chances are when peripheral clues have been correctly identified and there is a high clinical suspicion for ballotable kidneys.
> 2. Always palpate first – deeply enough, and pay attention not just to an obvious mass but to any sensation of flank fullness.
> 3. The kidneys are more medial than many think (remember that they are separated from the aorta only by relatively short vessels), so do not make the mistake of simply balloting lateral abdominal fat!
> 4. Pay attention to concomitant masses (e.g., a polycystic liver with polycystic kidney, renal allograft with a polycystic native kidney)!

You must be able to distinguish between a liver, spleen, and kidney. Examiners generally do not require you to pedantically justify why you think a mass is a liver, kidney, or spleen — as long as you get it right. Their classical characteristics are:

- Liver: a right hypochondrial mass that has no clear upper border (i.e., you cannot get over it), moves inferiorly with respiration, is dull to percussion, and is not ballotable.
- Spleen: as for a liver, except in the left hypochondrium. A notch may be palpable in a large spleen.
- Kidney: ballotable flank mass that you can get over and is resonant to percussion.

Pitfall: Uncertain large masses

> With large masses, it can be tricky to tell apart a kidney, spleen, or liver. A huge kidney mimics a liver or spleen in having no clear upper border (too large), becoming dull to percussion (displacing overlying bowel), and being non-ballotable (too large).
>
> Helpful differentiating factors include the following:
>
> - Dullness to percussion in Traube's space reliably signifies a spleen. A kidney, however large, is very unlikely to give dullness here.
> - Kidneys, however enlarged, never cross the midline. A mass that enlarges across the midline is a liver or spleen.
> - A well-defined lower border suggests a liver or spleen. The kidney tends not to have a clear lower border.
> - A palpable notch makes a spleen likely (this is only felt in massive spleens).
> - A mass with a nodular outline is likely a liver (polycystic or malignant) or kidney, unlikely a spleen.
> - Very large polycystic kidneys are likely to have failed. Hence, if there is no evidence of renal replacement therapy or transplant, a very large abdominal mass is less likely to be a kidney.

Shifting dullness. Do this step with finesse. Avoid abdominal masses as you percuss for dullness. Keep the non-striking finger aligned sagittally as you move laterally. If dullness is heard, turn the patient lateral while keeping the non-striking finger at the same spot, then check if the percussion note becomes resonant, which would signify ascites. While the patient is turned, look for posterior scars (especially a nephrectomy or bone marrow aspirate scar) and palpate for any sacral oedema. If there is gross ascites, fluid thrill is an alternative manoeuvre to shifting dullness.

Auscultate the abdomen in the right iliac fossa (for bowel sounds) and over the liver and renal arteries (for bruit). This carries little additional value but is quite routine

Finishing up

Sit the patient up. Standing behind the patient, palpate for cervical and supraclavicular **lymph nodes**. Inspect the **back** for scars (nephrectomy, splenectomy, bone marrow aspirate) and telangiectasia (there are often more spider naevi posteriorly than anteriorly). Check for pedal oedema and thank the patient.

Some additional steps can be performed (e.g., checking pronator drift in suspected polycystic kidneys) — see individual clinical syndromes for details.

Clinical Syndromes

Narrow down to one of these main clinical syndromes. Further interpretation of each syndrome is detailed in the subsequent pages.

Clinical syndrome	Key features
1. Hepatosplenomegaly/ splenomegaly	Splenomegaly Hepatosplenomegaly with predominant spleen Hepatomegaly with splenectomy scar Peripheral signs of 'liver' or 'haematological' abdomen
2. Isolated hepatomegaly	Hepatomegaly Peripheral signs of 'liver' abdomen
3. Ascites only	Ascites, often massive; no organomegaly
4. Ballotable kidney(s)	Ballotable kidneys Peripheral signs of 'renal' abdomen
5. Transplant kidney	RIF/LIF scar + underlying ovoid mass
6. Uncommon – Liver transplant – Simultaneous pancreas-kidney transplant – Luminal disease (e.g., Crohn's disease with multiple scars)	

For each syndrome, in addition to recognising the condition, you will need to:
- Suggest an aetiology.
- Look for complications.

Abdomen – Clinical Syndromes

5.1 | Hepatosplenomegaly/Splenomegaly (or splenectomy scar)

Hepatosplenomegaly (with predominant splenomegaly) or isolated splenomegaly points to chronic liver disease or haematological disease. The causes of hepatosplenomegaly is a long list — suggesting sensible differentials based on peripheral clues and patient profile requires some thought. One challenge is that the standard order of abdominal examination gives the aetiology of liver/haematological disease (peripheral clues) before detection of the key organomegaly, so be observant right from the start.

Recognise Pathology

Present key findings of:
- Abdominal scars.
- Hepatomegaly – including the size and characteristics of the liver.
- Splenomegaly – including the size of the spleen.

Examiners generally do not need a justification for why the mass is a liver or spleen (i.e., that it is dull to percussion, moves inferiorly with respiration, and you cannot get above it), which would be more appropriate in a medical school examination. However, you must get it correct and not mistake a kidney for a liver/spleen.

Suggest Aetiology

Peripheral clues will suggest an aetiology (Table A5.2). Be aware of the predictive value of each sign — some are specific, while others are merely suggestive.

- Hepatomegaly is unexpected in advanced chronic liver disease as the liver would be shrunken. If there is hepatomegaly, consider alcoholic hepatitis, non-alcoholic steatohepatitis, or the development of hepatocellular carcinoma superimposed on chronic liver disease.
- If the liver is not enlarged and there is no other obvious cause, begin by suggesting the most common causes (chronic viral hepatitis, alcoholic and non-alcoholic steatohepatitis), then less common causes (autoimmune hepatitis, metabolic disease i.e., Wilson's and haemachromatosis, primary biliary cholangitis, etc.).

Key diagnostic categories are:

1. Hepatosplenomegaly/splenomegaly with overt stigmata of chronic liver disease: chronic liver disease.
2. Hepatosplenomegaly/splenomegaly with pallor: myeloproliferative disease, chronic haemolytic anaemia, chronic liver disease.

Table A5.2. Common causes of hepatosplenomegaly/splenomegaly.

Category	Aetiology	Specific clues	Suggestive clues
Haematological	Myeloproliferative neoplasm (especially CML*, MF*)	Bone marrow aspirate scar	Pallor[#]
	Lymphomas, leukaemia (incl. hairy cell leukaemia*)	Bone marrow aspirate scar	Lymphadenopathy Hickmann line
	Chronic haemolytic anaemia (thalassaemia, hereditary sphereocytosis)	Splenectomy scar Prominent supraorbital ridge (frontal bossing) Dental malocclusion	Chelation marks Pallor Mild icterus
Hepatic	Chronic liver disease[^] - Chronic viral hepatitis - Alcoholic liver disease - Non-alcoholic steatohepatitis - Autoimmune hepatitis - Metabolic: Wilson's, haematochromatosis	Clubbing Palmar erythema Spider naevi (≥ 5 in superior vena caval distribution) Gynaecomastia Axillary hair loss Caput medusae Ascites ± drain scars	Scleral icterus
	Primary biliary cholangitis	As above, plus orbital xanthelasma	
	Wilson's disease	As above, plus tremor, chorea, dysarthria	
Infective	Chronic malaria* Kala-azar (leishmaniasis)* Viral: CMV, EBV, HIV Bacteria: endocarditis, typhoid, leptospirosis Splenic abscess Others (e.g., schistosomiasis)		Lymphadenopathy Fever
Endocrine	Acromegaly	Spade-like hands, macroglossia	
Rheumatological	Felty syndrome	Rheumatoid hands	
Infiltrative	Amyloidosis Storage disorders (e.g., glycogen storage disease)		

CML: chronic myeloid leukaemia; CMV: cytomegalovirus; EBV: Epstein-Barr virus; MF: myelofibrosis

*Causes of massive hepatosplenomegaly.
[#]There may be conjunctival suffusion instead of pallor in polycythemia vera.
This is not an exhaustive list. Rare cases or cases that are unlikely to present in PACES are not represented.
[^]In a case of chronic liver disease, you would be expected to suggest the underlying aetiology. Look for suggestion of the underlying cause, such as Dupuytren's contracture (alcohol), parotidomegaly (alcohol), intravenous needle track marks (viral hepatitis), extensive tattoos (viral hepatitis), or xanthelasma (primary biliary cholangitis).

3. Hepatosplenomegaly/splenomegaly with lymphadenopathy: lymphoma, viral infection.
4. Massive splenomegaly: chronic myeloid leukaemia, myelofibrosis, chronic malaria, and kala-azar.
5. 'Bland' hepatosplenomegaly/splenomegaly with no obvious clues of aetiology: suggest most common differentials first:
   - Old patient: myeloproliferative disease.
   - Young patient: lymphoproliferative disease, chronic haemolytic anaemia, infections.
   - Any age: chronic liver disease remains a differential (although chronic liver disease patients listed in PACES typically have clear stigmata).

Look for Complications

For each case, consider possible complications and present significant positive and negative findings. This must be tailored to the specific case, for example:

1. **Liver disease:** **Look for:**
   - Hepatic encephalopathy — Asterixes
   - Coagulopathy — Peripheral ecchymoses
   - Portal hypertension — Ascites, previous taps
   - Variceal bleed — Marked pallor, request for rectal exam
   - Hepatocellular carcinoma — Nodular, irregular hepatomegaly

2. **Myeloproliferative disease**
   - Thrombosis — Neurologic deficit – stroke
   - Cytopenias — Ecchymoses, infections
   - Transformation (to leukaemia, blast crisis) — Unwell patient, worsening cytopenias

3. **Chronic haemolytic anaemia**
   - Transfusion dependence — Cubital fossa marks
   - Developmental delay, growth stunting — Whether patient is well thrived
   - Hemochromatosis – heart failure — Pedal oedema
     – diabetes — Glucose check marks
     – hypogonadism — Axillary hair loss, testicular atrophy
   - Pigment gallstones — Cholecystectomy scar
   - Side effects of iron chelation — Visual or hearing impairment

Requests

Tailor the requests to your clinical suspicion — consider what could be helpful in searching for aetiology or in finding complications. For example:

1. **Liver diseases**
   - Examine external genitalia for testicular atrophy.
   - Rectal examination for melena (suggesting a variceal bleed) or impacted stools (increases risk of encephalopathy).

2. **Myeloproliferative/lymphoproliferative disease**
   - Examining the other lymph node stations.
   - Taking a history for fever, night sweats, and weight loss.
   - Taking a travel history (if suspecting malaria or kala-azar).
   - Doing a neurological examination (for complications of thrombosis).

3. **Chronic haemolytic anaemia**
   - Screening vision and hearing (potential side effects of iron chelation therapy).
   - Doing cardiac examination and ECG for signs of cardiomyopathy (from iron overload).
   - Examining external genitalia for signs of hypogonadism (due to iron overload).
   - Urine dipstick for glycosuria (endocrinopathy from iron overload).

Sample Scripts

Chronic liver disease

This gentleman has hepatomegaly with liver span of 15 cm. The liver is smooth, non-nodular, non-tender, and not craggy. The spleen is enlarged 3 cm below the costal margin. There is shifting dullness. In the peripheries, my findings include multiple stigmata of chronic liver disease including scleral icterus, clubbing, palmar erythema, gynaecomastia, spider naevi, axillary hair loss, and multiple scratch marks*. I also note conjunctival pallor but no asterixes. The likely diagnosis is chronic liver disease. His pallor makes me concerned about the possibility of variceal bleeding and I will like to do a rectal examination. Possible aetiologies of liver disease include chronic viral hepatitis and alcoholic and non-alcoholic steatohepatitis.

*Do not simply rattle off, but present what is found and omit what is not!

Myeloproliferative disease

This patient has massive splenomegaly with conjunctival pallor and an old bone marrow aspirate scar. There is no other organomegaly, cervical lymphadenopathy, or jaundice. My principle diagnosis is myeloproliferative disorder, in particular myelofibrosis or chronic myeloid leukaemia. A differential will be chronic infections such as malaria or kala-azar. Chronic liver disease is less likely in the absence of peripheral stigmata. I will like to complete my examination by doing a rectal exam to exclude rectal bleeding as a cause of pallor, and taking a travel history of visits to malaria-endemic countries.

Abdomen – Clinical Syndromes

5.2 | Isolated Hepatomegaly

Isolated hepatomegaly, in the absence of splenomegaly, is less likely to be haematological disease or late chronic liver disease (in which splenomegaly is typical). The characteristic of the liver is key to diagnosis.

Recognise Pathology

Present key findings of hepatomegaly and any peripheral signs. Be careful to not miss a spleen. Pay particular attention to describing the characteristics of the liver.

Suggest Aetiology

The main causes of isolated hepatomegaly can be distinguished by liver characteristics (Table A5.3) and include:

- Growths: Malignancy, cysts, adenomas, focal nodular hyperplasia.

Table A5.3. Common causes of isolated hepatomegaly, by liver characteristics.

Liver	Suggested diagnosis	Supporting signs
Hard, craggy	Neoplasm (hepatocellular carcinoma or metastases)	Jaundice, cachexia
Pulsatile	Tricuspid regurgitation	JVP: giant c-v waves
Nodular	Polycystic liver and kidney disease	Ballotable kidneys, renal failure
	Nodular growths (e.g., malignancy, focal nodular hyperplasia)	
Tender	Infective (e.g., viral hepatitis, CMV, EBV, HIV)	Lymphadenopathy

None of the above	Liver disease - alcoholic
	    - fatty liver
	    - viral hepatitis
	    - primary biliary cholangitis
	    - hepatic cysts, adenomas
		Dupuytren's, parotidomegaly
		Large body habitus, diabetes
		Tatoos, IV drug use marks
		Xanthelasma

	Cardiac – congestive hepatomegaly	Pedal oedema, raised JVP
	Infiltrative diseases, glycogen storage diseases	
	Rest of causes identified above	

- Liver diseases: alcoholic liver disease, viral hepatitis, fatty liver disease, primary biliary cholangitis (cirrhosis is less likely).
- Cardiac: tricuspid regurgitation.
- Infective.

Note: The cirrhotic liver is typically shrunken and isolated hepatomegaly would be unusual.

Look for Complications

Suggest important positives and negatives based on the clinical suspicion, such as:

- Absence of signs of portal hypertension (i.e., no splenomegaly, no ascites), which suggests early liver disease.
- Absence of signs of liver failure (no asterixes, peripheral ecchymoses).

Requests

Sensible requests may include:

- Checking temperature chart for fever (infective causes).
- Doing a rectal examination for masses (metastatic disease)/hard stools and melena (chronic liver disease).
- Examining the cardiovascular system (suspecting cardiac congestion).
- Examining all other lymph node stations (suspecting infection or malignancy).

Sample Scripts

Nonspecific hepatomegaly

This young lady has hepatomegaly with a liver span of 15 cm. The liver is smooth, non-tender, non-pulsatile, and not nodular. There was no palpable splenomegaly and no ascites. I did not note any peripheral stigmata of chronic liver disease, no scleral icterus, no conjunctival pallor, no cervical lymphadenopathy, and no parotidomegaly or Dupuytren's contracture. There is no suggestion of congestive cardiac failure. My differentials for her hepatomegaly include fatty liver disease, viral hepatitis, alcoholic liver disease, hepatic cysts or adenomas, and infiltrative diseases. I will like to complete the examination by checking a temperature chart, examining the rest of the lymph node stations, and auscultating the heart to exclude a tricuspid regurgitation murmur. I will also like to ask her for a history of contraceptive pill use which will predispose to hepatic adenomas.

Hard, irregular hepatomegaly

This elderly gentleman has 5 cm hepatomegaly. The liver is hard with an irregular outline and he is jaundiced. There is no splenomegaly or ascites, no palmar erythema, axillary hair loss, clubbing, no cervical lymphadenopathy, and no parotidomegaly or Dupuytren's contracture. The likely diagnosis is a neoplastic lesion which may be primary or metastatic. A differential is polycystic liver disease. He has no asterixes, peripheral ecchymoses, and no ascites. I will like to complete my examination with a rectal examination for masses, and examining all other lymph node stations.

Abdomen – Clinical Syndromes

5.3 | Ascites Only

Ascites may occur (1) along with cirrhosis, (2) with a craggy liver suggestive of malignancy, or (3) by itself without an obvious underlying cause. When ascites is massive and tense, underlying organomegaly may be present but difficult to palpate.

Recognise Pathology

Key signs

- Distended abdomen.
- ± Eversion of the umbilicus.
- Positive shifting dullness or fluid thrill (do not assume that a distended abdomen is due to ascites).
- Prior **abdominal tap** marks which could be diagnostic or therapeutic.

Cases with palpable organomegaly are discussed in the previous clinical syndromes.

Suggest Aetiology

The causes of ascites are classified based on the serum ascites albumin gradient (SAAG, >11 g/L suggests portal hypertension). However, you will not have access to this information and will have to make a best guess based on peripheral clues (Table A5.4).

Table A5.4. Common causes of isolated ascites.

Category	Cause	Supporting signs
Portal hypertension	Chronic liver disease Budd-Chiari syndrome Portal vein thrombosis	Stigmata of chronic liver disease (e.g., jaundice, clubbing, palmar erythema, axillary hair loss, gynaecomastia)
	Right heart failure Constrictive pericarditis	Peripheral oedema, giant c-v wave ± parasternal heave
Non-portal hypertension, exudative	Peritoneal carcinomatosis Infective (e.g., tuberculosis)	Cachexia Lymphadenopathy
Non-portal hypertension, transudative	Nephrotic syndrome	Anasarca Lower limb oedema
	Serositis (e.g., in lupus)	Raynaud's phenomenon, malar rash, arthropathy

Splenomegaly is typically present in ascites due to portal hypertension, but it may not always be palpable beneath tense ascites.

Look for Complications

1. Look for complications secondary to ascites
   - Hernias (paraumbilical, inguinal) – check cough impulse, reducibility of herniae.
   - Spontaneous bacterial peritonitis (SBP) – comment on the absence of abdominal tenderness (you are unlikely to have a patient with real SBP in PACES, but if the stem is 'this patient has abdominal pain', you must certainly raise this possibility).
2. Look for complications secondary to underlying disease

Sample Scripts

Chronic liver disease

This middle-aged gentleman has tense ascites with positive shifting dullness. Given the peripheral signs of jaundice, palmar erythema, gynaecomastia, spider naevi, loss of axillary hair, and caput medusa, his ascites is likely secondary to **portal hypertension from chronic liver disease**. I expect splenomegaly, but was unable to palpate a spleen beneath the tense ascites. There is no abdominal tenderness to suggest spontaneous bacterial peritonitis, and no obvious herniae. He is not encephalopathic, and there are no ecchymoses to suggest coagulopathy. I will like to complete the examination by doing a rectal examination checking for melena.

Abdomen – Clinical Syndromes

5.4 | Ballotable Kidney(s)

Mildly to moderately enlarged kidneys are not easy to ballot and can be missed — see the pitfalls on page 145. The key tasks in this station are

1. Identify the ballotable kidney(s).
2. Suggest their aetiology.
3. Comment on the patient's current renal function or modality of renal replacement therapy.
4. Look for complications of renal failure.
5. Look for complications of polycystic kidney disease.

Recognise Pathology

Key signs

- Peripheral clues of renal disease (dialysis fistulae, parathyroidectomy scar, previous temporary dialysis catheter sites).
- Unilateral or bilateral ballotable kidneys – distinguish from liver/spleen.
- Any nephrectomy scars.
- Concomitant presence of hepatomegaly (Figure A5.1).

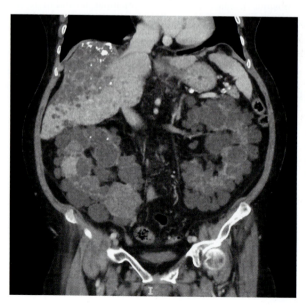

Figure A5.1. Polycystic kidneys and liver.

Q: How does one separately identify the right kidney and liver when they are so close as to be one contiguous mass?

A: Percussing upwards from the right iliac fossa, the percussion note changes from resonant (kidney) to dull (liver).

Suggest Aetiology

1. **Bilateral ballotable kidneys**

This is almost always autosomal dominant polycystic kidney disease (PKD). Differentials include:

- Bilateral hydronephrosis (e.g., from bladder outlet obstruction).
- Infiltrative disease (e.g., amyloidosis, sarcoidosis).
- Acromegaly.
- Bilateral angiomyolipomas in tuberous sclerosis (look for cutaneous stigmata; i.e., facial angiofibroma, subungual fibroma, shagreen patch, ash leaf macule).
- Early diabetic nephropathy (rarely ballotable).

2. **Unilateral ballotable kidney**

   a) Cause of bilaterally enlarged kidneys, but only one side is palpable
   - PKD with asymmetric enlargement (common).
   - PKD with ballotable kidney and contralateral nephrectomy.

   b) Causes of unilateral kidney enlargement
   - Tumour (e.g., renal cell carcinoma, angiomyolipoma).
   - Unilateral hydronephrosis.
   - Renal vein thrombosis.

Comment on Renal Function

State whether the patient is on renal replacement therapy, and through what modality. For example:

- Patient is not on renal replacement therapy and appears to be clinically euvolemic and not uremic.
- Patient is on haemodialysis via a right neck tunnelled dialysis catheter (note: temporary dialysis catheters imply that the patient is on active haemodialysis — they will be removed if not used).
- Patient has an immature, small left radiocephalic arteriovenous fistula. He/she may be being prepared for renal replacement therapy.
- Patient does not have evidence of ongoing renal replacement therapy, but he/she is sallow/in fluid overload with pedal and sacral oedema/is pruritic with multiple scratch marks, which could suggest renal insufficiency.

Look for Complications

1. **Complications of renal failure** — **Sign**
   - Fluid overload — Pedal oedema, lung crepitations
   - Anaemia — Conjunctival pallor
   - Tertiary hyperparathyroidism — Parathyroidectomy scar, fractures
2. **Complications/other manifestations of PKD** — **Sign**
   - Polycystic liver disease — Nodular hepatomegaly
   - Intracranial aneurysms, which may rupture — Pronator drift
   - Pain/renal cell carcinoma/complicated infection — Nephrectomy

Abdominal pain is a common stem in this scenario. The causes of abdominal pain in PKD include: infection, ruptured cyst, haemorrhage into cyst, and nephrolithiasis.

Requests

Many requests are possible and relevant
- For complications of renal disease – measure blood pressure, dipstick for proteinuria.
- For complications of PKD
  - Neurological examination for any residual deficits from a previous ruptured intracranial aneurysm.
  - Cardiac examination (for associated mitral valve prolapse or aortic regurgitation).
  - Checking temperature chart (for fever from urinary tract infection).
- Asking for a family history.

Sample Scripts

Polycystic kidney disease

This gentleman likely has polycystic kidney disease complicated by renal failure. Examination of the abdomen is significant for bilateral ballotable kidneys. He is on haemodialysis with a right arteriovenous graft that has a good thrill and evidence of recent needling. In terms of complications, he has conjunctival pallor and a neck scar consistent with parathyroidectomy for tertiary hyperparathyroidism. There is no palpable hepatomegaly to suggest polycystic liver, and no pronator drift to suggest ruptured intracranial aneurysms. I will like to complete my examination by checking his blood pressure, doing a neurological examination to look for any other neurological deficit, and listening for a mitral valve prolapse or aortic regurgitation murmur which may be associated with polycystic kidney disease. I will also ask for a family history.

Tip: A note on polycystic kidney disease

Polycystic kidney disease can be a true test of skill in abdominal examination. Remember that many combinations of masses are possible in this condition:
- Bilateral ballotable kidneys.
- Unilateral ballotable kidney (one side too small to ballot).
- Unilateral ballotable kidney + nephrectomy scar.
- Ballotable kidney(s) + nodular hepatomegaly ± nephrectomy.
- Renal transplant with any combination of the above.
- Explanted renal allograft (Rutherford-Morrison scar with no underlying mass) with any combination of the above.

Key takeaway: do not stop at identifying ballotable kidneys but look out for all the rest!

Abdomen – Clinical Syndromes

5.5 | Transplant Kidney

This is an easy abdominal case as long as you remember to expose the patient adequately so as not to miss a Rutherford-Morrison scar. The following points must be answered:

1. Identify the renal allograft.
2. Comment on current renal function or modality of renal replacement therapy.
3. Suggest possible aetiologies of end-stage renal failure.
4. Look for complications of (a) renal failure, (b) transplantation, and (c) underlying aetiology.

Recognise Pathology

Key signs

- Right and/or left iliac fossa Rutherford-Morrison scar*.
- Palpable bean-shaped mass beneath the scar.

*Note: The right iliac fossa is the first choice for implantation site, so if the allograft is in the left iliac fossa, search hard in the right iliac fossa for another kidney (dual transplant may be done if the donor kidney is marginal) or a graft nephrectomy (two old Rutherford-Morrison scars).

Think this through: Simultaneous transplants

> Simultaneous transplants may be encountered if you are taking PACES in a tertiary specialist centre.
>
> 1. **Dual kidney transplant** (left and right, or both same side) – two scenarios:
>   - Dual kidney transplant in expanded criteria donors (as these kidneys are expected to function more poorly, both kidneys are transplanted into the same recipient).
>   - Re-transplant after one kidney failed.
> 2. **Pancreas + kidney transplant**: a midline laparotomy scar* (instead of a Rutherford-Morrison scar) + palpable renal allograft. This is typically done for diabetes with diabetic nephropathy. If the pancreas transplant is working, patient should no longer be diabetic.
>
> *Note: A midline laparotomy can also be used for nephrectomy of a native polycystic kidney and implantation of a renal allograft in a single elective surgery.

(Cont'd)

3. **Liver + kidney transplant** – Mercedes-Benz (rooftop) scar with a midline laparotomy or Rutherford-Morrison scar. This may be simultaneous or sequential; indications include:
   - Liver transplant complicated by calcineurin inhibitor-induced nephrotoxicity.
   - Hepatitis C cirrhosis with cryoglobulinaemia.
   - Concomitant autoimmune hepatitis and renal disease.
   - Ischaemic liver + kidney injury (uncommon: ischaemic hepatitis usually recovers and does not require transplant).
   - Polycystic liver and kidney (uncommon: a polycystic liver does not usually fail.
   - Amyloidosis.

Comment on Renal Function

State whether the graft is functioning well, and if not, whether the patient is on renal replacement therapy and through what modality. For example:

- The graft appears to be functioning well. The patient is euvolemic and not uremic. There is an old left radiocephalic arteriovenous fistula which has no evidence of recent cannulation, but still has a good thrill.
- I note that the patient is in fluid overload and has uremic pruritus, which may suggest allograft dysfunction.
- The graft has failed and the patient is on haemodialysis via a left brachiocephalic arteriovenous fistula, which has a good thrill and evidence of active cannulation.

Suggest Aetiology

Key aetiologies to look for include:	Signs
- Polycystic kidney disease*	Ballotable kidneys
- Diabetic nephropathy	Capillary glucose check marks
	Diabetic dermopathy (may also suggest post-transplant diabetes)
- Glomerulonephritis	Signs of rheumatological disease (e.g., lupus)

*Note: Nephrectomy scars do not necessarily imply polycystic kidney disease as nephrectomies may also be done for native kidney renal cell carcinomas.

Look for Complications

1. **Complications of renal failure**   **Signs**
   - Anaemia   Conjunctival pallor
   - Tertiary hyperparathyroidism   Parathyroidectomy scar

2. **Complications/signs of transplant**
   - Infections   –
   - Malignancy   Surgical scars/skin excisions
   - Calcineurin inhibitor use   Fine tremor, gum hypertrophy, hypertrichosis
   - Steroid use   Cushing's *(uncommon with modern regimes)*

3. **Complications of underlying aetiology**
   - Polycystic kidney disease   See Section 5.4
   - Diabetic nephropathy   Vascular disease, amputations, etc.

Tip: Graft nephrectomies

> Failed allografts are not routinely removed. Indications for graft nephrectomies include:
> - Malignancy.
> - Refractory symptoms related to chronic allograft rejection.
> - To enable rapid withdrawal of immunosuppression (e.g., in a patient who is sick or who needs to initiate chemotherapy urgently).
> - To create space for new transplant.

Requests

Possible requests include:
- Measuring the blood pressure.
- Urine dipstick for proteinuria.
- Searching for complications of aetiology (as in polycystic kidney disease, see Syndrome 5.5).

Sample Scripts

Renal transplant

This young lady has had a renal transplant as evidenced by a right iliac fossa Rutherford-Morrison scar with an underlying bean-shaped mass. The graft appears to functioning well as she is clinically euvolemic; there is an old left radiocephalic fistula which has a good thrill but has no recent needle marks, suggesting that it is not currently in use. The most likely aetiology of renal failure in this young lady is chronic glomerulonephritis; she does not have any sign of systemic rheumatological illness, capillary glucose check marks to suggest diabetes, or ballotable kidneys suggesting polycystic kidney disease. In terms of complications, she is not cushingoid, and there is no conjunctival pallor. I will like to complete my examination by checking her blood pressure and performing a urine dipstick for proteinuria.

Abdomen

5.6 | Discussion Framework

This section provides a general framework to answer the examiner's questions. A large range of conditions can be encountered in the abdominal exam — stick to basic principles but tailor them to your patient and your list of differentials.

How Would You Investigate?

"I will investigate to confirm my diagnosis, establish an aetiology, and look for complications."

1. **Liver disease**

    (a) Confirm the diagnosis

    - Ultrasound or CT abdomen to confirm findings and identify cirrhotic liver outline.
    - Liver function tests for hyperbilirubinaemia, transaminitis, hypoalbuminaemia.

    (b) Establish aetiology

    - History of ethanol use, hepatotoxic drugs.
    - Viral hepatitis serology (hepatitis B, C).
    - Primary biliary cholangitis – antimitochondrial antibody.
    - Autoimmune hepatitis – antinuclear antibody, IgG.
    - Haemochromatosis – serum ferritin, transferrin saturations.
    - Wilson's disease – slit lamp exam for Kayser-Fleischer rings, serum ceruloplasmin (low), 24 h urinary copper (high).
    - Consider liver biopsy.

    (c) Look for complications

    - Full blood count for haemoglobin (low in bleed) and platelets (low in hypersplenism).
    - Check PT/aPTT for coagulopathy.
    - Consider esophagogastroduodenoscopy for esophageal varices.
    - If ascites, do abdominal tap to rule out spontaneous bacterial peritonitis.
    - Alpha-fetoprotein and ultrasound abdomen screening for cancer.
    - If suspect malignancy, consider triphasic CT or MRI liver.

2. **Haematological disease**

    (a) Confirm the findings

    - Ultrasound abdomen to confirm abdominal exam findings.

(b) Establish the aetiology (modify based on suspected aetiology)
- Take a history for symptoms.
- Full blood count and peripheral blood film (e.g., target cells and sphereocytes in haemolytic anaemias, leukocytosis with immature neutrophil precursors, elevated basophils and eosinophils in chronic myeloid leukaemia).
- Haemoglobin electrophoresis (if suspecting thalassaemia).
- PCR analysis for the BCR-ABL gene/Philadelphia chromosome (t9:22) (for chronic myeloid leukaemia).
- Bone marrow aspirate + trephine (state expected finding).
- Lymph node biopsy (if suspecting lymphomas).
- Viral serology (e.g., for EBV, CMV).

(c) Look for complications, for example in suspected chronic haemolytic anaemia:
- Ferritin for iron overload.
- MRI T2* for cardiac and hepatic iron overload.
- Screen for diabetes, hypothyroidism, hypogonadism, and other endocrinopathies.

3. **Renal abdomen**

    (a) Confirm diagnosis
    - Ultrasound to confirm polycystic kidneys and look for differentials such as bilateral hydronephrosis.

    (b) Evaluate renal function
    - Check serum urea, creatinine, and electrolytes.
    - Check urine protein/creatinine ratio or 24-hour urine protein.
    - Urine microscopy.

    (c) Look for complications
    - Of underlying disease (e.g., in polycystic kidney disease, ultrasound for polycystic liver, discuss screening for berry aneurysm; in diabetes, retinopathy and foot screening).
    - Of dialysis: calcium/phosphate/vitamin D/parathyroid hormone, haemoglobin, iron studies.
    - Of immunosuppression: check HbA1c (post-transplant diabetes), CMV, BK virus titres, malignancy screen, etc. (you will not be expected to know details).

4. **Ascites**
    - Ascitic tap with paired serum albumin looking at:
        ○ Serum ascites albumin gradient (> 11 g/L suggests portal hypertension).
        ○ Biochemistry: protein, glucose.
        ○ Cell count and differential, rule out spontaneous bacterial peritonitis.
        ○ Gram stain and culture if suspecting spontaneous bacterial peritonitis.

- Cytology if suspecting malignancy.
- Imaging: ultrasound abdomen looking for cirrhosis, splenomegaly.
- Bloods: liver function tests, renal function.
- Echocardiography if suspecting cardiac aetiology.

Don't forget: Tailor your answer to the scenario

> The stem or examiner might give a scenario/presenting complaint. Tailor your response to this scenario. For example:
>
> **This patient complains of abdominal pain, how would you investigate?**
> - Take a history for abdominal pain.
> - If ascites – ascitic tap with cell count, differential, gram stain and culture looking for spontaneous bacterial peritonitis (also send the other usual ascitic fluid studies).
> - If polycystic kidney disease
>   - Urine microscopy and culture (for infection).
>   - CT KUB for urolithiasis, cyst rupture, haemorrhage into cyst.

How Will You Manage?

"My patient will benefit from a multidisciplinary team approach to management involving the physician, nurse educator, dietician, and … with the goal of treating underlying disease, managing complications, and maximising function."

1. **Specific management of disease**
   - Renal disease: Renal replacement therapy, monitoring access patency, monitoring dry weight and dialysis adequacy, etc.
   - Renal transplant: immunosuppression, regular monitoring of graft function.
   - Chronic liver disease: antivirals for hepatitis B/C, ursodeoxycholic acid for primary biliary cholangitis, penicillamine for Wilson's disease, phlebotomy for haemochromatosis.
   - Chronic haemolytic anaemia: nil.
   - Myeloproliferative disease: cytoreductive therapy (e.g., hydroxyurea), targeted therapy (e.g., tyrosine kinase inhibitors for chronic myeloid leukaemia), chemotherapy.

2. **Management of complications**
   - Chronic liver disease:
     - Hepatocellular carcinoma surveillance with alpha-feto protein and ultrasound.

Abdomen 169

- ○ Variceal surveillance and variceal banding and/or beta blocker prophylaxis.
- ○ Spontaneous bacterial peritonitis prophylaxis (specific indications).
- ○ Ascites: low salt diet, spironolactone/furosemide.
- Renal disease:
  - ○ Treating anaemia with iron repletion and erythropoiesis stimulating agents.
  - ○ Blood pressure control.
  - ○ Management of mineral bone disease (e.g., phosphate binders, activated vitamin D).
- Chronic haemolytic anaemia: iron chelation therapy.
- Haematological disease:
  - ○ Supportive transfusions of blood and blood products.
  - ○ Aspirin for thrombosis prophylaxis (specific indications; e.g., most patients with polycythemia vera).

3. **Supportive management**
   - Patient education.
   - Prevent further hepatic/renal insult (e.g., avoid NSAIDs, alcohol).
   - Diet: fluid restriction, low-salt diet (in renal and liver disease), nutritional supplements.
   - Vaccinations (hepatitis A/B in liver disease, hepatitis B in dialysis patient, encapsulated organisms in splenectomy, COVID-19, influenza, and pneumococcal vaccinations for all).
   - Clear bowels (in cirrhosis).
   - Genetic counselling and family planning (in polycystic kidney disease, chronic haemolytic anaemia).

4. **Management of co-morbidities and preservation of overall function**

Physical Examination

6 | Respiratory

The respiratory examination is challenging to complete within 6 minutes. One's technique, particularly chest expansion and percussion, is very visible to examiners; therefore it is advisable to practice appearing smooth and effortless. On the bright side, only a few clinical syndromes and diagnoses are stable enough to appear in PACES (therefore pneumonias and pneumothoraxes tend not to appear). Aim to secure the diagnosis as early as possible, with hard signs that you can have confidence in.

Walk-Through and Tips

Listen to the stem

The stem usually provides the patient's presenting complaint. This can be very informative.
- Shortness of breath – non-specific.
- Cough – interstitial lung disease, bronchiectasis; occasionally also collapse (from lung malignancy), consolidation.
- Recurrent chest infections – bronchiectasis.
- Haemoptysis – bronchiectasis, lobectomy, pneumonectomy, lung cancer.

Inspection

Positioning. Position the patient at 45 degrees and expose the chest. Standing at the foot of the bed, visually scan the patient's surroundings (sputum mug, nebuliser, inhalers, supplemental oxygen, mucus clearance devices), the patient's face (microstomia, malar rash, pursed lip breathing, cyanosis, plethora in superior vena cava obstruction), and the general appearance (cachexia, respiratory distress). Listen for any cough (wet or dry), wheeze, or stridor and at the length of inspiration-expiration. Ask the patient to take deep breaths and observe for chest expansion (unilaterally reduced, bilaterally reduced, or hyperinflated) — inspection is quite sensitive for asymmetric chest expansion. Note any scar (but thoracotomies are typically only visible when examining the back).

171

Many conditions in the respiratory examination reveal themselves at this step:
- Hyperinflated chest, pursed lip breathing, nicotine stained hands – COPD until proven otherwise.
- Wet cough and copious purulent sputum in a mug – bronchiectasis.
- Bilaterally poor chest expansion – interstitial lung disease.
- Microstomia, malar rash, rheumatoid hands, or sclerodactyly – interstitial lung disease.
- Lobectomy scar – pneumonectomy, lobectomy, or lung transplant (less likely).
- Clamshell (bilateral subcostal) scar – lung transplant (can also be done via a sternotomy).

Observe the patient's work of breathing at the foot of the bed. Look for any oxygen use, tachypnea, prominent sternocleidomastoid, as well as any indrawing of intercostal muscles.

Peripheries

Hands. Examine the hands stretched out (for tremor) and wrists cocked up (asterixes), and have a close look at both the dorsum and palm. Pay particular attention to the nails (clubbing, nicotine stains), evidence of rheumatologic disease (rheumatoid arthritis, sclerodactyly, dermatomyositis), and wasting (possible T1 nerve root involvement from pancoast tumour). Clubbing is an important sign and occurs in pulmonary fibrosis, suppurative lung disease, and lung cancer — COPD is not a cause of clubbing. Asterixes and palmar erythema are rare in the exam. Feel the patient's pulse and count the respiratory rate — make a show out of counting with a stopwatch.

Go through the face and neck quickly – time is short and there are few high-yield signs here. Look in the conjunctivae for pallor, at the lips for cyanosis, and in the mouth for oral thrush. Go down to the neck and look for the jugular venous pressure (right heart failure secondary to lung disease, or as a cause of crepitations).

The trachea is important – don't rush here. Warn the patient: *"Sir/Mdm, I'm now going to feel your neck, it may be slightly uncomfortable. Please let me know if it is too uncomfortable and I will stop. Please look straight ahead."* Ensuring that the patient is positioned symmetrically and looking straight (or you may get an erroneous sign), place one finger in the jugular notch at the midline and inch upward. If the trachea is central, your finger should hit the middle of the trachea, and there should be an equal amount of space on either side. Very slight deviation to the right is physiologic. Palpate the trachea just above the jugular notch where it is fixed — *not too superiorly*, where the trachea is mobile and subtle head turning can give erroneous trachea deviation.

The combination of unilaterally reduced chest expansion (best observed from the foot of the bed, rather than palpated) and tracheal deviation can give you a diagnosis:
- Trachea deviated to side of reduced chest expansion: collapse, fibrosis, lobectomy or pneumonectomy (look for a scar).

- Trachea deviated away from side of reduced chest expansion: massive effusion or pneumothorax.
- Trachea central: consolidation.

Palpate the apex beat for evidence of mediastinal displacement. Check for signs of pulmonary hypertension — whether there is a parasternal heave or a palpable pulmonary component of the second heart sound. Do not spend too long here as it is not critical in the respiratory exam.

At this juncture, decide whether to examine the front or the back first. *If the trachea is central*, examining the back first is usually higher yield (in particular in picking up a lobectomy/pneumonectomy scar, and in hearing crepitations at the posterior lung bases) — examining the front first means you may only get the diagnosis in the last minute. On the other hand, if the trachea is deviated, examine the front first as an upper lobe pathology (e.g., collapse) becomes more likely.

Back and axillae

Sit the patient up and offer a pillow to hug "for comfort" — but more importantly, this moves the scapulae out of the way (an experienced patient may know how to position himself/herself without a pillow — if so, let the patient do so in his/her preferred way). Inspect very carefully for lobectomy scars and smaller scars (video-assisted thoracoscopic surgery, pleural biopsy, ex drain sites etc.). Notice any kyphoscoliosis as this may alter findings in chest expansion.

Palpate for chest expansion in three regions — first with palms flat over the upper chest, then with palms placed on either side of the chest (thumbs abducted and tips of thumbs meeting in the midline) at the middle and lower regions. Technique is important to transmit lung movements into movements of your hands: place palms on the chest when the patient is in full expiration, only then have the patient take a deep breath in. A common mistake is to place your fingers with the patient in mid-expiration. This decreases the chest excursion felt and therefore the sensitivity of this step. The side that does not expand is always the abnormal side.

Before **percussing**, warn the patient that you will tap lightly on his/her back. Percuss inferiorly enough or you may miss a small effusion; remember that the base of the scapulae marks T7 while the lung goes downwards all the way to T12. You can examine the axillae together with the back, or later on with the front — either is acceptable. Look out for dullness (consolidation) and stony dullness (effusion); if a stony dull note is found, determine the level of the effusion. Hyper-resonance (pneumothorax) is unlikely as such patients would not be left to sit around and wait to be examined.

Most diagnoses can be made before auscultation. If the examination has been completely normal up to this point, make sure to listen very carefully (and go inferiorly enough) for crepitations as bronchiectasis and interstitial lung disease may only reveal themselves here.

Auscultate in approximately 4 points on the back and 2 in each axilla. Ask the patient to take deep breaths, and listen to a complete breath at each point (i.e., let the patient fully exhale before lifting off your stethoscope). Listen first for the length and characteristic of the breath sounds — vesicular or bronchial (long, harsh expiratory phase, often separated from inspiration with a pause), and whether there is a prolonged expiratory phase (normal expiration is short and follows immediately after inspiration with no pause). Next listen for additional sounds. If crepitations are heard, decide if these are fine or coarse based on their characteristic (velco-like vs. deep, gurgling) and number (> 8 crepitations per breath is likely fine). Time the crepitations (pan-inspiratory, end-inspiratory) and ask the patient to cough (change in coughing in bronchiectasis). If a wheeze is heard, decide if it is polyphonic and diffuse (obstructive airway disease), or monophonic and localised (local obstruction; e.g., bronchial tumour).

Check for vocal resonance by asking the patient to say 'ninety-nine' at each position where you put down your stethoscope. This is generally of low yield except in the case of dull percussion note and reduced breath sounds — in which vocal resonance helps to distinguish consolidation (vocal resonance increased) from collapse (reduced).

Palpate for cervical lymph nodes before leaving the back.

Pitfall: Why respiratory signs may be missed

Know — and avoid — these pitfalls:
- Missing peripheral signs which clue in to the diagnosis — particularly clubbing of fingers/toes, peripheral stigmata of a rheumatologic cause of interstitial lung disease, and guttering of fingers (pancoast tumour).
- Missing signs in the lung bases (not going inferiorly enough posteriorly) and apices (due to lack of percussion/auscultation above the clavicle).
- Missing bronchial breath sounds. Bronchial breath sounds are subtle and easily missed if the candidate takes the stethoscope off the chest before full expiration is complete, or fails to pay attention to the length of inspiration vs. expiration.

Front

Lie the patient back down to examine the front. Proceed similarly as with the back, checking chest expansion, percussion, auscultation, and vocal resonance. Remember not to miss the supraclavicular fossae, and to examine the axillae if these were not examined posteriorly. It is less important to go all the way inferiorly here except in the case of COPD, in which you would want to look for a loss of cardiac and liver dullness on percussion.

Thank the patient and cover up.

Typical requests at the end of the respiratory examination are:
- Checking the oxygen saturation.
- Looking at the temperature chart.
- Taking a history (e.g., smoking history, occupational and recreational exposures, etc. — tailor to the underlying clinical syndrome).

Pitfall: Running out of time

> Among the physical examination stations, it is easiest to run out of time in the respiratory station. Some tips:
>
> - It is generally sufficient to percuss and auscultate at 4 points posteriorly, 2 points in the axilla, and 3 points anteriorly. Chest expansion can be done in 3 regions posteriorly and 2 regions anteriorly. Any more is a luxury.
> - Examine the back first. The only finding in a patient with early idiopathic pulmonary fibrosis may be fine crepitations right at the posterior lung bases — the candidate that starts with the front and runs out of time to reach the posterior lung bases will miss this diagnosis.
> - Know what to examine quickly — the face, apex beat, and for parasternal heave. These areas generally have few high-value signs for the respiratory examination.
> - If you are running out of time, skip the cervical lymph nodes and parasternal heave. Ideally these should be examined, but if you are out of time, it is better to and add it to the list of 'requests' at the end, than to not complete the back!

Clinical Syndromes

Key signs in the respiratory examination are summarised in Table A6.1. The main clinical syndromes in the respiratory examination are:

Clinical syndrome	Key features
1. Interstitial lung disease	Signs of rheumatologic disease in the limbs and face Clubbing Bilaterally reduced chest expansion Fine inspiratory crepitations
2. Bronchiectasis	Wet cough, purulent sputum, mucus clearance device at bedside Clubbing Coarse inspiratory crepitations, change on coughing
3. Pleural effusion	± Decreased chest expansion (unilateral) ± Tracheal deviation (away from side) Stony dull percussion note Reduced breath sounds
4. Lung resection	Thoracotomy or VATS scar ± Decreased chest expansion (unilateral) ± Tracheal deviation (towards side)

(Cont'd)

Clinical syndrome	Key features
5. Collapse	Decreased chest expansion
	Tracheal deviation (towards side)
	Dull percussion note
	Reduced breath sounds
6. Consolidation	± Decreased chest expansion (unilateral)
	± Dullness to percussion
	Bronchial/reduced breath sounds
	Increased vocal resonance
	± Monophonic, localised ronchi
7. Obstructive airway disease	Barrel chest, pursed lip breathing
	Prolonged expiratory phase
	Polyphonic, generalised expiratory ronchi

For each syndrome, in addition to recognising the condition, you will need to:
- Suggest an aetiology.
- Look for complications.

Table A6.1. Chest signs in dyspnoea.

	Collapse	Pneumothorax	Fibrosis	COPD	Bronchiectasis	Effusion	Consolidation
Trachea deviation	Towards affected side (if upper lobe)	Away from affected side (if tension)	Towards affected side (if upper lobe)	Nil. May have tracheal tug	Nil	Away from affected side (if massive)	Nil
Chest expansion	↓ On affected side	↓ On affected side	↓ On affected side	↓ Bilaterally Hyperinflated	—	↓ On affected side	↓ On affected side
Percussion	Dull	Hyperresonance	—	Hyperresonance	—	Stony dull	Dull
Added sounds	—	—	Fine crackles[a]	Expiratory wheeze ± coarse crackles	Coarse crackles, changes with cough[b]	Crackles if there is pulmonary oedema	Coarse late inspiratory crackles
Breath sounds	↓	↓	↓	↓ Or normal	Normal or bronchial[b]	↓	Bronchial
Vocal resonance	↓	↓	—	—	Normal or ↑[b]	↓	↑

[a] In severe pulmonary fibrosis, there may be traction bronchiectasis, leading to mixed fine and coarse crepitations.
[b] If there is superimposed consolidation, there may be bronchial breathing/increased vocal resonance.

Respiratory – Clinical Syndromes

6.1 | Interstitial Lung Disease

Interstitial lung disease (ILD) is a relatively straightforward case. You will need to present the signs of interstitial lung disease, suggest aetiology, and look for complications.

Recognise Pathology

While the diagnosis of ILD is only confirmed upon auscultation of fine crepitations, it must be strongly suspected in a patient with symmetrically reduced chest expansion and a dry cough, or who has peripheral signs of rheumatologic disease.

Key signs

- Bilateral, symmetrically reduced chest expansion.
- ± clubbing.
- Trachea central.
- Resonant percussion note.
- Fine pan-inspiratory/end-inspiratory crepitations that do not change with coughing (describe distribution of crepitations).

Suggest Aetiology

The causes of ILD may be summarised as idiopathic, secondary to connective tissue disease, environmental exposures, drugs, and other causes. Give examples of each category based on (i) the distribution of crepitations (Table A6.2), as well as (ii) peripheral signs, particularly of connective tissue disease.

Look for Complications

Comment on the presence/absence of:
- Respiratory distress.
- Oxygen use.
- Pulmonary hypertension (parasternal heave, loud pulmonary component of the second heart sound).

Table A6.2. Major causes of interstitial lung disease.

General rule	Upper lobe	Lower lobe
Connective tissue disease – *lower lobe fibrosis except ankylosing spondylitis*	Ankylosing spondylitis	Systemic sclerosis Dermatomyositis Rheumatoid arthritis Sjogren's syndrome
Environmental – *upper lobe fibrosis, except asbestosis*	Inorganic dusts (e.g., silicosis, coal worker's pneumonitis) Hypersensitivity pneumonitis, chronic (e.g., farmer's lung, bird fancier's disease) Vapours (e.g., hydrocarbons)	Asbestosis
Drugs – *generally lower lobe fibrosis*		Immunosuppressive: methotrexate, leflunomide, cyclophosphamide, everolimus Chemotherapy: bleomycin, gemcitabine, checkpoint inhibitors Cardiology: amiodarone Antibiotics: nitrofurantoin, isoniazid Antiepileptic: phenytoin, carbamazepine
Others	Sarcoidosis Old tuberculosis Radiation-induced lung injury Histiocytosis	Radiation-induced lung injury
Idiopathic*		Idiopathic pulmonary fibrosis (most common) Nonspecific interstitial pneumonia

*Other idiopathic interstitial pneumonias have characteristic distributions, such as patchy (as in cryptogenic organising pneumonia) or diffuse.

Sample Scripts

Idiopathic pulmonary fibrosis

My positive findings are peripheral clubbing, bilaterally reduced chest expansion, and bilateral fine pan-inspiratory crepitations, best heard in the lung bases posteriorly. The trachea is central. He is not on oxygen, but I note increased work of breathing with tachypnoea and accessory muscle use. The likely diagnosis is interstitial lung disease. I do not note any peripheral stigmata of rheumatologic disease. I will like to take a drug, occupational, and exposure history, and ask about symptoms of connective tissue disease. If these are negative, I will consider idiopathic causes of interstitial lung disease, most common of which is idiopathic pulmonary fibrosis.

Systemic sclerosis

The findings in this young lady are in the lower chest where there is reduced expansion and bilateral fine end-inspiratory crepitations. The trachea is central. Additionally, I note microstomia, sclerodactyly, digital infarcts over the right ring finger, and a salt and pepper rash over the upper chest. There is a prominent parasternal heave and loud pulmonary component of the second heart sound. She is neither in respiratory distress nor tachypnoeic. In summary, this young lady likely has systemic sclerosis complicated by interstitial lung disease and pulmonary hypertension.

Respiratory – Clinical Syndromes

6.2 | Bronchiectasis

Bronchiectasis is a reasonably straightforward case, but distinguishing coarse vs. fine crepitations can sometimes be tricky.

Recognise Pathology

Key signs
- Productive cough ± productive sputum (in mug at bedside).
- ± Clubbing.
- Trachea central.
- Generally normal chest expansion.
- Resonant percussion note.
- Coarse inspiratory crepitations which change on coughing. It is important to describe the distribution of crepitations, such as generalised, focal, or bibasal.
- Some patients may have expiratory ronchi (some element of airway obstruction is seen in bronchiectasis).

Tip: Distinguishing coarse vs. fine crepitations

The 'sound' of the crepitations (coarse and wet in bronchiectasis vs. 'velcro-like' in interstitial lung disease (ILD)) is critical, but some cases are genuinely difficult. If you are unsure, additional clues to consider include:

Peripheral clues
- A wet cough is more likely bronchiectasis, while a dry cough favours ILD.
- Thick sputum in a mug is almost always bronchiectasis.
- The presence of bronchodilators at the bedside suggests bronchiectasis (not absolute).
- Significantly reduced bilateral chest expansion favours ILD.
- The hands are important – stigmata of systemic sclerosis or dermatomyositis suggests ILD. Rheumatoid arthritis may be complicated by either ILD or bronchiectasis.
- Clubbing can occur in both bronchiectasis and ILD and does not distinguish the two.

Chest auscultation
- Number of crepitations per breath cycle – typically ≤ 5 in bronchiectasis vs. ≥ 10 in ILD.
- Whether the crepitations change in coughing (which occurs in bronchiectasis).

Note that crepitations in advanced ILD can sound coarse (possibly due to traction bronchiectasis). Fine crepitations are unlikely to be bronchiectasis.

Suggest Aetiology

The causes of bronchiectasis can be divided based on the location of crepitations:

a) **Focal crepitations**
- Upper chest
  – Post-tuberculous
  – Post-radiation
- Lower chest
  – Aspiration
- Any distribution
  – Infective and post-infective
  – Post-obstructive
    > Intraluminal (e.g., foreign body)
    > Luminal (e.g., endobronchial mass)
    > Extraluminal (i.e., extrinsic compression)

b) **Generalised crepitations**
- Any age:
  – Systemic immunodeficiency (e.g., hypogammaglobulinaemia)
  – Allergic bronchopulmonary aspergillosis (ABPA)
- Young patient, also
  – Cystic fibrosis (look for gastrostomy tube, insulin pen)
  – Ciliary dysfunction (e.g., Kartagener's syndrome (dextrocardia))

Note: Bronchiectasis may occur in rheumatoid arthritis and Sjögren's syndrome, but think twice before presenting a case of rheumatoid hands and pulmonary crepitations as bronchiectasis, as ILD is far more common in this population.

Requests: in addition to looking at the temperature chart, sputum mug, and oxygen saturation, it will be impressive to request for a history of asthma, which would prompt suspicion of ABPA.

Look for Complications

Comment on the presence/absence of:
- Respiratory distress.
- Oxygen use.
- Pulmonary hypertension (parasternal heave, loud pulmonary component of the second heart sound).

Sample Scripts

Focal bronchiectasis

This elderly gentleman has a wet cough, thick sputum in a pot, digital clubbing, and coarse pan-inspiratory crepitations which change on coughing and is best heard in the right lung base. The trachea is central and percussion note is resonant. He is not in respiratory distress, not on oxygen, and there is no evidence of pulmonary hypertension. The likely underlying diagnosis is bronchiectasis with lower lobe predominance. I note that he has a left hemiparesis and I wonder if recurrent aspiration due to dysphagia could be the cause of his bronchiectasis. Other possible causes of bronchiectasis include post-infective, post-obstructive, and congenital which is less likely for his age. Causes of post-infective bronchiectasis include previous bacterial or tuberculous infection. Causes of post-obstructive bronchiectasis include endoluminal causes such as mucous plugging or a foreign body, luminal causes such as neoplasm or endobronchial tuberculosis, and extraluminal causes such as bronchial obstruction.

Generalised bronchiectasis

This young gentleman has finger clubbing. He has a wet cough and diffuse coarse pan-inspiratory crepitations which change on coughing. The trachea is central and percussion note is resonant. He is not in respiratory distress, not on oxygen, and there is no evidence of pulmonary hypertension. The likely unifying diagnosis is cystic fibrosis as he also has a gastrostomy tube in situ and an insulin pen at the bedside. Other possible aetiologies in this young gentleman include ciliary dysfunction as well as congenital immunodeficiency.

Respiratory – Clinical Syndromes

6.3 | Pleural Effusion

This is not a difficult case as long as you remember to percuss inferiorly enough, and can identify the stony dull percussion note.

Recognise Pathology

Key signs in a unilateral pleural effusion:
- Unilaterally reduced chest expansion.
- ± Trachea and apex beat deviation to the opposite side (in a massive effusion).
- Stony dullness to percussion (state level until which percussion note is stony dull).
- Reduced/absent breath sounds.
- ± Area of bronchial breathing above the effusion.
- Reduced vocal resonance.
- ± Previous aspiration or chest tube scars.

Bilateral effusions are more challenging to pick up as one will not be able to compare chest expansion against the contralateral side.

Suggest Aetiology

Attempt to identify a possible aetiology for the pleural effusion based on (a) whether it is unilateral or bilateral, and (b) signs to suggest a specific cause (Table A6.3).

Look for Complications

Comment on the presence/absence of:
- Respiratory distress.
- Oxygen use.

Sample Scripts

Unilateral pleural effusion

The positive findings are in the right lower chest where there is decreased expansion, stony dullness to percussion up to the base of the scapula, reduced breath sounds, and reduced vocal resonance. The trachea was central. I also note a 2 cm by 2 cm hard, irregular lymph node in the right supraclavicular fossa. In summary, this lady has a right-sided pleural effusion, the aetiology of which may be neoplastic or tuberculous.

Table A6.3. Major causes of a pleural effusion.

	Causes	Key signs
Bilateral	Fluid overload	Pedal oedema, raised jugular venous pressure Other signs of cardiac or renal failure (e.g., displaced apex beat, temporary dialysis catheter in situ)
	Nephrotic syndrome	Pedal oedema, ascites
	Chronic liver disease	Peripheral stigmata (e.g., jaundice, clubbing, palmar erythema, spider naevi)
Unilateral	Malignant	Cachexia, cervical lymphadenopathy, hoarse voice, radiation marks, previous mastectomy scar, clubbing
	Tuberculous	Cachexia ± cervical lymphadenopathy
	Parapneumonic	Fever, IV antibiotics
	Connective tissue disease	Deforming polyarthropathy (rheumatoid arthritis) Malar rash (lupus)
	Pleuro-peritoneal fistula Hepatic hydrothorax	Right-sided effusion in patient with ascites/chronic liver disease or on peritoneal dialysis

Respiratory – Clinical Syndromes

6.4 | Lung Resection

A case of lung resection is easy *if one notices the thoracotomy scar*. This must not be missed. One can identify the diagnosis based on unilaterally reduced chest expansion and ipsilateral tracheal deviation alone, but these signs can be subtle and easily missed.

Recognise Pathology

Step 1: Identify lung resection
- Thoracotomy or video-assisted thoracoscopy scar (more challenging; some centres consider them unfair for PACES).
- Ipsilateral reduced chest expansion.
- Trachea deviation to the affected side (may be subtle, so examine carefully; on the other hand, the trachea may be central in lower lobe lobectomy, so present only what you find).

Step 2: Distinguish lobectomy vs. pneumonectomy. The keys to tell them apart are:
- The presence of tracheal deviation – the trachea is central in a lower lobectomy but deviated to the side of a upper lobectomy or pneumonectomy.
- Lobectomies have only a focal area of decreased breath sounds and dull percussion note (upper or lower chest, as the case may be). In contrast, pneumonectomies are likely to have absent breath sounds in the axilla, as well as decreased breath sounds and a dull percussion note in most of the hemithorax (although normal breath sounds may be heard closer to the midline due to hyperinflation of the contralateral lung).

	Pneumonectomy	Lobectomy Upper	Lobectomy Lower
Tracheal deviation	Yes	Yes	No
Extent of percussion dullness	Extensive	Small area	Small area
Breath sounds in axilla	None	Normal or slightly reduced	Normal or slightly reduced

Step 3 (optional): Consider uncommon differentials to a lobectomy or pneumonectomy
- Thoracoplasty for old tuberculosis: an older patient with missing ribs ± phrenic nerve crush scar.
- Unilateral lung transplant: consider if taking in a tertiary specialist hospital, the contralateral lung is very diseased (i.e., bronchiectasis or interstitial lung disease), and there are no signs of volume loss. Bilateral lung transplant is more likely performed through a clamshell subcostal incision.
- Other lung procedures: open lung biopsy, decortication, or pleurectomy.

- Non-respiratory procedures: oesophageal surgery, repair of coarctation of aorta, and mitral valve surgery. These would not be expected in the respiratory station.

Consider Aetiology

Common indications for lobectomy/pneumonectomy are:
- Lung cancer.
- Focal bronchiectasis complicated by pulmonary haemorrhage that has failed non-invasive treatment.
- Infection.
  - Historical treatment of tuberculousis.
  - Rarely used in difficult-to-treat infection (e.g., persistent disease despite medical therapy, resistant organism, or abcess).
- Lung volume reduction surgery in chronic obstructive pulmonary disease (lobectomy).

Look for Complications

The presence of respiratory distress or oxygen requirement will be unusual in a stable lobectomy or pneumonectomy.

Sample Scripts

Pneumonectomy

This elderly gentleman has a left thoracotomy scar with smaller secondary scars. The trachea is deviated to the left. The left chest has reduced expansion, an extensive area of dull percussion note, absent breath sounds, and reduced vocal resonance. The likely diagnosis is a left pneumonectomy. Functionally, he is comfortable at rest and not on oxygen. In terms of the underlying aetiology, I do not note any clubbing, cachexia, or cervical lymphadenopathy to suggest a mitotic lesion; the contralateral lung is normal. Possible causes for the lobectomy include a pulmonary neoplasm, abscess, or mycetoma.

Lobectomy

This gentleman has a left thoracotomy scar, tracheal deviation to the left, reduced left-sided chest expansion, as well as dullness to percussion, reduced breath sounds, and reduced vocal resonance in the left lower chest. There is a port-a-cath in situ. In summary, this gentleman is likely to have had a left lower lobectomy. The likely underlying aetiology for the lobectomy is pulmonary neoplasm, given the port-a-cath in situ.

Respiratory – Clinical Syndromes

6.5 | Collapse

Lung collapse is one of the harder respiratory cases as the signs of volume loss can be subtle, leading to a misdiagnosis of effusion or consolidation.

Approach

Recognise unilateral volume loss — decreased chest expansion and tracheal deviation to the same side. Ensuring that a lobectomy scar is absent, the remaining differentials are lung collapse, collapse-consolidation, and fibrothorax (pleural space inflammation leading to scarring which restricts lung expansion). They are not easy to tell apart and can be offered as differentials to each other.

Right upper lobe collapse

- Tracheal deviation to the ipsilateral side *(upper lobe collapse) – in a lower lobe collapse, the apex beat may be deviated instead.*
- Unilaterally decreased chest expansion.
- Dullness to percussion.
- Decreased breath sounds and vocal resonance.*
- There is no overlying scar *(This is critical! If there is a scar, think lobectomy).*

*Listen in the axilla — even in complete collapse, there may still be resonant percussion note and breath sounds medially because the contralateral lung hyperexpands.

Right lung collapse-consolidation/fibrothorax

- Tracheal deviation to the ipsilateral side – *in a lower lobe collapse, the apex beat may be deviated instead.*
- Unilaterally decreased chest expansion
- Dullness to percussion
- ± Bronchial breath sounds
- ± Crepitations
- ± Increased vocal resonance
- No overlying scar

} *Features of consolidation alongside those of collapse. Crepitations and bronchial breath sounds are also present in a fibrothorax.*

Suggest Aetiology

Look for physical signs that may give a clue on the underling aetiology, and consider intraluminal, luminal, and extraluminal causes (Table A6.4). Acute causes of lung collapse (e.g., mucous plugging, foreign body) are unlikely in PACES.

Table A6.4. Major causes of lung collapse.

	Causes	Possible signs
Extraluminal	Fibrothorax from old pleural inflammation (e.g., TB, empyema, haemothorax) Compression by extrinsic mass	
Luminal	Endobronchial tumour Endobronchial tuberculosis	Clubbing, cachexia, cervical lymphadenopathy, radiation marks, Horner's syndrome
Intraluminal	Secretions, mucus plugging Foreign body Aspiration	Expiratory wheeze (mucous plugging in allergic bronchopulmonary aspergillosis) Dysphagia/nasogastric feeding (aspiration)

Look for Complications

The presence of respiratory distress or oxygen requirement is unusual in a case of chronic lung collapse that appears for PACES.

Sample Script

Collapse

This lady is clubbed. The trachea is slightly deviated to the left. The findings are in the left chest in which there is reduced chest expansion, a dull percussion note, reduced breath sounds, and diminished vocal resonance. This appears to be complicated by moderate respiratory distress with tachypnoea and use of accessory muscles of respiration. She likely has a left lung collapse. Clubbing may suggest an endobronchial neoplasm as the underlying aetiology. Other causes of lung collapse include intraluminal causes such as mucous plugging, as well as extraluminal causes such as extrinsic mass compression.

Fibrothorax

This elderly lady has right-sided volume loss with reduced right chest expansion and trachea deviated to the right. There is dullness to percussion, reduced breath sounds, and coarse crepitations in the right hemithorax. There is no lobectomy scar, although I do note a small scar which may be an old chest tube. She is neither clubbed nor in respiratory distress. Differentials include fibrothorax (Figure A6.1) and lung collapse. Causes of fibrothorax may include old empyema, pleural tuberculosis, or a traumatic hemothorax.

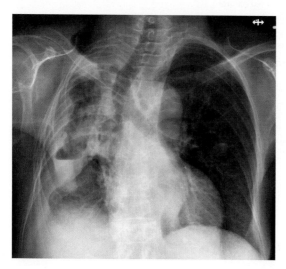

Figure A6.1. Fibrothorax from old empyema.

Remember this X-ray to visualise the physical signs that one will encounter here:
- Tracheal deviation to right
- Reduced right-sided expansion
- Dull percussion note
- Decreased breath sounds and coarse crepitations

Respiratory – Clinical Syndromes

6.6 | Consolidation

Consolidation is a challenging case. The diagnosis will be missed if one does not pay attention to an easily missed finding of focal bronchial breath sounds. Look also for any features suggestive of volume loss (decreased chest expansion, tracheal deviation) which would suggest a collapse-consolidation (see Syndrome 6.5).

Recognise Pathology

Right lower chest consolidation

- ± Clubbing (if neoplastic or chronic suppurative cause).
- Absence of volume loss i.e., symmetrical chest expansion, central trachea.
- ± Dull percussion note in right lower chest (absent if area of consolidation is small).
- Bronchial breath sounds in right lower chest.
- ± Focal monophonic wheeze (suggests fixed obstruction; e.g., cancer).
- Increased vocal resonance in right lower chest.

Tip: Identifying the bronchial breath sound

> The bronchial breath sound can be subtle. Some clues are:
> - Prolonged expiration (recall that in normal vesicular breath sounds, the inspiratory phase is longer than the expiratory phase).
> - Pause between inspiration and expiration.
> - Harsh, hollow character of sound.
>
> Bronchial breath sounds are uncommon and may be unfamiliar to some candidates. Try to look up some audio clips or online videos if you have not heard many!

Suggest Aetiology

The differentials for consolidation (Table A6.5) include pus (pneumonia), blood (alveolar haemorrhage), cells (neoplasm, inflammatory causes), water, and others (e.g., alveolar proteinosis, pulmonary infarction). Acute pathologies such as pneumonia or haemorrhage are less likely to appear in PACES as signs may resolve quickly with treatment, and patients may not be stable enough for repeated examination. However, inpatients pulled from the wards may still have acute pathologies.

Table A6.5. Major causes of consolidation in PACES.

	Causes	Possible signs
Cells	Neoplasm/mass	Clubbing, cachexia, cervical lymphadenopathy Monophonic wheeze
Pus	Pneumonia, abscess, Tuberculosis, aspergilloma	Fever, productive cough Inpatient pulled from ward
Other	Pulmonary infarct	–

Look for Complications

Comment on the presence/absence of:
- Respiratory distress.
- Use of supplemental oxygen.

Sample Script

Consolidation

The positive findings are in a focal area of the right lower chest, where there is a dull percussion note, bronchial breathing, and monophonic wheeze. The trachea is central and chest expansion is symmetrical. There is no clubbing, cachexia, or respiratory distress. There is a peripherally inserted central catheter in situ in the left arm. My principle diagnosis is a focal lung consolidation. In terms of underlying aetiology, the peripherally inserted central catheter may suggest chemotherapy for a neoplastic lesion, or prolonged antibiotics for a lung abscess or other chronic infection.

Respiratory

Respiratory – Clinical Syndromes

6.7 | Chronic Obstructive Pulmonary Disease

Many exam centres consider a vanilla case of chronic obstructive pulmonary disease (COPD) 'too easy' for PACES. Be alert for atypical features or complications.

Recognise Pathology

COPD should be diagnosed based on a barrel chest and a prolonged expiration phase; wheeze may not always be present. Key signs are:
- Pursed-lip breathing.
- Bronchodilators at bedside.
- Barrel chest with reduced bilateral chest expansion.
- Nicotine stains on the fingers suggesting underlying smoking.
- Tracheal tug.
- Prolonged expiratory phase.
- ± Polyphonic expiratory ronchi (not always present).

Two red flags suggest a diagnosis other than COPD:
- A monophonic wheeze present only at one area. The wheeze of COPD is polyphonic and diffuse; a monophonic wheeze suggests a fixed bronchial obstruction (e.g., cancer).
- Clubbing, which is not present in COPD and may suggest malignant change.

Asthma is unlikely to appear in the respiratory station as physical signs are transient, and patients in exacerbation would not be subjected to repeated examination.

Suggest Aetiology

This is almost always smoking, except in the young patient in whom alpha-1 antitrypsin deficiency may be considered.

Look for Complications

Comment on whether the patient is currently in exacerbation (unlikely, or you will not be allowed to examine the patient), and spend some time to look for complications:
- Respiratory distress: tachypnoea, use of accessory muscles.
- CO_2 retention: asterixes, palmar erythema. Also make a note that the patient is alert and not drowsy (as they would be in the exam).

- Pulmonary hypertension: parasternal heave, palpable pulmonary component of the second heart sound, secondary tricuspid regurgitation, cor pulmonale.
- Cancer: cachexia, clubbing, cervical lymphadenopathy, intrinsic muscle wasting and ptosis (Horner's syndrome), face and arm plethora and oedema (superior vena caval obstruction).
- Secondary pneumothorax (unlikely in exam): focal hyperresonance, breathlessness.

Sample Script

This elderly gentleman has chronic obstructive pulmonary disease as evidenced by pursed lip breathing, a barrel chest appearance, bronchodilators at the bedside, and a prolonged expiratory phase. The trachea is central, percussion note resonant, and air entry equal in both lungs. I note extensive nicotine stains of the fingers suggesting chronic smoking. I note finger clubbing which is unusual in COPD, and suspicious for a neoplastic lesion. There is no evidence of a parasternal heave or loud pulmonary component of the second heart sound to suggest pulmonary hypertension. He is comfortable and not having a COPD exacerbation at the moment.

6.8 | Discussion Framework

This section provides a general framework to answer the examiner's questions, which needs to be modified based on the suspected diagnosis. As the number of clinical syndromes in the respiratory examination is limited, the discussion tends to be very similar — aim to score here!

How Would You Investigate?

"I will investigate to confirm my diagnosis, establish an aetiology, and look for complications."

I. Discuss any potential emergency

If the patient appears to be in respiratory distress, explain how you will approach acute respiratory failure.

II. Confirm the diagnosis

1. **More history looking for…**
   - Interstitial lung disease: occupational and recreational exposures, drug history, symptoms of connective tissue disease.
   - Bronchiectasis: history of past respiratory infections, history of asthma (for allergic bronchopulmonary aspergillosis), etc.
   - Pleural effusion: history suggestive of acute infection vs. chronic cough, haemoptysis, weight loss.
   - COPD: smoking history
2. **Chest X-ray looking for…**
   - Interstitial lung disease: reticular changes (and to observe their distribution).
   - Bronchiectasis (tram-tracking, ring opacities).
   - Confirm other diagnosis: pleural effusion, lobar collapse, nodule, etc.
3. **CT scan looking for…** (specify high-resolution CT if looking for interstitial lung disease/bronchiectasis, CT thorax for most other applications)[24].

---

[24] Understand the difference between HRCT and standard CT thorax. HRCT images 1 mm-thin cuts at wide intervals (up to 1 cm); this gives high resolution to assess lung parenchyma, but will miss small masses if they happen to be between the imaged slices. CT thorax employs volume averaging, which ensures that nodules are not missed but impairs image resolution (i.e., parenchymal architecture is less clearly visualised).

- Bronchiectasis: bronchial dilation with lack of tapering towards the peripheries, dilated airways, signet ring sign, mucus plugging, air-trapping, and mosaicism.
- Interstitial lung disease (ILD): identification of specific patterns of ILD (e.g., usual interstitial pneumonia, nonspecific interstitial pneumonia) based on distribution and imaging characteristics. This is of diagnostic significance.
- Nodules/lung masses (as a cause of consolidation/collapse, beneath an effusion).
- Generally not helpful in COPD or in lung resection cases.
4. **Spirometry looking for...** (generally for interstitial lung disease/COPD cases)
    - Interstitial lung disease: reduced FEV1 and FVC but with normal FEV1/FVC ratio, reduced lung capacity, and reduced diffusion capacity.
    - COPD: a reduced FEV1/FVC ratio (diagnosis), degree of FEV1 reduction (severity grading in COPD), ± bronchodilator reversibility.
5. **Blood tests**
    - Asthma/COPD: full blood count and differential looking for eosinophilia.
    - Interstitial lung disease: serology for connective tissue diseases.
    - Bronchiectasis: full blood count for eosinophilia (e.g., in allergic bronchial pulmonary aspergillosis), immunoglobulin levels, sweat chloride (for cystic fibrosis), aspergillus precipitins, and others as indicated.
    - Bilateral pleural effusion: serum albumin, creatinine, and NT-proBNP looking for cause of fluid overload.
6. **Pleural tap in an effusion, sending**
    - Biochemistry: paired serum and pleural fluid protein and LDH (to determine exudative vs. transudative as per light's criteria), glucose, pH.
    - Microbiology (stain, culture, acid-fast bacilli smear and culture).
    - Adenosine deaminase (for tuberculosis).
    - Cytology/cell block (for malignancy).
7. **Other procedures**
    - Bronchoscopic studies (e.g., transbronchial lung biopsy of accessible nodule) to investigate an endoluminal obstruction, bronchoalveolar lavage for microbiological diagnosis, or endobronchial ultrasound.
    - CT-guided lung biopsy for peripheral nodule.
    - Sweat chloride (for cystic fibrosis; consider in young patients with bronchiectasis).

III. Look for complications

- Echocardiography for pulmonary hypertension, cor pulmonale.
- Sputum cultures for superimposed infections (e.g., in bronchiectasis).
- Arterial blood gas to look for Type 2 respiratory failure.
- Completion of staging scans if a malignancy is likely.

How Would You Manage?

"My patient will benefit from a multidisciplinary team approach to management involving the respiratory physician, nurse educator, and physiotherapist... with the goal of treating underlying disease, managing complications, and maximising function."

1. **Specific treatment**
   - COPD: long-acting bronchodilators (long-acting beta-agonists and long-acting muscarinic antagonist) ± inhaled corticosteroids.
   - Interstitial lung disease:
     - Secondary causes: stop exposures, treat underlying disease.
     - Idiopathic pulmonary fibrosis: discuss antifibrotics (nintedanib or pirfenidone).
   - Bronchiectasis: airway clearance (physiotherapy, mechanical or device clearance techniques), macrolides, bronchodilators for symptoms, treat gastroesophageal reflux.
   - Effusion: treatment of tuberculosis/malignancy.
   - Consideration of lung transplant.

2. **Supportive management**
   - Long term oxygen therapy if PaO_2 < 55 mmHg or SpO_2 < 88% (or 60 mmHg and 89% if there is cor pulmonale, right heart failure).
   - Treatment of infections.
   - Smoking cessation.
   - Vaccination – influenza, pneumococcal.
   - Pulmonary rehabilitation.
   - Patient education.
   - Palliative care.
   - Treat comorbids.

Sample Script

Malignant pleural effusion

I will like to take more history and examine the patient to identify if this is a primary lung malignancy or if these are lung metastases. I will like to begin investigation with a simple chest X-ray to confirm the effusion, followed by a CT thorax and a pleural tap. From the pleural fluid I will send paired serum, pleural fluid protein, and LDH to confirm an exudate, cell block for histological diagnosis, as well as gram stain and culture, mycobacterial stain and culture, and adenosine deaminase to look for differentials. If the cell block is inadequate for diagnosis, then biopsy will be required; this can be transthoracic or bronchoscopic depending on the location and accessibility of the tumour. I will also need to complete staging with a MRI brain and PET scan.

Management wise, the patient will benefit from a multidisciplinary team approach involving the respiratory physician, medical oncologist, radiation oncologist, and pathologist. The patient should be discussed at the multidisciplinary tumour board to consider options of chemotherapy, targeted therapy (if suitable mutations), and radiation therapy alongside good patient education, palliative care, and psychosocial support.

Remember that pleural effusion = stage 4 lung cancer, so do not offer surgery.

Section B: Consultations

Consultations

1 | Introduction and Walk-Through

The consultations station mimics an outpatient consult. You will need to assess the patient's complaint via history and examination, formulate a working differential, propose an investigation and management plan, and communicate this to the patient. Addressing patient concerns is mandatory; this may draw on communication skills as well as specific disease knowledge.

The consultations station is perhaps the most interesting and varied component of the PACES examination. You may encounter both stable clinic outpatients, as well as patients with an acute issue that would require urgent inpatient stabilisation. While any topic one would expect a General Medicine registrar to manage is fair game, rheumatology, endocrine, dermatology, and ophthalmology/neurology conditions are overrepresented because they are inadequately covered in the physical examination stations and lend themselves particularly well to the clinical consult format.

Preparing for this station will hone your diagnostic ability, particularly to always consider the breadth of differentials, uncover deeper issues, and apply knowledge about individual diseases to the specific patient. It will also give you confidence to manage a patient safely and holistically, while always maintaining good rapport and addressing the patient's questions.

Two Types of Consultation Cases

There are two general flavours in the consultations station — diagnostic cases and complications of disease cases.

Diagnostic cases

Example: A middle-aged man presents with muscle aches. Further history reveals loss of weight and difficulty getting up from a chair. You will need to recognise the syndrome of a systemic myositis, search for cutaneous signs of dermatomyositis, and elicit symptoms of underlying malignancy.

These stations begin with a (or several) presenting complaint(s) and require you to come to a unifying diagnosis and differential diagnosis, identify underlying aetiologies or risk factors, and look for complications. Sound clinical reasoning and a robust approach to differential diagnosis is key. It is important to have a well-oiled algorithm you are familiar with and use on a day-to-day basis, yet retain an intellectual flexibility to respond to unexpected curveballs.

Some stations may be rather straightforward, while others (depending on the whims of the question setters) may come with a 'catch'. The following three tips will put you in good stead:

(1) **Look for underlying secondary causes**. The trick is to keep asking 'why' as patients may not reveal underlying aetiologies unless asked specific questions. Examples:
   - Lady with rectal bleeding while on warfarin → why is she over-warfarinised? → drug-drug interaction; she was given ciprofloxacin for cystitis.
   - Lady with polyuria → why polyuric? → diabetes insipidus → what is the aetiology? → lithium toxicity.
   - Lady with biliary colic→ why biliary colic? (also, why is there a 'surgical' condition in a 'medical' exam?) → chronic haemolytic anaemia.
   - Gentleman with flank-to-groin colic → any cause for ureteric colic → hypercalcaemia → why hypercalcaemic? → causes of hypercalcaemia.

(2) **Search for a unifying diagnosis**. Always look for associated symptoms. Where patients have multiple active and unexplained symptoms, search for a unifying diagnosis — 'Occam's razor' applies often. Examples:
   - Pituitary tumour + prior 'neck surgery' + family history of 'pancreatic tumour' = multiple endocrine neoplasia (type 1), not a simple pituitary tumour.
   - Rectal bleeding + newly diagnosed diabetes = acromegaly with colonic polyps. The presence of sweaty palms may not be revealed unless you ask for it specifically.
   - Postural giddiness + lethargy + heat intolerance + loss of sexual drive = panhypopituitarism. Next step is to search for the cause of panhypopituitarism, especially examining the visual fields for bitemporal hemianopia.

(3) **Recognise pathognomonic clinical presentations**. You may not encounter them often in routine clinical work, but these have to be 'learnt' from the books. Examples:
   - Itch, without rash, that gets worse after a hot bath = aquagenic pruritus = polycythaemia rubra vera.
   - A young Asian lady with giddiness precipitated by upper limb movement = subclavian steal syndrome = Takayasu arteritis.

Complication of disease cases

Example: A patient with ankylosing spondylitis complains of shortness of breath. In addition to the usual causes of shortness of breath, you must consider specific complications of ankylosing spondylitis — pulmonary fibrosis, aortic regurgitation, anaemia from NSAID-induced gastrointestinal bleeding, and infections predisposed by immunosuppression.

Introduction and Walk-Through

In these cases, a patient with a known underlying condition presents with a new complaint. You will have to consider syndromes related to the existing condition, complications of the condition, and complications of treatment. On the other hand, the patient's current complaint may equally be unrelated to his prior diagnosis, so you must still consider general causes of the presenting symptom. Remember to exclude an emergency — the classic example will be the scleroderma patient who is found to have elevated creatinine. In PACES this will almost always be scleroderma renal crisis, but you must still explore other causes of kidney injury.

You may find out about the underlying condition in several ways:

(1) You may be informed in the question stem. Pay close attention if any past medical history is given, as this is likely significant.

(2) The patient may inform you of it when asked about his/her past medical history.

(3) You will not be directly informed – the question setters may expect you to recognise the underlying medical condition based on obvious physical signs, and indeed instruct the patient to deny having had any past medical history. This is tricky, but you must maintain a high index of suspicion for 'PACES favourites' which the following chapters will acquaint you with.

Walk-Through and Tips

This segment provides a walk-through of the consultations station, and your focus at each juncture of the station. Time discipline is critical here and it is helpful to have a stop-watch on hand (clip to your belt or dress so as to comply with hand hygiene policies).

Note that the consultations stations are calibrated in a similar manner to the physical exam stations (see page 10).

Preparation time

You will be provided a question stem and given time outside the room to prepare. You must read all information carefully. Some stems are unusually detailed and may even allow you to come to a unifying diagnosis. Other stems provide very little information — for example, "this patient complains of shortness of breath."

Whichever the case, you should use the information provided to brainstorm for differential diagnoses, jot down your approach/algorithm to the presenting symptom, and consider possible spot diagnoses that you need to be alert to. If laboratory data is provided, you should also use the time to interpret the data.

Pitfall: Misleading stems

> Some stems are intentionally misleading! Be wary when the stem seems to give away too much. For example, for the stem:

(Cont'd)

> *"Dear colleague, thank you for seeing this patient. He has a 3-month history of back pain and I am concerned about the possibility of ankylosing spondylitis."*
>
> Chances are that the diagnosis is not ankylosing spondylitis. However, you should explore why the GP had concerns that it might be ankylosing spondylitis.

Inspection

Having greeted the patient and examiner as you enter the room, your first task is not history taking but inspection. Unlike the physical examination station, you may not stand at the foot of the bed for ten seconds, but must make this quite seamless while introducing yourself.

Inspection is a critical step. Certain conditions tend to have vague histories that can mislead you, but the station becomes very easy once you can recognise the physical signs. For example, acromegaly is quite a far-fetched differential of headache, but if you can spot the diagnosis, you can immediately ask for a change in ring or shoe size and be on the home run! In a presenting complaint of rash or joint pain, ask the patient to show you the rash or swollen joint immediately — this will focus your history-taking. Some patients wear eye shades or caps; ask for these to be removed.

Tip: Common spot diagnoses in the consultation station

General habitus
- Acromegaly
- Cushing's syndrome
- Marfan's syndrome

Face and neck
- Thyroid: goitre, Graves' ophthalmopathy, thyroidectomy scar
- Rashes: cutaneous lupus, dermatomyositis, psoriasis
- Neurology: myotonic dystrophy, ptosis
- Hereditary haemorrhagic telangiectasia

Hands
- Rheumatologic hands: systemic sclerosis, rheumatoid arthritis, psoriasis, myositis
- Tremor: parkinsonism

Feet
- Skin conditions
- Neurology: foot drop, ankle-foot orthoses, Charcot's feet

History

Key components of history-taking are:

1. **Opening** – Begin with open-ended questions, both as a matter of good communication and because the patient may well feed you with information.

2. **History of presenting complaint** – This must demonstrate a systematic approach. Even if you recognise a 'spot diagnosis', you must show consideration of differentials. Be careful to rule out 'red flags' and emergencies.

3. **Past medical history** – It is often advantageous to ask for this early as it may completely change the differentials — some candidates choose to do this before (2); a smooth way to do so could be: "If I may get to know you better, may I ask if you have any previous medical conditions?"

4. **Medication history** – Pay attention to recent changes in medications and doses, as well as the potential for drug interactions. Ask about traditional and complementary medicine separately, as well as use of contraceptive pills.

5. **Drug allergy** – It is a sin to omit this in a case where you might need to prescribe antibiotics.

6. **Family history**

7. **Social, occupational, and travel history** – Be targeted here — think about what is important. For example, critical aspects include smoking history in a case of Grave's disease, travel history in an infection, and sexual history in a case of new-onset jaundice.

8. **Possibility of pregnancy/menstrual history (in females)** – You must exclude pregnancy especially if you may prescribe potentially teratogenic drugs, or if the suspected disease would have implications for pregnancy safety (e.g., pregnancy unadvisable in pulmonary hypertension).

Physical examination

History-taking and physical examination may be done in no particular order. It can be helpful to examine the patient before completing the history, particularly in cases of weakness, joint pain, and rashes. If you choose to complete the history first, move on to physical examination in a timely fashion.

Physical examination in the consultation station is targeted. You must identify, on history-taking, what are the key systems or areas you want to examine. Important aspects of physical examination include:

- Demonstrate physical signs of the underlying condition. For example, in a patient with breathlessness due to interstitial lung disease with underlying rheumatoid arthritis, do examine the hands. Marks are likely awarded for demonstrating the positive signs of rheumatoid arthritis, *even if the diagnosis of rheumatoid arthritis is given to you.*

- Look for signs of possible differential diagnoses.

- Look for complications in other systems, such as examining the eyes in a patient with ankylosing spondylitis.

- Look for suggestions of underlying aetiology, such as examining visual fields in a patient with Cushing's syndrome.

- Assess overall function.

Certain conditions (e.g., thyroid, rheumatologic hands) have set-piece examinations that you should rehearse for. Others will require you to make things up as you go — always know what sign you are looking for, as it is easy to miss signs when one examines without prior suspicion.

It must be emphasised that physical sign marks are crucial — many candidates fail PACES because of failing this skill. It is often far easier to bag marks for physical signs in the consult stations than in the physical examination stations, because many of the signs are overt on inspection and there are fewer signs demanded. These signs are calibrated in the same fashion as the physical exam stations.

Pitfall: Slipshod examinations

> You cannot perform 'full' examinations as in the physical examination station, but being targeted is not the same as being slipshod. Examiners' pet peeves include:
> - Auscultating heart and lungs through the clothes.
> - Examining the abdomen with the patient sitting in a chair (but it is acceptable to examine the heart, lungs, and upper limbs with the patient sitting).
> - Palpating a goitre from the front.
> - One-handed examination of rheumatoid hands (bimanual palpation is more orthodox and more sensitive).
> - Testing visual fields without first ensuring that the patient can see your red hat pin (or checking visual acuity in some form).

Addressing patient concerns

The last two minutes of the station should be dedicated to addressing patient concerns. Marks are specifically awarded for this task, and patients are briefed to raise one or two specific concerns to address. It is helpful to signpost that you are transiting into this segment. For example: *"Thank you for sharing all of this with me. Before I explain my thoughts, could I ask if you have any questions or concerns that you will like to raise?"* There are three key tasks to this section:

1. Address the patient's concerns.
2. Ensure safety.
3. Explain the management plan, including the disposition of the present consult (i.e., admit or follow up).

(1) **Address the patient's concerns**. It is important to answer the question *directly*. A common mistake is to explain your agenda instead! You may need to draw on your communication skills here. Examples:
  - Question: "What's wrong with me?" – explain the patient's diagnosis in lay terms.
  - Question: "Is this cancer?" / "Is this a stroke?"

- Reply: "You must be really worried given your dad's experience. I think that this is less likely a stroke, but instead [alternate diagnosis]. However, I want to make sure it is not a stroke by performing [test]."
- Reply: "You are right that cancer is a cause of [symptom], although it may also be [differentials]. We need to do [diagnostic tests] which will tell us what this is. This must be really worrying for you, but I want to tell you that if you do indeed have cancer, we are here for you and will start you on treatment as soon as possible".
- Question: "Is this condition serious?"
  - Reply: "I do think that a blood pressure of 200/120 is serious because [reason]. I will admit you for immediate treatment. With treatment, I think we have a good chance of getting on top of things and preventing [nasty consequences] from happening."
  - Reply: "You are right to worry that this could be serious because [reason]. The good news is that you have come to us early. We can start treatment immediately and with treatment we have a good chance to prevent these serious problems from happening."
- Question: "Can I be treated?" / "Am I going to become paralysed?"
  - Reply: "Yes, this is a treatable condition. You must have seen pictures of people with severe deformities from rheumatoid arthritis. Such deformities are less common nowadays because we have much better treatment. Many of our patients do well."
  - Reply: "It is scary to lose your independence and this must worry you a lot. It is true that some patients with multiple sclerosis become unable to walk, but there are also many patients who do well. I cannot promise that you will do well, but we will do everything we can to give you the best outcome."
- Question: "Can I get pregnant?" – This is a prompt to consider contraindications to pregnancy that may arise from the patient's diagnosis and its complications, as well as from medications (both existing and those that you will start).
  - Reply: "I hear your desire to have a child. Unfortunately, the drug you are on causes birth defects and is not safe in pregnancy. Additionally, as your condition is not stable now, it poses a risk to your baby, and pregnancy may pose a risk to your life. May I suggest that for now we first focus on getting your condition under control. When your condition is stable, I will discuss with your rheumatologist and obstetrician. We may be able to switch you to an alternative immunosuppressant that is safer in pregnancy."

(2) **Ensure safety**. You may need to address a safety issue, although this will be in much less detail than a communications scenario. For example:
- Driving – if you are suspecting a diagnosis that is incompatible with driving, advise the patient not to drive until fully worked up.

- Infectious disease – if you suspect HIV, inform the patient of the risk of transmission, and advise to abstain from sexual intercourse until test results are back.
- Advise the patient of the possibility of a serious medical condition and the need for inpatient admission or urgent investigation.

(3) **Explain management plan including disposition.** You will need to explain the possible differentials, disposition (admit or follow up), and management plan (further tests, treatment). Do so in layman terms. During questioning, the examiner may ask you in more detail.

Discussion With the Examiner

You must cover the following:

1. Positive physical findings. This cannot be underemphasised — present the physical signs upfront and score.
2. Diagnosis and differential diagnosis. Think broadly and have a range of differentials. If you feel that some differentials are less likely, explain why you think so. If the examiner prompts you with 'what else', chances are that you have either given too few differentials or have not offered the correct diagnosis yet.
3. How you will investigate and manage the patient. Always contextualise this to the specific patient you have seen. Explain (briefly) what you are looking for in each test. Show a thought process — for example, "I will do MRI. If MRI shows X, the next step is Y. If MRI shows A, the next step is B." Go for the money — you get little credit for giving a medical student-style presentation of "I will like to do full blood count, renal panel, inflammatory markers..." Rather, in an endocrine condition, say: "I will like to confirm my diagnosis by... If this is confirmed, I will like to localise the lesion by... I will like to assess other hormonal axes and look for complication by..."

Your answers should be succinct. You are marked on specific points that the examiners have agreed on in advance, so your aim is to hit these points AND show overall competency, rather than provide a detailed thesis on biologics used in the management of psoriasis (and lose marks because other points are not mentioned). Respond to the examiner and answer the questions (do not continue what you want to say!). Remember that if the examiner interrupts you, it is to help you hit the required marking points.

The worked cases provide sample discussions with the examiners.

Consultations

2 | Same Presentation, Different Conditions

These seven cases demonstrate the breadth of conditions that a single presenting complaint, breathlessness, can lead to. They illustrate the following key lessons:

1. The PACES consultation station requires lateral thinking. One cannot be too fixated on 'typical' or 'common' causes of each symptom, but must keep an inquisitive and open mind.
2. Begin each station not with specific questions about the presenting complaint, but by asking open-ended questions and having the patient share his/her story.
3. It is particularly helpful to elicit a 'symptom complex' (e.g., breathlessness with fever, breathlessness with chest pain, breathlessness with cough) as this quickly narrows down the range of differentials.
4. Elicit the patient's past medical history early as the present complaint is often related to the patient's existing conditions, such as a complication of the condition or a complication of treatment.

The cases in this section provide worked practice and are best attempted as mock stations, with a colleague or tutor simulating the patient's role. Each case comes with information for the candidate and a detailed patient's brief, and is followed by a discussion of the relevant approach and clinical reasoning, a suggested answer to the patient's concerns, and a possible presentation to the examiners. The cases are designed to be slightly more difficult than average so that you will be prepared for more challenging cases, which some exam centres are fond of.

Practice with a colleague or tutor. Use the pull-out 'candidate information' booklet, which gives the candidate's information for all practice scenarios, to blind yourself to the patient's brief and discussion.

Consultation Case 01

Mdm Ruby Toh (Dyspnoea)

Use this case as practice! The pull-out booklet contains the candidate's information.

Information for the Candidate

Patient Details: Mdm Ruby Toh, 37 years old

Your Role: Rheumatology Clinic SHO

Referral Letter:
> Dear Colleague,
>
> Thank you for seeing Mdm Toh who has been on your follow up. She has brought forward her appointment because she is short of breath.
>
> Sincerely,
>
> Dr Germaine Loo, GP

Vital Signs: BP 145/87 mmHg, HR 70/min, RR 16/min, SpO2 95% RA, T 37.0°C

Patient's Brief

Synopsis: *A patient with rheumatoid arthritis presents with subacute-onset breathlessness, cough, and reduced effort tolerance. The differentials are broad and include infections, low blood counts, lung fibrosis, and others.*

Open the consult with: I've been feeling more breathless over the past 3 weeks. *In addition to this opening line, volunteer the history of rheumatoid arthritis.*

History of current problem:
- This breathlessness started 3 weeks ago, and has gradually gotten worse since then.
- You do not feel overtly breathless at rest; however, you get very breathless on even minor exertion. You are no longer able to walk to the bus stop (some 400 m away).
- You have had a dry, hacking cough for the past 6 months. This is mild and does not bother you too much. You do not cough out any sputum or blood. The cough is not worse lying down, and you do not have any stuffy or blocked nose.
- You do not have any fever, night sweats, or weight loss.
- You do not have any lumps in your neck or armpit.
- Your breathlessness is not worse lying down. You do not have any chest pain or palpitations.
- You do not have any blood or bubbles in your urine, and no leg pain or swelling.

- You have been feeling lethargic and light-headed, especially on exertion. You do not have any blood in your stool, black and sticky stools, heavy menses, abnormal bleeding, or easy bruising.
- You have been going about your usual daily activity and have not been bedbound or otherwise immobile.

Past medical and surgical history:
- Rheumatoid arthritis. This was diagnosed 2 years ago when you presented with pain in the small joints of your hand. Your joint pains have been controlled with medication. You do not have any rashes, mouth ulcers, dry mouth or eyes, red or painful eyes, hand numbness or weakness, or neck pain. You have not been told that rheumatoid arthritis has affected your lungs or any other organs.
- You do not have any history of tuberculosis, lung nodules, or other lung problems.

Medication list:
- Folic acid 1 mg daily
- Methotrexate 20 mg weekly
- Naproxen 550 mg BD PRN, you take this approximately every alternate day
- Paracetamol 1 g QDS PRN
- Supplements and herbal remedies: a daily multivitamin
- Drug allergy: nil

Family history:
- No family history of autoimmune disease, joint problems, lung problems, lung cancers, or tuberculosis.

Relevant personal, social, occupational, and travel history:
- You are a primary school teacher.
- You are married with no children. After having had 5 miscarriages, you no longer hope for a child. You have not had unprotected sexual intercourse since starting methotrexate 2 years ago, as you were told that methotrexate is toxic to any foetus.
- You do not smoke or drink.
- No relevant travel history. You have not been on a long flight in the past year.
- No relevant occupational or recreational exposures to toxic chemicals, construction, farming/animals, or baking.

Relevant physical examination findings:
- Look: ulnar deviation, subluxation at metacarpophalangeal joints (worse on left), swan neck deformity of left ring and little finger (Photos 1 and 2).
- Feel: mildly swollen proximal interphalangeal and metacarpophangeal joints, some bogginess on palpation.
- Move: full range of motion of hands.

- Able to hold a pen and write with some difficulty, able to unbutton shirt.
- Bilaterally restricted chest expansion. Fine end-inspiratory crepitations at both lung bases.
- Parasternal heave and loud pulmonary component of second heart sound.
- No pedal oedema, jugular venous pressure not elevated.
- No cervical lymph nodes.
- Conjunctival pallor.
- Digital rectal examination – examiner instructs not to proceed.

Photo to be shown to candidate upon request (use colour plates for full-colour photos).

Photo 1   **Photo 2**

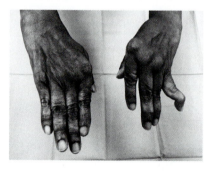 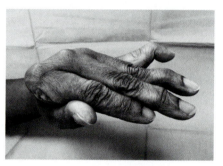

Clinical photo generously provided by Dr Stanley Angkodjojo, Sengkang General Hospital

You have some specific questions for the doctor at this consultation:
- What is happening to me doctor? Is this serious?

Approach and Clinical Reasoning

Mdm Toh presents with dyspnoea on a background of rheumatoid arthritis. It will be advantageous to briefly ask for the past medical history before delving into the history of presenting complaint — this will allow you to specifically consider the causes of dyspnoea in rheumatoid arthritis. A smooth way to do so might be: *"Mdm Toh, before I ask you more about your breathlessness, I will like to get to know you better. Do you have any past medical problems?"* (See also page 205.)

Table B2.1 lists the important causes of breathlessness to consider in systemic rheumatologic illnesses (this table will be applicable to most rheumatologic conditions, not just rheumatoid arthritis).

Table B2.1. Common causes of breathlessness in systemic rheumatologic illness.

Cause	Underlying aetiologies	Important features
Infection	Pneumonia Tuberculosis Atypical (e.g., pneumocystis pneumonia)	Fever, cough Weight loss, haemoptysis Exercise desaturation
Interstitial lung disease (ILD)	Secondary to underlying disease Secondary to drugs (e.g., methotrexate)	Dry cough, fine inspiratory crepitations
Pulmonary hypertension	Group 1: Independent of ILD Group 3: Due to ILD Group 4: Chronic thromboembolic pulmonary hypertension	Parasternal heave, loud P2 on examination Any ILD, recurrent pulmonary embolism
Fluid overload	Due to heart failure Due to glomerulonephritis Acute kidney injury from NSAIDs Scleroderma renal crisis	Orthopnoea, pedal oedema Haematuria, proteinuria
Anaemia	Cytopenia from underlying disease Drug-induced myelosuppression Gastrointestinal bleed from NSAID use	Other symptoms of anaemia, cytopenias Pallor
Pulmonary embolism	May be related to a hypercoagulable state (e.g., in antiphospholipid syndrome)	Hypercoagulable state, immobility, leg swelling
Pulmonary haemorrhage	Diffuse alveolar haemorrhage (e.g., ANCA vasculitis)	Haemoptysis
Causes of breathlessness in general (e.g., myocardial infarct, anaphylaxis).		
Rheumatoid arthritis is associated with additional pulmonary manifestations (e.g., rheumatoid pleural effusions, bronchiectasis).		

ILD: interstitial lung disease

Important considerations for Mdm Toh include:

- Infection, particularly pneumocystis pneumonia given the immunocompromised state, history suggestive of exercise desaturation, and subacute presentation.
- Anaemia – including macrocytic anaemia due to methotrexate, normocytic anaemia due to chronic disease, microcytic anaemia due to iron deficiency. However, this will not explain the cough.
- Pulmonary embolism – the history of recurrent miscarriage might suggest antiphospholipid syndrome.

- She may well have interstitial lung disease (due to rheumatoid arthritis itself or as a consequence of methotrexate) or pulmonary hypertension; however, breathlessness due to either of these is likely to be more insidious in onset. Mdm Toh's rapid progression of breathlessness over 3 weeks suggests another reason for decompensation.

Certain encounters are designed to have a clear-cut 'most likely' diagnosis, while others do not. This scenario falls into the latter category, and her breathlessness may well be multifactorial. Your priority is to rule out emergencies, recognise that the patient may be unwell, and make plans to investigate and manage further.

Physical examination serves two purposes: (1) to demonstrate the physical signs of rheumatoid arthritis — you should have a sleek routine for examining rheumatoid hands, and will be duly awarded marks for this, and (2) to look for causes of breathlessness — including examining the lungs for fine crepitations, checking for pulmonary hypertension, and looking at the conjunctivae for pallor and the calves for swelling (unilateral suggesting venous thromboembolism, bilateral suggesting fluid overload).

Practice makes perfect: The rheumatological hand examination

> Practice the steps of hand examination, using the look-feel-move schema. This should look sleek and practiced. Pay specific attention to the palpation of the metacarpalphalangeal and interphalangeal joints, which tends to be poorly performed.

Question and Answer

Suggested answer to the patient's concerns:

Mdm Toh, the exact reason why you are feeling more breathless is not clear at the moment, so we need to do more tests to find out. Possibilities include an infection, lung or heart disease from rheumatoid arthritis, low blood count, blood clots, and others. These are indeed potentially serious and I am thankful that you have come to us early for evaluation. I would like to admit you to do some blood tests, X-rays, and a scan of your lungs and heart. When we are clearer about why you are feeling so breathless, we will be able to treat you.

Suggested presentation to the examiner:

Mdm Toh presents with a subacute history of dyspnoea, dry cough, and reduced effort tolerance on a background of rheumatoid arthritis. Examination is remarkable for peripheral signs of rheumatoid arthritis including symmetrical small joint polyarthropathy affecting the metacarpophalangeal joints and proximal interphalangeal joints, ulnar deviation of fingers, and swan neck deformities. Disease is active as indicated by boggy and tender joints. Functionally, she is able to write and button her shirt. Extra-articular signs include fine end-inspiratory lung crepitations, loud pulmonary component of the second heart sound and a parasternal heave suggesting pulmonary hypertension, and conjunctival pallor.

Causes of breathlessness in Mdm Toh may include infection, particularly pneumocystis pneumonia, anaemia due to disease, methotrexate or gastrointestinal bleeding from NSAIDs, as well as interstitial lung disease and pulmonary hypertension. I will also like to evaluate for possibility of pulmonary embolism. Breathlessness may be multifactorial and thus due to a combination of all these.

Don't forget: Looking for complications of disease

> In a patient with an underlying systemic disease, you must specifically look for complications of that disease, instead of merely the causes of breathlessness in general.

I will admit Mdm Toh to the general ward after ensuring that her airway, breathing, and circulation are stable. Initial investigations include:

- Bloods: full blood count for anaemia, iron studies, B12 and folate levels, inflammatory markers, renal biochemistry, and a blood gas.
- Imaging: beginning with a chest X-ray, subsequently a high resolution CT looking for interstitial lung disease, and considering a CT pulmonary angiogram for pulmonary embolism.
- Echocardiogram looking at pulmonary pressures.
- Spirometry.
- Sputum for culture, acid fast bacilli, and pneumocystis microscopy/PCR.

She should be managed by a multidisciplinary team including the rheumatologist, pulmonary physician, and allied healthcare professionals. This will depend on the cause of breathlessness found and may include treatment of an infection, correction of anaemia, and immunosuppression to mitigate progression of interstitial lung disease.

Consultation Case 02

Mrs Puff (Dyspnoea)

Use this case as practice! The pull-out booklet contains the candidate's information.

Information for the Candidate

Patient Details: Mrs Puff, 30 years old

Your Role: Respiratory Medicine Clinic SHO

Referral Letter:
> Dear Colleague,
>
> Thank you for seeing Mrs Puff for her asthma. I have stepped up her treatment to a Budesonide/Formoterol (Symbicort®) inhaler, but she still complains of persistent symptoms.
>
> Thank you.
>
> Dr Wilbert Ho, GP

Vital Signs: BP 155/95 mmHg, HR 70/min, RR 10/min, SpO2 99% RA, T 37.0°C

Patient's Brief

Synopsis: *A patient with poorly controlled asthma and new-onset nephritis and neuritis. The unifying diagnosis is eosinophilic granulomatosis with polyangiitis.*

Open the consult with: I have had asthma since I was a child, but it had always been mild. I don't understand why my asthma has become so bad in the last 6 months. *Do not volunteer any other information unless asked.*

History of current problem:

- For the past few months, you have been having at least 2–3 exacerbations of breathlessness and wheeze per week. You feel somewhat breathless even now.
- During these episodes of breathlessness and wheeze, you also experience persistent non-productive cough (especially at night) and difficulty completing your usual 20 min jogs in the evenings.
- You do not find any specific triggers for these symptoms. They do not come together with a flu and are not better on weekends/holidays.
- Your symptoms improve whenever you are given a course of oral steroids, but the moment the steroids are stopped, the breathlessness and wheeze recur.

- You had to visit the emergency department multiple times when the usual inhaler failed to relieve your symptoms. On two occasions, you required admission but not high dependency care or intubation.
- You use your inhaler dutifully every morning and whenever you have symptoms. You know how to use the inhaler and the GP has said that your technique is acceptable.
- You have noticed small amounts of blood in your urine for the past 2 months. You have no discomfort on passing urine, urge or frequency, abdominal/flank pain, urethral discharge, decrease in urine output, or abdominal or leg swelling.
- In the past 3 weeks, you have been experiencing vague patchy numbness over your left leg. You were wondering if this is due to a pulled muscle, but you have not had much physical activity.
- You wake up most mornings with a blocked and stuffy nose.
- Your appetite has been poor and you have lost 5 kg in the past 3 months.
- You have no rash, leg swelling, chest pain, fever, coughing of blood, headache, giddiness, rash, or neck swelling.

Past medical and surgical history:
- You have had asthma since childhood. You do not recall if you had any formal 'breath' tests. You keep a salbutamol inhaler but use it at most twice or thrice in a year.
- In particular, you have no prior history of high blood pressure, kidney problems, urinary stones, bladder or prostate problems.

Medication list:
- Budesonide 160 ug/Formoterol 4.5 ug (Symbicort) inhaler, twice daily and as needed for symptoms.
- You have had various courses of oral prednisolone.
- Supplements and herbal remedies: nil
- Drug allergy: nil

Family history:
- Nil

Relevant personal, social, occupational, and travel history:
- You work as a computing systems analyst. This is a sedentary, desk-bound job.
- You have no exposure to farm material, industrial chemicals, or other allergens. You have no pets.
- You are a lifelong non-smoker. You do not have any exposure to second-hand smoke.
- You have been married for a year. You have no children.
- No relevant travel history.

Relevant physical examination findings:

This station may be run with a real patient (who would have been treated, and instead instructed to recreate an acute presentation) or a surrogate.

- General condition well, not in respiratory distress.
- No clubbing, cyanosis, or pallor.
- Lungs clear.
- No rashes or palpable purpura.
- Non-specific numbness to pinprick sensation over left lower limb, no weakness.
- No pedal oedema, jugular venous pressure not elevated.
- Device technique, if checked, is good.

You have some specific questions for the doctor at this consultation:
- I'm trying to get pregnant. Will my asthma affect pregnancy?
- Can I go home?

Approach and Clinical Reasoning

Mrs Puff presents with persistent asthma symptoms in spite of treatment with an inhaled corticosteroid and long-acting bronchodilator. The key questions are therefore (1) is this really asthma, and (2) if this is asthma, why is it poorly controlled? (Table B2.2).

Table B2.2. Questions to ask in 'poorly controlled asthma' (ABCDE).

Question	Consideration
Asthma? – Is this really asthma?	Look for asthma mimics: • Chronic obstructive pulmonary disease (COPD): smoker, breathlessness between flares, chronic sputum production • Eosinophilic granulomatosis with polyangiitis (or Churg-Strauss): multi-system involvement with eosinophilia, haemoptysis, sinusitis/nasal polyps, neuropathy, vasculitic rash, nephritis • Bronchiectasis: prominent purulent sputum, coarse inspiratory crepitations • Central airway obstruction: inspiratory stridor rather than expiratory wheeze, large goitre, history of lymphoma or mediastinal tumour • Fluid overload with 'cardiac wheeze' The following mimic asthma, but are hard to identify on history and examination alone: • Allergic bronchopulmonary aspergillosis (ABPA): recurrent asthma exacerbations, eosinophilia, ± X-ray features (central bronchiectasis, mucus plugging, upper or middle lobe consolidation). Diagnosis requires demonstration of elevated IgE and aspergillus sensitisation.

(Cont'd)

Question	Consideration
	• Paradoxical vocal fold motion: diagnosis is on laryngoscopy
	If the complaint is 'breathlessness' alone without wheeze, then more general causes of breathlessness must be considered.
Bronchial triggers	Untreated allergic rhinitis
	Smoking
	Drugs (e.g., beta blockers, NSAIDs)
Compliance	Check compliance with prescribed inhaled corticosteroids (ICS). High bronchodilator: ICS prescription ratio is associated with asthma mortality.
Device technique	Assess inhaler technique
Environment	Allergen exposure (particularly occupation, hobbies, and pets)
	Look out for occupational asthma (better on weekends or holidays)

Pitfall: Pay attention to the stem

> Careful candidates will note two clues given in the stem:
> - The given blood pressure is 155/95 mmHg. This is unexpected in a young 30-year-old lady — an early clue that this may be something more than asthma.
> - Mrs Puff "complains of persistent symptoms" — this is a bait for you to explore what exactly these symptoms are.

Mrs Puff has good compliance and technique, and no significant asthma triggers. However, in addition to asthma, she has hypertension and haematuria suggestive of nephritis, leg numbness suggestive of mononeuritis, and prominent otolaryngological involvement. The unifying diagnosis is eosinophilic granulomatosis with polyangiitis (Churg-Strauss disease). Realise that these additional symptoms must be elicited specifically as she will not volunteer the information.

The key tasks on physical examination are to:
- Ensure that she is stable and not in respiratory distress.
- Auscultate the lungs for crepitations (bronchiectasis, fluid overload), consolidation, or wheeze.
- Examine for fluid overload (nephritic syndrome) and objective evidence of a neuritis.

Question and Answer

Suggested answer to the patient's concerns:

Mrs Puff, I hear how much you will like to have a baby. Unfortunately, this may not be the best time to get pregnant. I worry that your condition is not just asthma but something more. I am suspecting a disease called Churg-Strauss syndrome, which is an autoimmune disease meaning that your immune cells are attacking these various organs. Your lungs, nerves, and kidneys have been affected. It is probably unsafe to get pregnant until the disease is under control. Additionally, some of the medicines that we use for this condition may not be safe for babies.

I will like to admit you. I will check your X-ray and lung function, do some blood tests, and likely carry out a biopsy. I will involve the rheumatologist, lung doctor, and kidney doctor. If this confirms what we think, we will start medications to control your immune system. We will walk with you and you should get better. Subsequently when you are more stable, we are more than happy to discuss pregnancy and help you get pregnant safely.

Suggested presentation to the examiner:

Mrs Puff presents with poorly controlled asthma, nephritis, and neuritis. The unifying diagnosis is eosinophilic granulomatosis with polyangiitis (Churg-Strauss syndrome), although poorly controlled asthma remains a differential. On examination, she is stable and not in respiratory distress. Her lungs were clear. There is no pedal oedema.

I would like to admit her as she has active disease and appears moderately unwell. I will investigate to confirm my diagnosis, assess for multi-organ involvement, and guide treatment. These include:

- Chest X-ray looking for patchy opacities
- Bloods: full blood count for eosinophilia, renal and liver biochemistries, autoantibodies particularly anti-neutrophil cytoplasmic antibody (MPO/p-ANCA)
- Urine microscopy and protein
- Spirometry looking for airway obstruction with bronchodilator response
- Nerve conduction study of the lower limb
- She may require a biopsy to confirm the diagnosis. I would favour a skin biopsy over kidney biopsy, if possible, as skin biopsy is less invasive and lower risk.

She will benefit from treatment with a multidisciplinary team including the rheumatologist, respiratory physician, nephrologist, and allied healthcare professionals. I will stabilise her acutely and ensure that her airway and breathing are stable. She will need systemic immunosuppression, such as with steroids and cyclophosphamide. Prior to starting immunosuppression, I will ensure that she is a suitable candidate with no active infection or malignancy.

Tip: Pregnancy and immunosuppression

Know which immunosuppressants may and may not be used in pregnancy.

Safe in pregnancy	Unsafe in pregnancy
Corticosteroids	Cyclophosphamide
Hydroxychloroquine	Methotrexate
Ciclosporin	Mycophenolate
Azathioprine	Leflunomide
TNF-alpha inhibitors	
Sulfasalazine	

Consultation Case 03

Ms G. Mao (Dyspnoea)

Use this case as practice! The pull-out booklet contains the candidate's information.

Information for the Candidate

Patient Details: Ms Gan Mao, 28 years old

Your Role: Emergency Department SHO

Referral Letter:
> Dear A&E,
>
> Thank you for seeing Ms Mao. She started having flu symptoms a few days ago, and on review today, she is complaining of difficulty breathing. Please assist to manage her.
>
> Sincerely,
>
> Dr Guo Weiwen, GP

Vital Signs: BP 110/60 mmHg, HR 81/min, RR 11/min, SpO2 95% RA, T 37.9°C

Patient's Brief

Synopsis: *A young lady with known myasthenia gravis presents with worsening shortness of breath, weakness, and diplopia. She has a myasthenia flare precipitated by an upper respiratory tract infection as well as levofloxacin.*

Open the consult with: I think I caught a cold. The cough has become chesty and I'm finding it hard to breathe. *Do not volunteer any other information unless asked.*

History of current problem:
- You started having a fever, cough productive of yellow sputum, runny nose, and sore throat 3 days ago.
- You saw a GP and were given some medicine, but the symptoms only got worse. Therefore, you went back to the GP today and he sent you to the A&E department.
- You are also feeling slightly short of breath in the past 24 hours. This is not worse when exerting yourself or on lying down.
- You have been feeling completely well prior to these 3 days. In particular, you do not have any lightheadedness, decreased effort tolerance, or bleeding.
- You have no wheeze, chest pain, or palpitations.

- You have no leg swelling. Your urine output is normal and there are no bubbles or blood in your urine.
- You feel slightly weaker than normal — you struggled to climb up the stairs the past 2 days, but you think this is due to you being 'under the weather'. The weakness feels somewhat more noticeable at the end of the day.
- You notice intermittent double vision when looking to the left and right, particularly in the evenings.
- Nobody has commented on whether you have a droopy face or eyelids.

Past medical and surgical history:
- You were diagnosed with myasthenia gravis four years ago when you experienced double vision and difficulty climbing up the stairs. Your disease is well controlled and you experienced no flares in the past year. There were no recent dose adjustments and you are fully compliant with your medications for myasthenia gravis.
- You electively underwent a caesarean section 5 years ago.

Medication list:
- Azathioprine 200 mg OM (started 1 year ago)
- Pyridostigmine 60 mg TDS
- Levofloxacin 750 mg OM × 5 days (given by the GP 3 days ago)
- Dextromethorphan 15 mg TDS × 5 days (given by the GP 3 days ago)
- Loratadine 10 mg OM × 5 days (given by the GP 3 days ago)
- You also take a daily contraceptive pill
- No drug allergy

Family history:
- Your mother was also being treated for myasthenia gravis, and currently enjoys good control of symptoms.

Relevant personal, social, occupational, and travel history:
- You are the regional sales manager for a Japanese cosmetics brand.
- You travelled to Tokyo (Japan) last week for a business meeting.
- You are married with a 1-year-old child.
- You are currently having your menstrual period.

Relevant physical examination findings:

This encounter will use a real patient.
- Non-toxic, not in respiratory distress
- Lungs clear
- Bilateral fatigable ptosis, non-conforming ophthalmoplegia (Photo 3)
- Proximal muscle power 4/5, fatigable. Neck flexion power 5/5.

- Calves supple and not swollen
- No conjunctival pallor
- Euvolaemic

Photo to be shown to candidate upon request (use colour plates for full-colour photos).

Photo 3

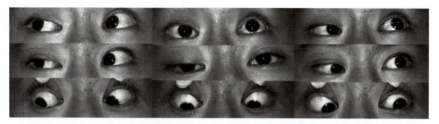

Clinical photo generously provided by Clin Assoc Prof Sharon Tow, Singapore National Eye Centre

You have some specific questions for the doctor at this consultation:
- I have a major presentation tomorrow and the deal might fall through if I back out. I wish to be discharged tomorrow and get back to work! Is this okay?

Approach and Clinical Reasoning

The stem is only tangentially helpful. Obviously in PACES it will not be a simple case of upper respiratory tract infection or pneumonia, so you must dig deeper for 'something more'. The critical step is to identify her history of myasthenia gravis, and consider how this might be related to her breathlessness. If she has obvious ptosis (she may be instructed to omit pyridostigmine on the examination day), the observant candidate may make a spot diagnosis of myasthenia gravis.

Important differentials to consider for Ms Mao include:

- Myasthenic crisis with respiratory muscle weakness – especially given the history of new/worsening proximal weakness.
- Pneumonia – particularly since she is taking immunosuppressants.
- Pulmonary embolism – she has had a recent long flight and is taking oral contraceptive pills.
- Other differentials include asthma, pneumothorax, anaemia, and cardiac causes of breathlessness.

Look for a precipitant for a myasthenia flare:
- Medications – the medications known to exacerbate the symptoms of myasthenia gravis (myasthenic flare) include aminoglycosides, fluoroquinolones, macrolides, beta blockers, hydroxychloroquine, and neuromuscular blocking agents. Ms Mao has had levofloxacin, which may explain her current symptoms.
- Infections.

- Dose reduction of immunosuppressants.
- Recent physical 'stressors' (e.g., surgeries or pregnancies).

Don't forget: Taking the drug history

> When taking the drug history, always ask for new medications, recent changes in dose, and compliance. Drug-drug and drug-disease interactions are commonly tested themes in the PACES exam.

The physical examination strategy will be to:

- Elicit the positive signs of myasthenia gravis, such as proximal weakness, ophthalmoplegia, fatigable ptosis, and fatigable speech. Neck flexion must be assessed — weak flexion heralds the onset of respiratory muscle weakness.
- Examine the chest for the clinical features of pneumonia. However, it is unlikely for a patient with active pneumonia to participate in the PACES exam.
- Examine clinical features of differential diagnoses such as anaemia, fluid overload, etc.

Question and Answer

Suggested answer to the patient's concerns:

Ms Mao, I hear that tomorrow's presentation is really important to you, but your breathlessness worries me. I am concerned that your myasthenia gravis has flared. You may continue to worsen and become too weak to breathe on your own, and that will endanger your life. I don't think that it is safe for you to go back to work tomorrow.

You need to be admitted urgently for treatment. Your oxygen levels will be monitored during your stay. Additionally, we will need you to blow into a meter to check if you already have difficulty breathing on your own. Also, a chest X-ray, blood tests, and an ECG will be arranged. Depending on the findings from the assessments, you may need to be admitted to a high dependency unit. If your weakness continues to worsen, you may need help to breathe through a breathing tube. Meanwhile, you will receive medications to treat both your infection and your myasthenia gravis, so that you will get better soon.

Regarding your presentation tomorrow, would it will be possible for you to participate remotely over a video conference? We can help to explain your situation to your employers, so that other work arrangements may be made. Let us know how else we can help.

Suggested presentation to the examiner:

Ms Mao presents with fever, dyspnoea, and increasing weakness. She is known to have myasthenia gravis, which was otherwise well-controlled over the past year. Examination findings were significant for bilateral fatigable ptosis, ophthalmoplegia, and proximal weakness. Her lungs were clear on auscultation. She is likely suffering a myasthenia flare, precipitated by the respiratory infection and recent fluoroquinolone use. In view of recent travel and oral contraceptive use, pulmonary embolism is a differential consideration. Asthma and cardiac causes of breathlessness are less likely.

Ms Mao should be admitted urgently. I will do an arterial blood gas test for hypercapnia, as well as bedside spirometry tests — forced vital capacity (FVC) and negative inspiratory force (NIF). In the event of respiratory failure, FVC less than 20 ml/kg, or NIF weaker than −30 cm H_2O, I will consider intubating the patient and escalating the level of care.

Further investigations and treatment measures include:

- Chest X-ray, ECG, and infective work up (blood cultures, full blood count, and inflammatory markers).
- Treating the infection with appropriate antibiotics other than fluoroquinolones.
- Requiring rapid immunomodulatory treatment (i.e., intravenous immunoglobulin or plasma exchange) if weakness worsens and especially if there is respiratory failure.
- Multidisciplinary management with neurologists, respiratory therapists, and physiotherapists.
- Nearing discharge, counselling on avoidance of triggers, sick day advice, and vaccinations.

Pitfall: Not every autoimmune condition is treated with steroids

Steroids and immunosuppressants (mycophenolate mofetil, azathioprine, etc.) have little role in the acute treatment of myasthenic crisis. In fact, starting high dose steroids in patients with myasthenic flares can worsen neuromuscular weakness. Intravenous immunoglobulin and plasma exchange are the therapeutic mainstays for treatment of a myasthenia flare.

Consultation Case 04

Mdm Miles (Dyspnoea)

Use this case as practice! The pull-out booklet contains the candidate's information.

Information for the Candidate

Patient Details: Mdm Miles, 37 years old

Your Role: Medical Admissions Unit SHO

Scenario: Mdm Miles presents with breathlessness and nausea after returning from a holiday in New Zealand.

Vital Signs: BP 155/91 mmHg, HR 161/min, RR 23/min, SpO2 94% RA, T 37.7°C

Patient's Brief

Synopsis: *This patient presents in thyroid storm with new-onset atrial fibrillation and cardiogenic pulmonary oedema.*

Open the consult with: It is our ten-year wedding anniversary and New Zealand was breath-taking. But I don't know why I started feeling somewhat breathless mid-trip. I had difficulty walking as much as I wanted to. I held out for a week till I returned home before seeing a doctor. *Do not volunteer any other information unless asked.*

History of current problem:

- Your breathlessness started a week ago; it was initially mild but gradually got worse.
- You have had difficulty exerting yourself — you had always been very fit but unexpectedly struggled with short treks this time.
- The breathlessness seems worse when you lie flat. Your husband bought return Business Class tickets which came with a lie-flat bed, but you found yourself having to prop yourself up at an angle.
- You have also been feeling nauseous in the past 3 days. You did not vomit and do not have abdominal pain. You have been passing three loose stools a day for the past 3 months.
- You feel generally warm and have been having a low-grade temperature.
- You have mild leg swelling of both legs, which you first noticed 3 days ago. This swelling is not painful.
- You have also felt your heart beating quite quickly. If asked to tap out a rhythm, you will tap out an irregular rhythm.

Consultation Case 04

- You have noticed hand tremors for the past month.
- You love the cold winter weather in New Zealand and you cannot stand the British summer/Singapore weather. You generally feel warm all the time.
- You have no cough, sore throat, runny nose, chest pain, or wheeze.
- You do not have any abdominal pain, jaundice, or dark-coloured urine.
- You do not have any headache, giddiness, or confusion.
- You have not noticed any change in appearance, neck lump, double vision, or blurred vision.

Past medical and surgical history:

- Nil. You go for yearly checkups and recall that your blood pressure has always been normal.

Medication list:

- Nil
- No known drug allergy.

Family history:

- Nil

Relevant personal, social, occupational, and travel history:

- You are a full-time church worker.
- You are married with two children.
- You do not smoke or drink.
- You are sure that you are not pregnant. Your periods have been irregular and spotty for as long as you remember.

Relevant physical examination findings:

This encounter will use a real patient although he/she may have been treated.

- Irregularly irregular pulse.
- Basal coarse lung crepitations, bilateral pitting pedal oedema, elevated jugular venous pressure – may be euvolemic post treatment.
- Small, smooth goitre without retrosternal extension ± thyroid bruit.
- Rest tremor + or nil tremor post treatment.
- Exopthalmosis present. Extraocular eye movements normal.
- No proximal myopathy.

You have some specific questions for the doctor at this consultation:

- What is causing my breathlessness?

Approach and Clinical Reasoning

You will be familiar with the important differentials in acute dyspnoea, which include:
- Acute pulmonary oedema/fluid overload.
- Acute coronary syndrome.
- Pulmonary infection.
- Pulmonary embolism.
- Obstructive airway disease.
- Other pulmonary pathology: pleural effusion, pneumothorax, etc.
- Non-pulmonary disease: anaemia, phaeochromocytoma, metabolic acidosis, etc.

Reading the stem, however, three important pieces of information stand out:

(i) Mdm Miles is a returning traveller who has just taken a long flight. This predisposes her to pulmonary embolism and infection.

(ii) She is hypertensive. In the context of acute dyspnoea, this quite commonly suggests pulmonary oedema or an acute coronary syndrome rather than sepsis or haemodynamically significant pulmonary embolism (which will cause hypotension).

(iii) She is *very* tachycardic.

Asking around these clues will reveal that Mdm Miles has new-onset atrial fibrillation causing congestive cardiac failure, presenting as symptoms of exertional breathlessness, orthopnoea, and pedal oedema. Do not stop here:

1. *Why does she have new-onset atrial fibrillation?* Triggers for atrial fibrillation can be divided into (i) systemic – thyrotoxicosis, infection, electrolyte disturbances, (ii) cardiac – myocardial ischaemia, cardiothoracic surgery, and (iii) pulmonary – pulmonary embolism. In this case, Mdm Miles is thyrotoxic with tremors, heat intolerance, and fever.

2. *Are there any other acute complications?* Recognise that she is in thyroid storm with cardiac failure, gastrointestinal symptoms, tachycardia, and fever.

3. *What is the cause of hyperthyroidism and contributory factors?*
   – Graves' disease – look for Graves' ophthalmopathy
   – Thyroiditis – ask for any history of neck pain (however thyroid storm is unusual)
   – Drugs – ask specifically about lithium and amiodarone
   – Take a family history and ask about associated autoimmune conditions

4. How do we manage her going forward? Ask about:
   – Any contraindications to anticoagulation
   – Pregnancy status and any plans for pregnancy

- Are there any children at home that she cannot avoid for 2 weeks? (caution for radioactive iodine)
- Does she use her voice professionally? (relative caution for surgery)

Tip: Search for a unifying diagnosis

> When a patient has multiple symptoms or multiple organ derangements, look hard for a unifying diagnosis — possible thyroid storm in this case. Do not stop at diagnosing a condition (new-onset atrial fibrillation), but also search for an underlying cause (thyrotoxicosis)! Many PACES stations do have an elegant unifying diagnosis.

Examination should aim to:

- Elicit signs of the hyperthyroid state (tremor, lid lag, tachycardia, atrial fibrillation).
- Elicit signs suggestive of a cause of hyperthyroidism (goitre, exophthalmos, Graves' ophthalmopathy).
- Confirm the suspicion of acute pulmonary oedema (lung crepitations, pedal oedema) and examine the heart.
- If time permits, also to screen neurology (embolus from atrial fibrillation).

Question and Answer

Suggested answer to the patient's concerns:

Mdm Miles, I think that you are feeling breathless because you have too much water in your lungs. Your heart does not seem to be pumping very well and your heartbeat is irregular. I suspect that this is because you have too much thyroid hormone, which is also causing your shaky hands, diarrhoea, and constant feeling of being very warm.

You are quite unwell, so I need to admit you. We will check your blood test, ECG, and X-ray, and start you on medicine to bring down your thyroid hormone levels and slow your heart rate. I will also need to talk to you about blood thinners because there is a risk of stroke when you have an irregular heartbeat like this.

Suggested presentation to the examiner:

Mdm Miles has new-onset atrial fibrillation and cardiogenic pulmonary oedema secondary to undiagnosed hyperthyroidism. I am concerned about thyroid storm as she is febrile and tachycardic, and has evidence of cardiac and gastrointestinal dysfunction.

I will ensure that her airway, breathing, and circulation are stable and admit her to a high dependency unit. I will confirm my diagnosis by performing thyroid function tests, an electrocardiogram, and a chest X-ray looking for pulmonary oedema and to rule out pneumonia. Other blood tests include a full blood count for raised total whites, electrolytes in view of her atrial fibrillation, troponins, and blood cultures. Investigation for an underlying cause of hyperthyroidism such as TSH receptor antibody or thyroid uptake scans can be done, but is not the priority in the acute setting.

Management plan will include:
- Admission to high dependency (or other monitored setting).
- Start beta blocker, propylthiouracil, and IV hydrocortisone.
- One hour later, Lugol's iodine to block the release of thyroid hormone.
- Diuretics and nitrates as treatment of pulmonary oedema.
- Cover with broad spectrum antibiotics in view of possible pulmonary infection.
- Consideration of anticoagulation in view of atrial fibrillation.

Consultation Case 05

Ms Chuan (Dyspnoea)

Use this case as practice! The pull-out booklet contains the candidate's information.

Information for the Candidate

Patient Details: Ms Chuan, 33 years old

Your Role: Emergency Department SHO

Referral Letter:
> Dear Colleague,
>
> Thank you for seeing Ms Chuan. She is complaining of worsening shortness of breath in the past month.
>
> Thank you.
>
> Dr Eugene Gan, GP

Vital Signs: BP 125/80 mmHg, HR 81/min, RR 14/min, SpO2 95% RA, T 36.2°C

Patient's Brief

Synopsis: *This patient with recurrent pulmonary embolism on long-term warfarin presents with breathlessness due to chronic thromboembolic pulmonary hypertension, and possibly new pulmonary emboli precipitated by subtherapeutic INR levels due to the drug interaction between warfarin and carbamazepine.*

Open the consult with: I have been slightly breathless, especially when I exert myself, for a year now. But the last month has been worse. *Do not volunteer any other information unless asked.*

History of current problem:
- Your breathlessness started a year ago. You used to be a yoga enthusiast, but you have had to give this up because even slight exertion would make you breathless, although you were still able to get about your daily life.
- The breathlessness is steadily worsening in the past month; it is now affecting even your walk home from the train station (a 10-minute walk).
- The breathlessness is not episodic and you do not have intermittent flares.
- Breathlessness is not worse lying down. You have neither leg swelling nor blood or bubbles in your urine.
- You have no cough, blood in the sputum, wheeze, fever, or weight loss.

- You have no chest pain or palpitations.
- There is no history of a long flight, immobilisation, surgery, or trauma.
- You have no joint pain, swelling, or rashes.
- You have no bleeding in the stools and no lightheadedness when you stand up.
- You have no weakness of arms, legs, or double vision.

Past medical and surgical history:
- You were admitted twice — once last year, and once 4 years ago for 'clots in the lung'. Both times you presented with sudden-onset breathlessness. The causes of these 'clots in the lung' was not found despite extensive work-up. After the second episode, you were put on long term warfarin.
- Two months ago, you experienced bad shooting pain which you were told was due to a facial nerve problem (trigeminal neuralgia). The neurologist started you on carbamazepine for this.

Medication list:
- Warfarin 5 mg OM. There have been no recent dose changes. Your last INR check was 3 months ago and you were told that it was acceptable. You are fully compliant and never miss a dose.
- Carbamazepine 200 mg OM.
- You have recently started taking oral contraceptive pills in the past month.
- No drug allergy.

Family history:
- Nil

Relevant personal, social, occupational, and travel history:
- You are married without children. You have had 3 miscarriages.
- You work as a customer service manager in the airport.
- You smoke socially — approximately 5 sticks a day, since you were 15 years old. You have been finding it difficult to find a place to smoke especially at work.
- You do not take alcohol.
- There is no recent travel history.

Relevant physical examination findings:

This encounter will use a real patient with the physical signs below, but the acute complaint will be simulated.

- Not in respiratory distress.
- Lungs clear.
- Heart: S1, S2, loud P2, parasternal heave. May have tricuspid regurgitation.
- No pedal oedema.

- Fluid status euvolemic.
- No obvious stigmata of rheumatologic illness.

You have some specific questions for the doctor at this consultation:
- What is happening? I have been taking my warfarin so diligently. Am I doing something wrong?

Approach and Clinical Reasoning

Pay attention to the temporal sequence of breathlessness. Ms Chuan has a 1-year history of chronic dyspnoea, which has gradually worsened in the past month. The key differentials in chronic dyspnoea, as well as key symptoms and signs to explore, are given in Table B2.3.

Table B2.3. Differentials in chronic progressive dyspnoea.

Differential	Important features
Fluid overload: heart failure, renal insufficiency, cirrhosis, etc.	Leg swelling, orthopnoea History of heart disease, renal failure, etc.
Respiratory disease - Progressive COPD - Interstitial lung disease - Lung cancer ± pleural effusion	Chronic cough, wheeze, haemoptysis Smoking history Prior exposures, rheumatologic disease, etc. Weight loss, abnormal chest examination
Infective: particularly mycobacteria, fungal and pneumocystis	Fever, weight loss, chronic cough, haemoptysis Contact history, underlying immunocompromise Sexual history may be suggestive for pneumocystis
Anaemia	Conjunctival pallor, pre-syncopal symptoms History of blood loss, iron deficiency, chronic disease or renal impairment
Vascular disease - Pulmonary hypertension - Thromboembolic disease - Superior vena cava obstruction	Parasternal heave, loud P2, known predisposition History of deep vein thrombosis, predisposition History of cancer, facial and upper limb swelling
Neuromuscular weakness	Muscle weakness, bulbar weakness, diplopia

COPD: chronic obstructive pulmonary disease; P2: pulmonary component of second heart sound

The key to diagnosis lies in Ms Chuan's medical history of two unprovoked pulmonary embolisms for which she is on warfarin. What might be causing the recent worsening of symptoms? Consider *what has changed*:

- Recurrence – pulmonary embolism
  - Non-compliance to warfarin or INR check.
  - Recent decrease in warfarin dose.
  - Drug-drug interaction.
- Complications of pulmonary embolism
  - Chronic thromboembolic pulmonary hypertension (CTEPH)*[1].
  - Right heart failure.*
  - Tricuspid regurgitation.*
- Complication of treatment
  - Anaemia – bleeding while on warfarin.*
- Unrelated condition (e.g., pneumonia)

*Note that the physical examination is critical to confirm or refute these differentials.

While Ms Chuan has been compliant to warfarin and INR checks, she has had two recent drug changes:

- Started carbamazepine. This is an enzyme inducer that increases warfarin metabolism and reduces INR.
- Started oral contraceptive pills (OCP). This drug should ring alarm bells — Ms Chuan has had thromboembolic disease and should not be on OCPs in the first place. OCPs may have a prothrombotic effect and an unpredictable effect on INR.

Physical examination should focus on:

- Demonstrating the presence of pulmonary hypertension, which will confirm a diagnosis of CTEPH — this can be subtle and easily missed if not specifically looked for.
- Looking for new deep vein thrombosis (check if the calves are supple).
- Looking for differentials of breathlessness — in particular, examine for fluid overload and auscultate the lungs.

Question and Answer

Suggested answer to the patient's concerns:

Ms Chuan, I appreciate the effort you put in to take your warfarin so diligently. Please do not blame yourself; I don't think this is your fault. I am wondering if the clots in your lung has made your heart pump at higher pressures to deliver blood to the lungs. On top of that, I am wondering if you have gotten any new clots in your lung. The new medications you are on for your facial pain may interact with warfarin so that warfarin becomes less effective. Whatever it is, I will try my best to get you better.

---

[1] Note that the history of previous pulmonary embolism may not always be so forthcoming as haemodynamically insignificant pulmonary embolism is quite commonly missed; patients may instead describe only a prolonged atypical pneumonia or a period of atypical chest pain.

I think it will be necessary to admit you. I will do blood tests, an X-ray, and lung scans to look at the blood vessels of your lungs. I will also do an echocardiogram to look at your heart, and refer you to the cardiologist and lung doctor.

Suggested presentation to the examiner:

Ms Chuan has chronic progressive dyspnoea, which has worsened in the past month, on a background of recurrent pulmonary embolism. Physical examination is significant for findings of pulmonary hypertension. I am concerned about chronic thromboembolic pulmonary hypertension possibly with a superimposed new pulmonary embolus. I note that she has recently started carbamazepine and oral contraceptive pills, which could interact with warfarin and predispose to thromboembolism. My differentials include anaemia due to occult gastrointestinal bleeding while on anticoagulation, heart failure, and pneumonia.

I will like to admit her. I will first ensure that her airway breathing and circulation are stable. I will check her bloods in particular the INR, haemoglobin, platelets, and inflammatory markers. I will do a chest X-ray for fluid overload and ECG looking for right heart strain. I will organise a ventilation/perfusion scan looking for chronic thromboembolic pulmonary embolism[2] and/or a CT pulmonary angiogram looking for a new pulmonary embolus. I will do an echocardiogram for right heart strain and consider referral for right heart catheterisation.

In terms of management, she will benefit from multidisciplinary team management including a cardiologist, cardiothoracic surgeon, respiratory physician, and haematologist.

- Acutely, I will adjust her warfarin dosing to ensure it is in the therapeutic range.
- For CTEPH, she should be:
  - Referred for consideration of pulmonary endarterectomy.
  - Be on lifelong anticoagulation with regular INR monitoring.
- Other aspects of management include:
  - Warfarin diet counselling.
  - Patient education on drug-drug interaction.
  - Ensuring that the work-up for prothrombotic disorders has been done (particularly antiphospholipid syndrome in view of recurrent pregnancy loss).

---

[2] The most sensitive test for diagnosis of CTEPH is a ventilation/perfusion scan (more sensitive than CT pulmonary angiogram).

Tip: Drug interactions with warfarin

Drug-drug interactions are a favourite in PACES. Warfarin is notorious for having many drug interactions, of which some of the more important ones are listed below:

Enzyme inducer (↓ INR)	Enzyme inhibitor (↑ INR)
Carbamazepine	Antibiotics: fluoroquinolones, bactrim, macrolides, metronidazole, augmentin (unreliable)
Phenytoin	
Phenobarbitone	Antifungals: azoles
Rifampicin	TB drugs: isoniazid
St John's wort	Selective serotonin reuptake inhibitors: fluvoxamine, sertraline
	Amiodarone
Ethanol (chronic use)	Ethanol (acute intake)

Consultation Case 06

Mr Freddie (Dyspnoea)

Use this case as practice! The pull-out booklet contains the candidate's information.

Information for the Candidate

Patient Details: Mr Freddie, 40 years old

Your Role: Respiratory Medicine Clinic SHO

Referral Letter:
> Dear Colleague,
>
> Mr Freddie has been complaining of cough and dyspnoea which did not respond to a course of clarithromycin. Could you please see him?
>
> Thank you.
>
> Dr Hutton, GP

Vital Signs: BP 109/63 mmHg, HR 71/min, RR 13/min, SpO2 93% RA, T 37.2°C

Patient's Brief

Synopsis: *Mr Freddie has a non-resolving respiratory infection, exercise desaturation, and weight loss on a background of high-risk sexual behaviour. The likely underlying diagnosis is pneumocystis pneumonia or tuberculosis with underlying retroviral infection.*

Open the consult with: I have been feeling slightly breathless for the last 2 months. The GP said that I should see you because I'm not getting better. *Do not volunteer any other information unless asked.*

History of current problem:
- Your breathlessness started out 2 months ago as a cough. The GP said that this was a 'flu', gave you some paracetamol and antihistamines, and told you to take a few days off work. You did not get better and went back to the GP 2 weeks later complaining of some breathlessness. This time he gave you a 5-day course of clarithromycin which you have completed, but this did not work. You do not recall doing any chest X-ray.
- You currently still feel mildly breathless, especially when you exert yourself. For instance, you tried to run to catch the train earlier today but had to stop halfway for a lack of breath, and ended up taking the next train. You have stopped going to the gym in the last 2 months.

- The breathlessness is not worse lying down.
- You have no history of asthma, no variation in symptoms with time of day, and no identifiable triggers for breathlessness.
- You have a chronic dry cough for the last 3–4 months. There is no phlegm or coughing out of blood. The cough is not worse at any particular time of day, when lying down, or after a heavy meal.
- You have unintentionally lost about 5 kg in the last 3 months.
- You occasionally feel 'warm' but do not routinely check your temperature.
- You had a bit of 'white stuff' coating your tongue and use a mouthwash each morning to get this 'cleaned'. You occasionally feel slight pain on swallowing, but this is mild.
- At the present moment, you have no sore throat, runny nose, lumps in the neck or groin, diarrhoea, penile discharge, or headache.
- You do not have any leg swelling, chest pain, palpitations, rashes, blood or bubbles in the urine, or decreased urine output.
- You do not have any stuffy nose in the mornings, reflux, or heartburn symptoms.

Past medical and surgical history:
- Nil. You have been well until this episode.
- You do not recall any childhood respiratory infections or personal history of tuberculosis.

Medication list:
- PO Codeine 30 mg TDS PRN for cough.
- PO Clarithromycin 250 mg BD × 1 week (completed).

Family/contact history:
- You have no family or contact history of tuberculosis.
- You have no family history of lung problems, cancer, or autoimmune conditions.

Relevant personal, social, occupational, and travel history:
- You were born and grew up locally.
- You are the regional sales director in an aerospace engineering company. Your job involves frequent (weekly or fortnightly) travelling to countries in the region.
- You are married with two young children. You have frequent sexual intercourse with your spouse.
- *Only if asked* – during your frequent travels, a number of entertainment sessions have ended in one-night stands with local hostesses. You typically use a condom but have forgotten a couple of times.
- You do not smoke or drink.
- You do not use intravenous drugs.

Relevant physical examination findings:

This encounter is likely to use a surrogate patient.

- Comfortable, not in respiratory distress, no asterixes.
- No clubbing.
- Lungs – clear.
- No pedal oedema.
- No lymphadenopathy.
- No oral thrush.
- Offer to walk the patient and check oxygen saturation after (looking for exercise desaturation).

You have some specific questions for the doctor at this consultation:

- Do I have lung cancer?
- (If told that it is not lung cancer) – Okay, what is wrong with me then?

Approach and Clinical Reasoning

This scenario is a PACES classic and one that is often kept as a 'standby' in case any patient is unable to make the exam at short notice (the other common standby case being a transient ischaemic attack, as both can be played by patient surrogates).

Mr Freddie presents with chronic cough, exertional breathlessness, and weight loss despite antibiotic treatment. The vitals provided indicate mild hypoxia. Recognise the clinical syndrome of a non-resolving respiratory infection (Table B2.4) which must prompt consideration of differentials and suspicion of an immunocompromised state. Common causes of an immunocompromised state in PACES include HIV (see Box), drugs (e.g., immunosuppression, chemotherapy, agranulocytosis as a side effect of anti-thyroid medication), and bone marrow failure syndromes.

Don't forget: Suspect HIV

> Cases of suspected HIV are a PACES favourite. Be attuned to scenarios in which you might be required to take a sexual history — for instance, chronic cough/breathlessness, chronic diarrhoea, weight loss, prolonged fever, lymphadenopathy, or sterile pyuria. Additionally, pay attention to stereotyped occupational histories such as long-distance truck drivers, travelling businessmen, or entertainment industry professionals — this is an unfair stereotype, but is also often the question setter's hint that you should consider taking a sexual history. See Table C5.5 for tips on taking the sexual history.

Table B2.4. Causes of 'non-resolving respiratory infection'.

Category	Cause	Important clinical features
Nonbacterial infection	Tuberculosis (TB)	Night sweats, fever, weight loss May have haemoptysis and epidemiologic risk (e.g., family history) May be immunocompromised
	Pneumocystis pneumonia (PCP)	Prominent exercise desaturation HIV or other immunocompromised state
	Fungi (e.g., aspergillosis)	Immunocompromise (e.g., chemotherapy)
Noninfective causes	Lung cancer	Haemoptysis, weight loss, chronic cough
	Inflammatory: - Vasculitis (incl. ANCA) - Sarcoidosis - Drug-induced	Other organ features (e.g., haematuria, arthralgia, rash, Raynaud's phenomenon) Examination: fine crepitations
	Pulmonary embolism	Unilateral leg swelling, sudden onset, predisposition (e.g., immobility, cancer).
	Obstructive airway disease	Wheeze, smoking history Examination: hyperinflated chest, coarse crepitations
	Heart failure	Bilateral leg swelling, raised jugular venous pressure
Complicated and recurrent infection	Bronchiectasis	Longstanding chronic cough, previous pulmonary infections Examination: coarse crepitations
	Recurrent aspiration	Dysphagia, old stroke, neuromuscular weakness, extrapyramidal disease
	Lung abscess	High spiking fevers, purulent sputum
	Pleural effusion, empyema	Examination: hemithorax stony dullness Unlikely in exam – patient will be sick

The clincher in this scenario is Mr Freddie's sexual history. Along with weight loss, oral thrush, and odynophagia suggestive of esophageal candidiasis, HIV must be strongly suspected. The key differentials in a patient with HIV who complains of pulmonary symptoms are PCP, TB, and other fungal infections. The latter two must be considered although PCP would be slightly favoured in view of resting hypoxia, prominent exercise desaturation, and the absence of productive cough or haemoptysis.

Examination should focus on:
- Ensuring that the patient is stable and not in respiratory distress.

- Chest examination. This may be normal as untreated PCP or TB will not appear in PACES. However, be alert for differentials (fine or coarse crepitations, or an effusion).
- Examine for other features of HIV (e.g., oral candidiasis or lymphadenopathy).

Question and Answer

Suggested answer to the patient's concerns:

Mr Freddie, this prolonged episode of cough and breathlessness and the thought that you could have lung cancer must be very frightening to you. I don't think that lung cancer is the most likely reason why you are feeling unwell, but you are right that we must rule this out. I plan to admit you for further tests and treatment.

There is something else that I am worried about and I'm not sure if it is good news. You seem to be having a somewhat unusual lung infection, along with white stuff coating your tongue and weight loss. I am concerned that your immune system might not be working so well — in particular, I must consider the possibility of HIV. [Pause]. If it is indeed what I fear, it is very important that we start you on treatment right away so that we can get you better.

Tip: Breaking bad news in a consultation station

> You may have to break bad news in a consultation station. This must be done with appropriate lead-ins and empathy (see communications section). At the same time, you do not have the luxury of time that the communication task offers, and must be succinct. Ensure that you answer the patient's question directly as failure to do so will certainly be penalised.
>
> Note that the presence of opportunistic infection suggests that Mr Freddie is likely to have AIDS rather than early HIV. Your response must reflect such an understanding and cannot be overly reassuring. For instance, a comment like "nowadays HIV has a very good prognosis as long as you take medications" is inaccurate in advanced AIDS.

Suggested presentation to the examiner:

Mr Freddie presents with the clinical syndrome of a prolonged respiratory infection with cough, breathlessness, and rest hypoxia. Additionally, he has weight loss, suggestion of oral and oesophageal candidiasis, and a worrisome sexual history. I am concerned about pneumocystis pneumonia or tuberculosis with underlying retroviral infection.

I will admit Mr Freddie. After ensuring that he is stable, I will investigate by:
- Obtaining a chest X-ray, blood gas, and basic laboratory investigations.
- Sending a HIV test.
- Confirming the diagnosis of TB or PCP by sending sputum for:

- TB: Acid fast bacilli smear, culture, and PCR.
- PCP: PCP microscopy and PCR.

as well as consideration of diagnostic bronchoscopy.

- If HIV is confirmed, additional tests include a CD4 count, as well as screening for other opportunistic infections and sexually transmitted diseases.

Management: Mr Freddie will require multidisciplinary team care including an infectious disease and respiratory physician.

- In the case of PCP, the first-line treatment is co-trimoxazole (Bactrim) after ensuring that he is not G6PD deficient. He may require steroid coadministration depending on the severity of PCP.
- In the case of TB, he will be started on antituberculous therapy typically a 4-drug combination.
- He should be started on combination antiretroviral therapy[3].

---

[3] This may not be started immediately as immune reconstitution inflammatory syndrome (IRIS) would be a concern. You would not ordinarily be expected to discuss IRIS in PACES, but should be aware that the timing of antiretroviral therapy initiation is not straightforward.

Consultation Case 07

Mr Nafas (Dyspnoea)

Use this case as practice! The pull-out booklet contains the candidate's information.

Information for the Candidate

Patient Details: Mr Nafas, 49 years old

Your Role: Medical Admissions Unit SHO

Referral Letter:
> Dear Colleague,
>
> I will appreciate if you could kindly review Mr Nafas. He presents today with a 2-day history of dyspnoea and looks moderately unwell.
>
> Thank you.
>
> Dr Ed. Mitt, A&E Consultant

Vital Signs: BP 128/70 mmHg, HR 100/min, RR 26/min, SpO2 100% RA, T 36.5°C

Investigations:
ECG: Sinus tachycardia
Capillary blood glucose: 11.3 mmol/L
Chest X-ray: Normal
Blood investigations: Pending

Patient's Brief

Synopsis: *Mr Nafas presents with dyspnoea, vomiting, and a normal chest X-ray. He also has polyuria and polydipsia while on dapagliflozin. Euglycaemic ketoacidosis is a key concern.*

Open the consult with: I don't know why I feel so breathless. *Do not volunteer any other information unless asked.*

History of current problem:

- You have been breathless the past few days. It got really bad yesterday and today, so you came in to Emergency.
- You have also been feeling nauseous. You vomited out the contents of your dinner last night.
- You have been feeling unusually thirsty and passing large amounts of urine.
- You are lethargic and did not manage to go to work the past 3 days.

- You have no chest pain, palpitations, or unusual sweating.
- You have no cough, wheeze, sore throat, loud breathing sounds, or fever.
- You do not have any abdominal pain, diarrhoea, or bleeding.
- You have no weakness, numbness, headache, or drowsiness.
- You have been well up to the past week and would consider yourself to be physically active.
- You have not lost weight. However, you have been trying to do a 'low-carbohydrate' diet ever since you saw your GP a month ago (see below).

Past medical and surgical history:
- Hypertension.
- Hyperlipidemia.
- Type 2 diabetes, diagnosed 5 years ago. Your control has been poor with a HbA1c of 8.7% (72 mmol/mol) a month ago. Your GP has advised you to start insulin, but you have bargained for 'one more chance' — promising to diet and exercise, while your GP adds on 'one extra diabetes medicine' (dapagliflozin). You have agreed to start insulin if your HbA1c still remains above 8% (64 mmol/mol).
- Gout, for which you get 2–3 flares a year.
- No history of asthma, blood clots, or heart problems.

Medication list:
- Atorvastatin 20 mg ON
- Dapagliflozin 10 mg OM (started 1 month ago)
- Diclofenac 50 mg TDS as needed for gout
- Glipizide 20 mg BD
- Metformin 850 mg TDS
- Nifedipine 60 mg OM
- Valsartan 160 mg BD (increased from 160 mg OM / 80 mg ON a month ago)

Family history:
- Your father passed away from a heart attack in his 60s.

Relevant personal, social, occupational, and travel history:
- You do not smoke or drink.
- You work as a taxi driver.
- You are not married and have a longstanding male partner.

Relevant physical examination findings:
This encounter may use either a real but treated patient or a trained surrogate.
- Volume status – no peripheral oedema, JVP not raised.

- Heart S1S2.
- Lungs clear.
- Abdomen soft non tender.
- No conjunctival pallor.

You have some specific questions for the doctor at this consultation:
- Am I having a heart attack?

Approach and Clinical Reasoning

The stem is fairly informative. The approach required is that to acute dyspnoea with a normal chest X-ray (Table B2.5). The normal chest X-ray makes fluid overload (including acute heart failure), parenchymal diseases (pneumonia, interstitial lung disease), and pleural disorders (effusion, pneumothorax) less likely. Differentials such as pulmonary embolism, metabolic acidosis, and anaemia are easily forgotten as causes of dyspnoea.

Table B2.5. Causes of acute dyspnoea and tachypnoea with a (fairly) normal chest X-ray.

Category	Cause	Possible clinical features
Cardiac	Coronary ischaemia	Chest pain, diaphoresis, ECG changes
	Arrhythmias	Palpitations, ECG changes
Respiratory	Upper airway obstruction	Stridor
	Bronchoconstriction (COPD/asthma)	Wheeze (may be 'silent chest' if severe) History of atopy, precipitant
Vascular	Pulmonary embolism	Unilateral leg swelling, hypercoagulable state
Metabolic	Metabolic acidosis	Air hunger. Causes of acidosis include: - Severe sepsis (lactic acidosis) - Vomiting, polyuria/polydipsia (ketoacidosis) - Poisoning/toxic alcohol ingestion
	Anaemia	Giddiness, pallor, blood loss
Other	Hypoventilation	Peripheral (LMN) weakness (e.g., myasthenia gravis) Drowsiness, sedation, or intoxication
	Anxiety	Diagnosis of exclusion

In addition to dyspnoea, Mr Nafas has been generally unwell with nausea, vomiting, polyuria, and polydipsia in the past week. Given that he has recently initiated dapagliflozin, a sodium-glucose co-transporter 2 (SGLT2) inhibitor, the current presentation is worrisome for euglycaemic ketoacidosis. This is a phenomenon of diabetic ketoacidosis but with normal blood glucose, as SGLT2 blockade results in glycosuria and prevents frank hyperglycaemia.

Reasonable differentials for Mr Nafas' presentation, assuming normal lung findings, include:

- Pulmonary embolism, which must always be considered in otherwise unexplained dyspnoea or sinus tachycardia.
- Anaemia given his history of postural giddiness, lethargy, and use of NSAIDs. This should be excluded on physical examination. In the absence of acute blood loss, anaemia is more likely to present insidiously rather than acutely.

Physical examination should achieve the following:

- Assess fluid status – looking for dehydration which will typically be seen in ketoacidosis (obviously Mr Nafas will not have untreated ketoacidosis in the exam).
- Auscultate the chest – rule out bronchoconstrictive disorders.
- Look for conjunctival pallor.
- Examine the calves for unilateral calf swelling, which would increase the probability of pulmonary embolism.
- If time permits, palpate the abdomen in view of nausea and vomiting.

Pitfall: A normal physical exam

> Since the introduction of Station 5 (brief clinical consult) in 2009, surrogates and treated patients with no positive physical signs have been used in the consultation station, particularly in acute medicine scenarios. Do not be surprised if the physical examination is entirely normal — *and do not make up signs!*

Question and Answer

Suggested answer to the patient's concerns:

Thank you for sharing all this with me; this breathlessness must be very worrying for you. I don't think you are having a heart attack at the moment, although I will not be able to conclusively rule this out until we do some blood tests. I am worried, however, that you may be developing accumulation of acid in the body, which may be related to the new diabetes medicine that you have been taking. I think it's best that we admit you for some blood tests and treatment. I think I will be able to get you feeling better soon.

Suggested presentation to the examiner:

Mr Nafas presents with dyspnoea, tachypnoea, vomiting, and osmotic symptoms on a background of newly initiated SGLT2 inhibition. Given a normal ECG and chest X-ray, I am most concerned about the possibility of euglycaemic ketoacidosis and a differential of pulmonary embolism.

I will admit him. Initial investigations will include:

- Serum ketones, bicarbonate, and a blood gas.
- Urea, creatinine, and electrolytes.
- Blood count.
- Cardiac enzymes.
- Liver function, amylase, and septic work-up in view of vomiting and looking for a precipitant for ketoacidosis.
- CT pulmonary angiogram if ketones are negative or breathlessness does not resolve with treatment.

Management includes:

- Stopping dapagliflozin.
- IV insulin to suppress ketosis, and dextrose as needed to prevent hypoglycaemia.
- Hydration and potassium replacement as guided by initial electrolyte values.
- Subsequently, to optimise diabetes management in particular consideration of insulin therapy.

Consultations

3 | Same Condition, Different Presentations

This section illustrates how individual disease conditions can give rise to a whole range of presenting complaints.

Exam coordinators often begin by identifying patients who are suitable to come for exams, and then writing an appropriate clinical scenario. A number of 'favourites' appear in the consultations station because (i) conditions with positive physical signs are favoured, (ii) only patients who are stable are listed for exams, and (iii) it is desired to cover conditions poorly represented in the physical examination stations — that is, endocrinology, rheumatology, dermatology, and ophthalmology.

It is helpful to think through the presenting complaints that can be set for each of these patients. The Royal College explicitly discourages listing patients with obvious, longstanding chronic conditions as if newly diagnosed — for example, the diagnosis of Graves' disease in a patient with overt goitre and exophthalmos is considered 'too easy'. Such patients are meant to be put up as a 'complication of disease' case instead.

Knowledge of the underlying medical condition may or may not be revealed to you. Possible permutations include:

1. The underlying condition is given in the stem.
2. The underlying condition is revealed in the past medical history.
3. The patient affirms that they have been seeing a specialist, but are unsure of their exact diagnosis. Some exam centres consider this unrealistic, while others deem it fair game — especially if the drug list contains giveaways (such as methotrexate or cabergoline) that point to the diagnosis.
4. The past medical history is hidden and instead a 'fresh case' is simulated. For example, a patient could claim to have no past medical history but when asked specifically about joint pain, he could say, "now that you mention it, indeed the small joints of my hand have been hurting and stiff for a long time, but isn't this just old age doctor?" This could also be a 'spot diagnosis' with obvious physical signs that you are expected to pick up upon entering the room.

In (1) and (2), the station very clearly becomes an exploration of complications of disease. (3) and (4) are more tricky in that you must diagnose the underlying condition and consider what complications of disease the patient is now facing.

As a general strategy, it is often wise to:

- Look out for possible spot diagnoses.

- Obtain the past medical history early.
- Pay attention to the drug list.

Example 1: Graves' Disease

Diagnostic cases

Possible stems include:

1. Chronic diarrhoea
2. Weight loss
3. Palpitations
4. Diplopia

These patients are likely to have less obvious features of Graves' disease. Note that for patients with hyperthyroidism but without Graves' ophthalmopathy, the differential of Hashimoto's thyrotoxicosis should be offered.

Complications of disease cases

Symptom	Possible considerations *in addition to general causes unrelated to thyroid disease*
1. Breathlessness	Cardiac: atrial fibrillation, heart failure (± thyroid storm)
	Infection – agranulocytosis secondary to thioamides
	Compressive goitre with upper airway obstruction
2. Difficulty seeing	Graves' ophthalmopathy (± worsened by radioiodine) – can manifest as diplopia, chemosis, exposure keratitis
	Amaurosis fugax, occipital infarct (± atrial fibrillation)
3. Weakness	Thyrotoxic periodic paralysis
	Stroke/transient ischaemic attack (± atrial fibrillation)
	Myasthenia gravis (associated with Graves' disease)
4. Jaundice	Hepatitis from thioamides
	Thyroid storm with cholestasis

Example 2: Acromegaly

As the physical changes of acromegaly do not diminish after treatment, patients who have previously undergone transphenoidal surgery are often asked to return for exams.

Classic presentations include change in appearance, bitemporal hemianopia, and sweaty palms. Less obvious presentations include:

Symptom	Possible considerations *in addition to general causes unrelated to acromegaly*
1. Headache	Acromegaly (new diagnosis) Pituitary apoplexy Hypertensive urgency (associated with acromegaly)
2. Constipation	Colonic malignancy (acromegaly increases risk; number of colonic polyps is proportional to the number of skin tags) Hypercalcaemia (multiple endocrine neoplasia type 1 with pituitary and parathyroid adenomas)
3. Fatigue	Adrenal insufficiency (from panhypopituitarism) Obstructive sleep apnoea Anaemia – rectal bleeding from colonic polyps
4. Hand numbness	Diabetic peripheral neuropathy Carpel tunnel syndrome
5. Rectal bleeding	Colonic malignancy

Example 3: Rheumatoid Arthritis (RA)

Symptom	Possible considerations *in addition to general causes unrelated to RA*
1. Joint pain	Disease flare Non-compliance to therapy Septic arthritis If joint pain occurs at a site atypical for RA, also consider – Osteoporotic fracture (e.g., vertebrae) – Avascular necrosis (of hip)
2. Breathlessness	Interstitial lung disease secondary to disease or drugs Anaemia Infection – pneumonia, tuberculosis, pneumocystis Pulmonary hypertension Fluid overload – acute kidney injury from NSAID use Other pulmonary manifestation of RA: effusion, bronchiectasis Pericardial effusion

(Cont'd)

Symptom	Possible considerations *in addition to general causes unrelated to RA*
3. Anaemia	Anaemia of chronic disease Gastrointestinal bleeding from NSAID use Folate deficiency as a side effect of methotrexate use Marrow suppression from immunosuppression Cytopenia from viral infection (e.g., CMV)
4. Fatigue	Poorly controlled disease Hypocortisolism due to steroid withdrawal Anaemia
5. Weakness	UMN: atlantoaxial subluxation, cervical spine instability with myelopathy Neuropathy: – Peripheral neuropathy – Mononeuritis multiplex – Entrapment neuropathy (e.g., Carpal tunnel syndrome) Myopathy – Myositis (overlap syndrome) – Steroid-induced myopathy Anaemia
6. Difficulty seeing	Red eye, eye pain - Scleritis - Secondary Sjögren's syndrome Blurring of vision – Hydroxychloroquine toxicity (bull's eye maculopathy) – Cataract (due to steroid use) – Glaucoma (predisposed by steroid use) Diplopia – mononeuritis multiplex of extraocular muscles
7. Nephrotic syndrome	NSAID use (associated with membranous GN) Amyloidosis Reactivation of hepatitis B/C

Example 4: Hereditary Haemorrhagic Telangiectasia (HHT)

The classic stem for this case is epistaxis. Other possible presentations are:

Symptom	Possible considerations *in addition to general causes unrelated to thyroid disease*
1. Breathlessness	Anaemia (from epistaxis, gastrointestinal bleeding) Pulmonary arteriovenous malformation (AVM) with right-to-left shunt High-output cardiac failure from pulmonary or hepatic AVM Pulmonary embolism (HHT is associated with increased venous thromboembolism risk)
2. Stroke/giddiness	Paradoxical emboli through a pulmonary AVM Rupture of intracranial arteriovenous malformation Hypercoagulable state Hypoperfusion/watershed infarct from anaemia

Consultations

4 | Worked Practice

This section provides deliberate practice for the PACES consultation station. Each case comes with information for the candidate and a detailed patient's brief, and is followed by a discussion of the relevant approach and clinical reasoning, a suggested answer to the patient's concerns, and a possible presentation to the examiners. We suggest attempting each case as a mock consultation with a colleague or tutor simulating the patient's role. Simply reading through the station will be of diminished learning value. The purpose of this section is to provide practice — not details about individual conditions (look up a reference text if required) or a framework to approach presenting complaints (some flowcharts from Algorithms in Differential Diagnosis[4] are reproduced — refer to Algorithms for a more detailed walk-through). Most cases are written to be of above-average difficulty so that you will be prepared for more challenging cases, which some exam centres are fond of.

You may wish to revisit key points and lessons at some point. The Index to cases will allow you to quickly search for the relevant content.

For practice with a colleague or tutor: Use the pull-out 'candidate information' booklet, which gives the candidate's information for all practice scenarios, to blind yourself to the patient's brief and discussion.

---

[4] Fong N. 2019. *Algorithms in Differential Diagnosis: How to Approach Common Presenting Complaints in Adult Patients, for Medical Students and Junior Doctors.* Singapore: World Scientific.

4 | Worked Practice

Consultation Case 08

Mr Ee Chee (Rash)

Use this case as practice! The pull-out booklet contains the candidate's information.

Information for the Candidate

Patient Details: Mr Ee Chee, 59 years old

Your Role: Dermatology Clinic SHO

Referral Letter:
> Dear Colleague,
>
> Mr Ee Chee presents with a 2-month history of rashes. Please see and manage.
>
> Thank you.
>
> Dr Lydia Chuah, GP

Vital Signs: BP 146/87 mmHg, HR 57/min, RR 15/min, SpO2 99% RA, T 35.8°C

Patient's Brief

Synopsis: *A middle-aged gentleman has a psoriatic flare precipitated by alcohol, steroids, and beta blocker exposure. He also has psoriatic arthropathy.*

Open the consult with: These rashes flared 2 months ago and I can't bear the itch. Is this because of stress at work? *Do not volunteer any other information unless asked.*

History of current problem:
- Your rashes are very extensive, covering both legs, the back of both arms, your trunk (especially near the umbilicus), back, scalp, and pubic region. Your hands and feet are not affected, but there is some nail discolouration.
- You have always had mild rash over the same areas for many years. However, it never really bothered you until 2 months ago when things became much worse.
- You do not have childhood eczema.
- The GP gave you some moisturiser and antifungal creams, but these did not work.
- You have tried some herbal scrubs over your entire body, but they did not make the rashes any better. The last time you applied these herbal scrubs was a month ago.
- The pruritus has been unbearable; disrupting your daily life and your sleep.

- You have been having bilateral finger and knuckle pain for some time. This is worse in the morning and gets better as you move about during the day. There is morning stiffness lasting 2 hours. You do not have pain or swelling of any other joints. You have no back pain.
- You do not have any difficulty breathing, palpitations, red eye, painful eye, or swollen joints or tendons.
- You have no weight loss, fever, night sweats, urethral discharge, unexplained diarrhoea, or neck/groin lumps.

Past medical and surgical history:
- Angina. You have been experiencing intermittent exertional chest pain since 3 months ago. A cardiologist had done some tests and advised you to take medication as needed for chest pain.
- Asthma. You have had asthma since childhood. You have been off regular inhalers for many years; however, you had a flare-up 1 month ago. It resolved after your GP gave you a course of oral steroids.
- Hyperlipidaemia.

Medication list:
- Aspirin 100 mg OM
- Bisoprolol 5 mg OM – started 3 months ago
- Atorvastatin 20 mg ON
- Salbutamol inhaler PRN
- You had a course of PO prednisolone 30 mg OM × 1 week a month ago
- Supplements and herbal remedies: herbal scrubs (see above)
- Drug allergy: nil

Family history:
- Nil

Relevant personal, social, occupational, and travel history:
- You are a salesman; work has been stressful.
- You are married with two teenage children.
- You smoke 2 packs a day, and have done so since your teenage years.
- You drink frequently due to the need for business entertainment. Most weekdays, you take up to 4–5 glasses of wine plus a few shots of hard liquor.

Relevant physical examination findings:
- Extensive scaly, excoriated erythematous plaques over the trunk, extensor surfaces of upper and lower limbs (Photos 4 and 5), umbilicus, gluteal cleft, scalp, and post-auricular regions. There is no annularity, central clearing, or satellite lesions. There are no foot ulcers, and no pustules. Approximately 30% of the body's surface area is affected.

Consultation Case 08

- Hands and nails: onycholysis and nail pitting (Photo 6). There is synovitis of the metacarpophalangeal joints, but no deformities.
- Back – normal range of motion, no sacroilitis (negative sacroiliac compression test).
- Achilles tendon not swollen.
- No red eye.

Photo to be shown to candidate upon request (use colour plates for full-colour photos).

Photo 4 **Photo 5**

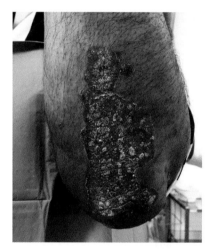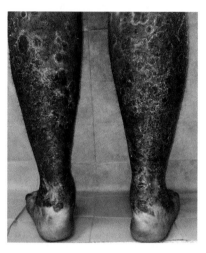

Clinical photos 4 and 5 generously provided by Dr Stanley Angkodjojo, Sengkang General Hospital

Photo 6

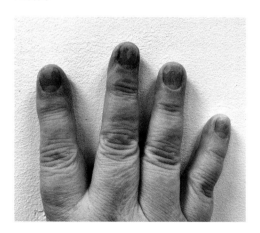

Clinical photo 6 generously provided by Dr Jon Yoong Kah Choun, Singapore General Hospital

You have some specific questions for the doctor at this consultation:
- Is this rash infectious? Can I spread it to my wife and children?
- Will it go away?

Approach and Clinical Reasoning

It is wise to deviate from the typical history taking and physical examination sequence, and instead ask to view the rash right at the start.

Pitfall: Additional questions in a simple 'psoriasis' case

> A straightforward case of psoriasis that poses neither diagnostic nor management difficulty may be considered too easy for PACES. Many exam centres incorporate additional issues such as extra-cutaneous manifestations or precipitants of psoriasis. Look out for these.

1. **Establish the diagnosis of psoriasis**. This should be a spot diagnosis.

   Important differentials include:
   - Allergic contact dermatitis from the 'herbal scrubs' – these can persist after cessation of use of herbal scrubs.
   - Tinea corporis.
   - Eczema.
   - Less likely possibilities:
     - Cutaneous lupus.
     - Mycosis fungoides (cutaneous T-cell lymphoma).

2. **Look for a precipitant**. Important precipitants of psoriasis include:
   - Drugs: beta blockers, steroids, lithium, antimalarials.
   - Infections: bacterial (streptococcal), HIV.
   - Metabolic risk factors: smoking, alcohol, obesity.

   Mr Ee Chee has had exposure to beta blockers, steroids, and alcohol.

3. **Look for extra-cutaneous manifestations and associations**
   - Arthropathy – both axial and appendicular skeleton can be affected. Mr Ee Chee does have inflammatory small joint arthropathy.
   - Dactylitis.
   - Tendinitis.
   - Uveitis.
   - Psoriasis is associated with the metabolic syndrome. Consider screening for obesity, hypertension, and diabetes.

4. **Assess severity and complications**
   - Body surface area >10% denotes severe disease.

- Pustular psoriasis (crops of pustules on flexures, trunk, palms and soles) or erythroderma denotes unstable disease.
- Secondary bacterial infection.
- Complications from treatment (e.g., steroid skin atrophy, systemic therapies such as ciclosporine, methotrexate)

As you move to physical examination, systematically examine all areas affected by the psoriatic rash — ask to examine the umbilicus, gluteal cleft, and scalp, which are favourite areas affected by psoriasis. Examine for other manifestations of psoriasis in the nails (pitting, onycholysis), joints (psoriatic arthropathy), tendons (enthesitis), and eyes (uveitits).

Question and Answer

Suggested answer to the patient's concerns:

Mr Ee Chee, I don't think this rash is something that can spread by touch from one person to another. I think you have psoriasis, which happens when the skin cells are triggered to grow too fast. It may have been triggered by some of the medications you are on. I will need to consider other causes of this rash, such as allergic reaction to the herbal scrubs.

I will get some tests organised. Once we get these out of the way, I will start you on treatment. I do think that with treatment, we have a good chance of controlling the rash. There is no cure for this, but it can certainly be treated by aiming for the rashes to resolve and maintaining control subsequently.

Suggested presentation to the examiner:

Mr Ee Chee has psoriasis, as evidenced by scaly erythematous plaques over the trunk, limbs, gluteal cleft, and perineal region, associated with onycholysis and nail pitting. There is inflammatory joint pain and synovitis, indicative of psoriatic arthropathy. There is no dactylitis, enthesitis, or uveitis. Possible triggers for psoriasis include beta blocker and steroid use. Differentials include allergic contact dermatitis from herbal scrubs, eczema, and fungal infection.

Investigations:
- Psoriasis is a clinical diagnosis, but I will like to perform a skin scraping for fungal microscopy to exclude tinea.
- I will do an X-ray of the hands and feet, looking for erosions such as a pencil-in-cup appearance and keeping in view spine imaging if any back pain develops.
- I will also check baseline labs including a blood count, CRP, ESR, and renal and liver function.
- I will look for associated metabolic diseases by checking fasting glucose and lipids.
- Prior to starting immunosuppression, I will check hepatitis viral serology, HIV, chest X-ray, and tuberculosis interferon gamma release assay.

Treatment:

- Remove precipitants – discuss with the cardiologist whether the beta blocker could be switched to another anti-anginal agent, stop corticosteroids, and insist on smoking cessation.
- Systemic therapy will be indicated in view of psoriatic arthropathy. First-line therapy will be a nonbiologic DMARD (e.g., methotrexate, sulfasalazine, azathioprine, or cyclosporine). If response is suboptimal, biologic therapy (TNF-alpha or IL-17 inhibitor) will be indicated.
- Note: Topical therapy (steroids, retinoids, calcipotriol) or phototherapy will be ineffective for arthritis. They remain useful adjuncts, but would not be appropriate sole therapy in this scenario.
- Note: Nonbiologic DMARDs are not used if arthritis is axial (vs. peripheral). Axial disease is managed along the lines of ankylosing spondylitis – physiotherapy and NSAIDs for mild disease, or biologics for moderate to severe disease.
- Adjuncts include antihistamine for itch, patient education, and support groups.
- Treat comorbids including metabolic syndrome.

Consultation Case 09

Mrs Lump (Rash)

Use this case as practice! The pull-out booklet contains the candidate's information.

Information for the Candidate

Patient Details:	Mrs S. Lump, 40 years old
Your Role:	Dermatology Senior House Officer
Scenario:	Mrs Lump complains of lower limb rash.
Vital Signs:	BP 100/70 mmHg, HR 50/min, RR 10/min, SpO2 97% RA, T 36.0°C

Patient's Brief

Synopsis: *A middle-aged lady presents with erythema nodosum, migratory polyarthralgia, and cough suggestive of sarcoidosis (Lofgren syndrome).*

Open the consult with: I have been having this rash on my legs for the past 2 weeks. *Do not volunteer any other information unless asked.*

History of current problem:
- These lumps started suddenly and grew larger and more painful over the last 2 weeks.
- They are not pruritic. The lumps are limited to both shins and you do not have any other rashes.
- You have also been having a low grade fever for the past 2 weeks.
- You have had intermittent joint pain. Earlier this week, your right shoulder and left knee were painful. Yesterday, your left hand and right knee were painful. Today, both ankles are painful. The pain is nonspecific, not worse with movement or with rest. There is no joint swelling.
- You have also had a dry cough for the last 1–2 weeks, which is not worse at any particular time of day or with any particular activity, and not worse lying down. You have not seen any physician or taken any medication for this complaint.
- You do not have any chronic cough, weight loss, night sweats, personal or family history of tuberculosis, or lumps in your neck or groin.
- You have no abdominal pain, diarrhoea, blood in your stools, or mouth ulcers.

- You have no constipation and no increase in urinary frequency or volume.
- You do not have any red eyes or blurred vision.

Past medical and surgical history:
- Nil
- No past medical history or contact history of tuberculosis.

Medication list:
- Nil
- Supplements and herbal remedies: combined oral contraceptive pill.
- Drug allergy: nil

Family history:
- No relevant family history including tuberculosis, bowel problems, etc.

Relevant personal, social, occupational, and travel history:
- You are married with 2 daughters.
- You work as a childcare teacher.
- Your last menstrual period is 1 week ago and you are certain that you are not pregnant.
- No relevant travel history.

Photo 7

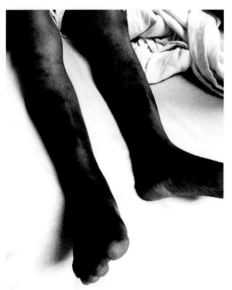

Relevant physical examination findings:
- Multiple 2 × 2 cm tender nodules on both anterior shins.
- No joint swelling, tenderness, or enthesitis; gait normal.
- Tongue moist, not dehydrated.
- Chest clear.
- No lymphadenopathy.

Photo to be shown to candidate upon request (use colour plates for full-colour photos)

Clinical photo generously provided by Assoc Prof Derrick Aw, Sengkang General Hospital

You have some specific questions for the doctor at this consultation:
- What is happening to me, is this cancer?
- Will I get better?

Approach and Clinical Reasoning

You should recognise the typical appearance and distribution of erythema nodosum. Ulceration should be absent. Any atypical features must prompt consideration of differentials (Table B4.1).

Table B4.1. Differentials for shin lumps.

Cause	Important clinical features
Erythema nodosum	Tender, well-defined lumps on anterior shins
Erythema induratum (nodular vasculitis)	Ulcerated nodules, typically on posterior calves Associated with tuberculosis
Lupus panniculitis	Tender nodules and plaques, which tend to develop on the face, upper arms, hips and trunk; less likely on lower limbs
Medium vessel vasculitis (e.g., polyarteritis nodosa)	Palpable purpura, ulcers, subcutaneous nodules, or peripheral gangrene. May be accompanied by constitutional symptoms (fever, myalgia).
Infection – abscesses, carbuncles	Bacterial, fungi or non-tuberculous mycobacteria. Typically, solitary. May be fluctuant and ulcerate.

Do not stop at the diagnosis of erythema nodosum (EN), but search for an underlying cause (Table B4.2). Mrs Lump presents with EN, migratory polyarthralgia, and pulmonary symptoms, which is highly suggestive of Lofgren's syndrome, a form of sarcoidosis. Differentials include:

Table B4.2. Associations with erythema nodosum ('*NODOSUMM*').

Association	Comment
NO cause – idiopathic	Idopathic in up to 50–60% of patients
Drugs	Penicillins, sulphonamides, NSAIDs
Oestrogen	Pregnancy, oral contraceptives
Sarcoidosis	Look for other manifestations of sarcoidosis (see below)
Ulcerative colitis and Crohn's	Bloody diarrhoea, oral ulcers
Microbes – infections	Streptococcal throat infection Tuberculosis Others: chlamydia, gastroenteritis, viral illnesses
Malignancy	Lymphoma (most often Hodgkin's lymphoma) Leukaemia, other carcinomas

- EN associated with streptococcal throat infection, in view of the history of cough and fever.
- EN due to oral contraceptive pill use.

Don't forget: Always look for underlying causes

> Do not stop at clinching the obvious diagnosis, but look for underlying causes and disease associations!

Finally, if time permits, screen for other manifestations of sarcoidosis. The manifestations of sarcoidosis include:
- Pulmonary – cough, bilateral hilar adenopathy, reticular opacities, or consolidation.
- Musculoskeletal – polyarthritis (acute or chronic).
- Cutaneous – papular or nodular sarcoidosis, lupus pernio, erythema nodosum.
- Hypercalcaemia – polyuria/polydipsia, constipation, renal colic, lethargy.
- Eye – red eyes, blurring of vision, eye pain.
- ENT – sinusitis, hoarseness of voice.
- Hematologic – lymphadenopathy, hepatosplenomegaly.
- Others – mononeuritis multiplex, cardiac atrioventricular conduction block.

Physical examination should focus on evaluating the shin nodules and demonstrating the other features of sarcoidosis (i.e., examining joints, chest, eyes, lymph nodes, and hydration status).

Question and Answer

Suggested answer to the patient's concerns:

Thank you for sharing your concern with me. I don't think this is cancer. You have 'erythema nodosum', which is basically a fancy term for saying 'red lumps'. This sometimes occurs without any good reason, sometimes after a throat infection, or in people who are taking contraceptive pills. In your case, I am also suspecting sarcoidosis, which can affect the lung, joints, and skin. The cause of sarcoidosis is debated, but it is not cancerous.

I will need to do some tests for you, including a chest X-ray and some blood tests, which will help me rule out other causes of these lumps and see if there are any other organs involved in sarcoidosis. Let's do the tests now and I will review you in my afternoon clinic.

Most patients with this condition get better within weeks to a few months, although there is a risk of it coming back later. I will start you on some medicine if these tests confirm what I think. Please stop your contraceptive pills and use another form of contraception, as the pills can worsen the lumps. I will have to review you in a few weeks. If you are not better, we will refer you to a dermatologist for further treatment.

Suggested presentation to the examiner:

Mrs Lump presents with erythema nodosum, migratory polyarthralgia, pulmonary symptoms, and fever. Examination is significant for erythema nodosum; there is no active arthritis and her chest is clear. My diagnosis is sarcoidosis, more specifically Lofgren's syndrome. Erythema nodosum secondary to contraceptive pills or streptococcal throat infection are differentials.

Investigations:

- I will like to confirm my diagnosis and look for other manifestations of sarcoidosis by doing:
  - Chest X-ray for bilateral hilar lymphadenopathy.
  - Serum angiotensin converting enzyme (elevated in sarcoidosis but can be normal in Lofgren's syndrome).
  - Serum electrolytes, particularly calcium.
  - Skin biopsy to confirm diagnosis and elucidate type of panniculitis (although classic Lofgren's syndrome does not require a biopsy for diagnosis; in practice skin biopsy is typically offered to the patient as part of work up).
- Checking for differentials including:
  - Chest X-ray for tuberculosis
  - Anti streptolysin O titre
  - Full blood count for infection or malignancy

Management wise, I will involve a multidisciplinary team including dermatology, respiratory medicine, and rheumatology specialists.

- First-line treatment for erythema nodosum is removal of underlying precipitating causes (e.g., stopping offending drugs) and treatment of sarcoidosis with oral steroids.
- Other treatment methods include NSAIDs, colchicine, and potassium iodide (watch for hypothyroidism).

Consultation Case 10

Mrs Sweet (Rash)

Use this case as practice! The pull-out booklet contains the candidate's information.

Information for the Candidate

Patient Details: Mrs C. Sweet, 35 years old

Your Role: Dermatology SHO

Referral Letter:

Dear Colleague,

Mrs Sweet is on follow up with me for diabetes mellitus. She has recently had an infected right lower limb wound. I have given two 1-week courses of co-amoxiclav without much improvement.

Please help with her management. Thank you.

Dr Nicholas Hong, GP

Vital Signs: BP 130/83 mmHg, HR 67/min, RR 10/min, SpO2 97% RA, T 37.0°C

Patient's Brief

Synopsis: *A 35-year-old has pyoderma gangrenosum, along with inflammatory small joint polyarthropathy suggestive of underlying rheumatoid arthritis.*

Open the consult with: The GP's medicine was no good. This wound is getting from bad to worse. *Do not volunteer any other information unless asked.*

History of current problem:

- One month ago, you sustained a minor scratch over your right shin while working in the garden. You did not think too much about it at the time. A small pimple developed at the site of injury. This broke to leave a small ulcer, which rapidly grew in size.
- The wound is painful but not pruritic.
- Apart from the wound, you do not have any lower limb pain at rest or on walking.
- Your legs are not swollen and do not feel heavy at the end of the day.
- You do not have any numbness in your feet, and have never had foot ulcers.
- For the past year, you have been having mild joint pains in the small joints of both hands, which is relieved by paracetamol. Joint pain seems to be worse with rest, but gets better with movement. This is associated with morning stiffness that lasts

1–2 hours. You have never had joint swelling. Your back and other joints are unaffected. You believe that these joint pains are due to 'rheumatism' as you age, and they do not affect you too much.

- No abdominal pain, diarrhoea, or rectal bleeding.
- No weight loss, neck/groin swelling, night sweats, or fevers.
- No red eye/eye pain, breathlessness, or chronic cough.

Past medical and surgical history:

- Diabetes mellitus, diagnosed 2 years ago while you were pregnant. Your latest HbA1c is 6.7%. You do not have any heart, eye, or kidney complications from diabetes.

Medication list:

- Metformin 500 mg TDS
- Dapagliflozin 5 mg OM
- Paracetamol 1000 mg QDS PRN for your joint pains
- Supplements and herbal remedies: nil
- Drug allergy: nil

Family history:

- Your mother had ulcerative colitis, which required a colectomy.

Relevant personal, social, occupational, and travel history:

- You work at a bus terminal which involves long hours of standing.
- You are married with one child, aged 2 years old. You are trying for a second child.
- You do not smoke or drink.
- Two months ago, you travelled to tropical Indonesia. You spent a night at a farm and learnt about rice planting in a paddy field.

Photo 8

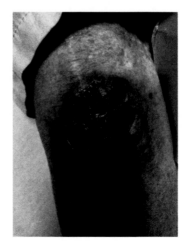

Relevant physical examination findings:

- 5 cm × 7 cm ulcer over the right distal shin. This has a violaceous rim, undermined edges, and sloughy base.
- Skin over lower limb is otherwise normal. No other ulcers, lipodermatosclerosis or hyperpigmentation, or shiny appearance.

Photo to be shown to candidate upon request (use colour plates for full-colour photos).

Clinical photo generously provided by Assoc Prof Derrick Aw, Sengkang General Hospital

- No pedal oedema.
- Dorsalis pedis pulse well felt.
- Pinprick sensation in the toes normal.
- Hands – no joint swelling or deformity. No rheumatoid nodules.

You have some specific questions for the doctor at this consultation:
- Is this ulcer related to my diabetes? My GP told me that diabetes can cause leg ulcers that heal poorly. But I have been controlling my diabetes so well. This is so unfair.
- My husband and I are trying for a child. Will this affect my ability to get pregnant?

Approach and Clinical Reasoning

Glance at the 'wound' at the beginning of the consult. Pyoderma gangrenosum is a spot diagnosis you should recognise, but it is important to consider differentials to a lower limb ulcer (Table B4.3). Note that Mrs Sweet has a significant exposure history 'learning about rice farming', which typically involves waterlogged paddy fields, and is at risk of nontuberculous mycobacterial infection.

Table B4.3. Differentials to a lower limb ulcer.

Cause	Important clinical features
Arterial insufficiency	Atherosclerotic risk factors, absent peripheral pulses, shiny hairless skin
Venous insufficiency	Leg swelling worse with prolonged standing, venous skin changes (venous eczema, lipodermatosclerosis), varicosities
Neuropathic ulcer	Longstanding diabetes, loss of pinprick sensation. Typical location on pressure points of the sole
Infective	Exposure to nontuberculous mycobacteria and fungi (e.g., soil and water exposure)
Inflammatory	Pyoderma gangrenosum: painful ulcer with undermined edges, history of pathergy
Malignant	Slow growing, painless, heaped up edges; may arise in a longstanding venous ulcer

Next, look for systemic associations with pyoderma gangrenosum including:
- Inflammatory bowel disease.
- Rheumatoid arthritis and other inflammatory arthritis.
- Myeloproliferative disorder, myeloma, or other malignancy.

Mrs Sweet does give a history of inflammatory small joint polyarthropathy, suggestive of rheumatoid arthritis. Screen quickly for other systemic manifestations of rheumatoid arthritis, of which she has none.

Examination should cover:

- The presenting complaint, her ulcer. Appreciate the typical features of pyoderma gangrenosum.
- The differentials to lower limb ulcers particularly in a diabetic — examine lower limb pulses and sensation, and look for signs of venous insufficiency.
- Her hands, looking for active synovitis (tenderness, joint swelling) and deformities typical of rheumatoid arthritis. Be aware that modern treatment of rheumatoid arthritis, particularly the early use of disease-modifying anti-rheumatic therapy, has made textbook deformities (e.g., ulnar deviation, swan neck deformity) relatively uncommon.
- Consider offering a rectal examination for rectal bleeding from inflammatory bowel disease.

Question and Answer

Suggested answer to the patient's concerns:

Mrs Sweet, I am very thankful that you have been so conscientious about controlling your diabetes. Indeed, diabetes is a common cause of leg ulcers, but I think that what you have is quite different and not related to diabetes. I suspect that you have this condition called pyoderma gangrenosum, which is a type of inflammation that causes ulcers. Your joint pains and stiffness also make me wonder if you have rheumatoid arthritis, which is associated with this type of ulcer. I will arrange for some blood tests and a biopsy of the rash.

As for pregnancy, this ulcer and the arthritis are both unlikely to affect your ability to conceive. However, pregnancy does affect the treatment of rheumatoid arthritis because some of the medications used are potentially harmful to a foetus. There are medications that are safer in pregnancy, and I think you would do well on them as your disease is relatively mild. It may be best to ensure that you are stable on these medications before trying for a baby. I will refer you to a rheumatologist who will be able to come up with a treatment plan bearing your desire for a child in mind.

Suggested presentation to the examiner:

Mrs Sweet has pyoderma gangrenosum as evidenced by a lower limb ulcer with violaceous rim, sloughy base, and undermined edges. This may be due to underlying rheumatoid arthritis, although examination of her hands does not find any typical rheumatoid deformities or active synovitis. A differential for the lower limb ulcer includes chronic infection with non-tuberculous mycobacteria or fungi, as Mrs Sweet has an exposure history to rice paddies. Her diabetes is well controlled and there is no evidence of neuropathy or peripheral arterial disease.

Investigations:

- I will confirm my diagnosis by doing a skin biopsy and send it for:
  - Histopathology.
  - Tissue culture.
  - Acid-fast bacilli stain and cultures.
- I will do blood tests including:
  - Erythrocyte sedimentation rate and C-reactive protein for inflammation.
  - Auto-antibodies including rheumatoid factor and anti-cyclic citrullinated peptide.
  - Full blood count, peripheral blood film, and myeloma panel for haematological disease.
  - Renal and liver biochemistries in view of the intent to start immunosuppression.

Management: Mrs Sweet will benefit from multidisciplinary team management involving the dermatologist, rheumatologist, and allied health professionals. This includes:

- Topical measures such as dressings, topical steroids and topical calcineurin inhibitors.
- After exclusion of infection, a consideration of disease-modifying anti-rheumatic drugs such as ciclosporin or infliximab.
- Patient education.
- Analgesia.

Consultation Case 11

Ms McDonald (Weight Gain)

Use this case as practice! The pull-out booklet contains the candidate's information.

Information for the Candidate

Patient Details: Ms McDonald, 40 years old

Your Role: Endocrine Clinic SHO

Referral Letter:
> Dear Colleague,
>
> Ms McDonald was referred from the GP for bariatric surgery. I agree that this is strongly indicated, but could I please have you on board to optimise her diabetic control? Her latest hbA1c is still 8.2% despite three oral hypoglycaemic agents.
>
> Thank you.
>
> Dr Kentucky, General Surgery

Vital Signs: BP 148/92 mmHg, HR 80/min, RR 13/min, SpO2 99% RA, T 37.1°C

Patient's Brief

Synopsis: *This lady with weight gain and poorly controlled diabetes has underlying Cushing's syndrome.*

Open the consult with: I've been putting on quite a lot of weight. My GP referred me for bariatric surgery, but the surgeon has asked me to see you first. *Do not volunteer any other information unless asked.*

History of current problem:

- You have always been on the plump side, but your weight has increased from 80 kg (176 lb) half a year ago to 96 kg (211 lb) at present.
- You tend to binge-eat when stressed or upset, and you take fast food at least 3 times a week. This has been your diet since your early adult years.
- You are also concerned about your appearance — your acne is worsening, and you have unsightly abdominal stretch marks.
- You have a number of bruises over your skin, and you noticed that your skin is becoming thinner.
- You do not have any cold intolerance or constipation.

- Your periods are regular and neither spotty/light nor excessively heavy.
- You have bilateral leg swelling, most pronounced at the end of a long day on your feet and associated with a dull ache in both legs. You do not have any breathlessness, frothy urine, jaundice, or change in urine colour.
- You have no muscle weakness.
- You do not have difficulty seeing; you do not complain of bumping into things on your sides or getting into car accidents. You have no headaches.
- You do not have balding, deepening of voice, or increased pubic hair growth.
- You do not have chronic cough or breathlessness.

Past medical and surgical history:
- Asthma. This is well controlled on a daily puff. You have not needed oral steroids for many years.
- Diabetes, diagnosed 9 months ago. Your latest HbA1c is 8.2%. Control has not been optimal despite your GP adding on multiple drugs.
- Hypertension, diagnosed 7 months ago.
- Depression, diagnosed 4 years ago after your divorce.

Medication list:
- Amitryptyline 10 mg ON
- Budesonide 50 mcg inhaler, 2 puffs BD
- Dapagliflozin, 5 mg OM
- Gliclazide modified release 60 mg OM
- Losartan 50 mg OM
- Metformin 850 mg BD
- Salbutamol 100 mcg inhaler, PRN
- Supplements and herbal remedies: nil
- Drug allergy: nil

Family history:
- Nil

Relevant personal, social, occupational, and travel history:
- You work as a clothing salesperson. This involves standing for long hours. You are concerned that your physical unattractiveness will compromise your job.
- You do not smoke or drink.
- You are divorced with no children.
- Your last menstrual period was 1 week ago. You are certain that you are not pregnant.

Relevant physical examination findings:

- Centripedal obesity with dorsocervical and supraclavicular adiposities.
- Facial plethora, acne.
- Thin skin, occasional bruising.
- Abdominal distension with violaceous striae (Photo 9), no abdominal masses.
- Visual fields and eye movements normal.
- Muscle power normal.
- No pedal oedema, jugular venous pressure not elevated.

Photo 9

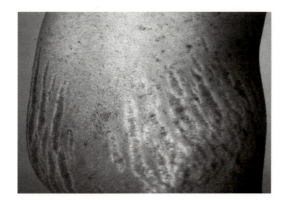

Reproduced with permission from DermNet NZ www.dermnetnz.org

You have some specific questions for the doctor at this consultation:

- My friend told me that I could be gaining weight because of the asthma inhalers. Is this true?

Approach and Clinical Reasoning

The candidate information in this scenario comes close to giving away the diagnosis of Cushing's syndrome — weight gain, poorly controlled diabetes, and hypertension. Consider the causes of weight gain (Table B4.4).

Key differentials for Ms McDonald's weight gain are:

- Cushing's syndrome – in view of worsening acne and abdominal stretch marks.
- Fluid overload – in view of bilateral leg swelling; however, her description of leg swelling is more characteristic of venous insufficiency.
- Drug-induced due to amitriptyline or gliclazide.

The next step is to look for an aetiology of Cushing's syndrome (Table B4.5). Ms McDonald does not have any clear suggestion of a specific cause of Cushing's syndrome.

Table B4.4. Common causes of/associations with weight gain.

Cause	Important clinical features
Fluid retention	Pedal oedema, symptoms of congestive heart failure/nephrotic syndrome/renal insufficiency/cirrhosis
Hypothyroidism	Cold intolerance, menorrhagia, constipation
Cushing's syndrome	Centripetal obesity, skin thinning, abdominal striae
Polycystic ovarian syndrome	Oligomenorrhoea, hirsuitism, subfertility
Drug-induced weight gain	Drug history: corticosteroids, antipsychotics, antidepressants, antiepileptics, sulphonylureas, insulin
Pregnancy	Amenorrhoea
Psychiatric	Binge eating, often associated with anxiety, depression, or post-traumatic stress disorder
Diet and lifestyle	Exclusion of all other secondary causes

Table B4.5. Localisation of Cushing's syndrome.

Localisation	Important clinical features
Exogenous steroid use	Drug history, including supplements and herbal remedies
Pituitary adenoma (Cushing's disease)	Bitemporal hemianopia, headache, suppression of other endocrine axes, hyperpigmentation (from ACTH excess). The absence of these features does not rule out Cushing's disease, which is often due to a microadenoma.
Adrenal tumour	Signs of androgen excess (hirsutism, virilization e.g., frontal balding, deepening voice, clitoral hypertrophy)
Ectopic ACTH production	Symptoms of underlying malignancy, most commonly lung. There may be weight loss rather than gain. Due to rapid disease progression, physical signs of Cushing's syndrome may be absent.

Consider the complications of Cushing's syndrome. She already has new-onset diabetes and hypertension. Look out for proximal myopathy, neuropsychologic symptoms, cataracts, sleep apnoea, and so on.

Examination should focus on:

- Demonstrating the features of Cushing's syndrome. Note that extremely florid signs are unlikely as the patient would have been treated.
- Looking for a cause of Cushing's syndrome.
- Checking for differentials (i.e., looking for a thyroidectomy scar, pedal oedema).

Consultation Case 11

Practice makes perfect: The Cushing's examination

Prepare a 'set-piece' examination routine for the Cushing's syndrome patient. The only way to be smooth in the exam is to have rehearsed! A possible routine could include:

- Inspection for centripetal obesity, limb wasting, hyperpigmentation (suggests ACTH access)
- Face – hirsutism, acne, plethora, rounded countenance (do not say 'moon face')
- Eyes – visual fields (bitemporal hemianopia), eye movements
- Neck – dorsocervical and supraclavicular fat pads
- Arms – thin skin, easy bruising, proximal weakness
- Abdomen – violaceous striae, abdominal masses, surgical scars

Question and Answer

Suggested answer to the patient's concerns:

Ms McDonald, you are right that steroids can cause weight gain. However, low-dose inhaled steroids for asthma are unlikely to lead to this complication. I suspect that your weight gain may be caused by the hormone glands in your body overproducing steroids. It may also be due to the diabetes and depression medicine that you are taking.

I don't need to admit you, but let's do some tests to confirm the diagnosis. I will give you a tablet to take overnight. The next morning, come in exactly at 8am to do a blood test. I will also ask you to collect a 24-hour urine sample. Depending on these test results, I may need to order some scans to see which of your hormone glands are enlarged. In the meantime, it is important that you continue to take your asthma inhalers and do not stop them.

Suggested presentation to the examiner:

Ms McDonald presents with weight gain. Physical examination is significant for features of Cushing's syndrome such as violaceous abdominal striae, proximal weakness, thin skin and easy bruising, centripetal obesity, dorsal cervical adiposity, acne, and facial plethora. In terms of the aetiology of Cushing's syndrome, there is no bitemporal hemianopia to suggest a pituitary tumour, no history of virilisation to suggest an adrenal tumour, and no cough or haemoptysis to suggest lung cancer and ectopic ACTH production. There is no exogenous steroid use. Differentials to Cushing's syndrome include drug-induced weight gain from sulphonylureas and antidepressants.

Investigations:

- I will like to confirm my diagnosis by doing a low-dose dexamethasone suppression test, 24 h urine free cortisol, and/or midnight salivary cortisol (2 positive tests required to confirm the diagnosis).
- Next, I will localise the lesion with a basal ACTH level (differentiate ACTH-dependent vs. ACTH-independent Cushing's syndrome).

- If ACTH is high, the next step is a high dose dexamethasone suppression test (differentiates between Cushing's disease and ectopic ACTH secretion), MRI pituitary, formal visual field testing, and checking the rest of the anterior pituitary hormones.
- If ACTH is low, I will do a CT of the adrenal glands.

She will benefit from a multidisciplinary team approach to management involving the endocrinologist, pituitary surgeon, and allied health professionals.

- The first principle is to treat the underlying disease.
    - If she has Cushing's disease, the gold standard is transphenoidal resection of pituitary tumour, although radiotherapy and medical treatment with ketoconazole are alternatives.
    - If she has an adrenal tumour, adrenalectomy is the option of choice. Subsequently she will require replacement hydrocortisone and fludrocortisone.
- Complications need to be managed. I will optimise her sugar and blood pressure control.
- Adjuncts include patient education and support groups.

Consultation Case 12

Mdm Grumps (Headache)

Use this case as practice! The pull-out booklet contains the candidate's information.

Information for the Candidate

Patient Details: Mdm Grumps, 50 years old

Your Role: Neurology Clinic SHO

Referral Letter:

> Dear Colleague,
>
> I've been seeing Mdm Grumps for migraine. However, her headaches have gotten worse recently and doesn't respond completely to analgesia. Think it's best if you have a look at her.
>
> Thank you.
>
> Dr Linus Chua, GP

Vital Signs: BP 120/80 mmHg, HR 70/min, RR 14/min, SpO2 99% RA, T 36.0°C

Patient's Brief

Synopsis: *A 50-year-old lady presents with a new headache, transient visual disturbances, jaw claudication, lethargy, and polymyalgia. The diagnosis is giant cell arteritis.*

Open the consult with: I've always had migraines, but the headaches have been terrible over the past month. I'm just not feeling like my usual self. *Do not volunteer any other information unless asked.*

History of current problem:

- You usually have 2–3 migraine headaches a month. These headaches are typically unilateral, severe (pain score 8/10), and associated with nausea, flashing lights, and sensitivity to light. They are usually triggered by poor sleep. They usually resolve within 24 hours with painkillers and rest in a dark and quiet environment.

- You have been having near-continuous headaches over the past month, which started insidiously and gradually worsened with time. This headache is left-sided, severe (pain score 8/10), and constant. It is not worse during a particular time of day.

- If prompted by the candidate, you will realise that the current headache feels different from your usual migraine headaches.
- You have taken painkillers daily over the past month, but the headache has only gotten worse. You feel restless due to the headache.
- This headache is not exacerbated by sneezing, coughing, or lying down.
- Additionally, you have noticed intermittent darkening of your left eye's vision, without concomitant pain, redness, drooping of the eyelid, or double vision.
- You have been having jaw soreness over the past week, which was particularly noticeable when chewing tough meat.
- You have no scalp tenderness when combing your hair.
- You have been feeling lethargic, and your muscles feel achy and sore. However, your joints feel fine and you experienced no weakness or numbness in your limbs.
- You have lost 3 kg over the past month and your appetite is poor.
- You have no fever, neck stiffness, rash, head injury/trauma, slurring of speech, facial weakness, facial droop, limb weakness, or numbness.

Past medical and surgical history:
- Migraine, as above.
- You are of normal habitus.
- Your health was screened several months ago by your company doctor, and you do not have diabetes mellitus, high cholesterol, or hypertension.

Medication list:
- Paracetamol 1 g QDS PRN (Taken daily for past month).
- Diclofenac 75 mg BD PRN with Omeprazole 20 mg BD PRN (Taken daily in past month).
- Cafergot (ergotamine tartrate 1 mg/caffeine 100 mg), 1 tab PRN (12 tablets taken in past week).
- Supplements and herbal remedies: nil
- Drug allergy: nil

Family history:
- Nil

Relevant personal, social, occupational, and travel history:
- You are the senior partner of a legal firm. The nature of work is highly stressful. You are concerned that these headaches may affect your work.
- You are unmarried and without children.
- You did not travel recently.
- You do not smoke or drink.
- You do not drive (you have a chauffeur).

Relevant physical examination findings:

This station can be run with either a real patient (who has been treated) or a surrogate.

- Conjunctiva appears normal bilaterally.
- Visual acuity is normal bilaterally.
- Both pupils are equal and reactive to light.
- Swinging torch test was negative for relative pupillary afferent defect.
- The visual fields are normal.
- Cranial nerve findings were unremarkable.
- Examination of the limbs was negative for sensorimotor and cerebellar deficits.
- Temporal arteries were well felt and non-tender.
- Fundoscopy (provide finding, need not attempt): swollen left optic disc.

You have some specific questions for the doctor at this consultation:

- Do I have a brain tumour?
- Can you make this headache go away?

Approach and Clinical Reasoning

Mdm Grumps presents with a new headache superimposed on a history of typical migraine. You have to be careful and specific with this history — many candidates fall into the trap of eliciting the features of her headache in general, and either failing to recognise that her new headache is quite distinct from usual migraine or mashing up features of the two. Your main aim is to look for features suggesting life-threatening causes of headache, such as thunderclap onset, neurological deficits, and fever and neck stiffness (Figure B4.1), and to specifically consider the headache syndromes which have associated concomitant visual disturbances (Table B4.6).

The important differentials for Mdm Grump's headaches will include:

- Giant cell arteritis, given visual symptoms, jaw claudication, and systemic features of polymyalgia rheumatica.
- Medication overuse headache, as she has taken painkillers daily for the past month.

Think this through: Headache in systemic illnesses

> Which systemic illnesses can present with headaches? Some examples to get you started include polycystic kidney disease (subarachnoid haemorrhage) and scleroderma (renal crisis with hypertensive urgency). You will see that the differential net has to be cast very wide indeed.

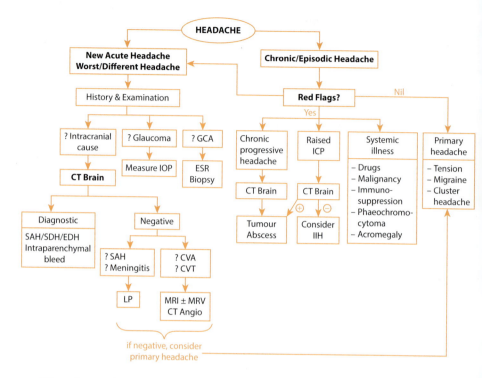

CVA: cerebrovascular accident; CVT: cerebral venous thrombosis; EDH: extradural haemorrhage; ESR: erythrocyte sedimentation rate; GCA: giant cell arthritis; IIH: idiopathic intracranial hypertension; IOP: intraocular pressure; LP: lumbar puncture; MRV: magnetic resonance venogram; SAH: subarachnoid haemorrhage; SDH: subdural haemorrhage

Figure B4.1. Approach to headache.

The key tasks on physical examination are to:

- Look for features of giant cell arteritis – examine for temporal artery tenderness and decreased visual acuity.
- Consider differentials – check for red eye (uveitis), fixed mid-dilated pupils (glaucoma), and bitemporal hemianopia[5] (pituitary adenoma).
- Screen for any neurological deficits.
- Fundoscopy may support the diagnosis by showing optic disk swelling (anterior ischaemic optic neuropathy) or cotton wool spots (retinal ischaemia).

Fundoscopy is vital in the examination of a patient with headaches, especially when atypical or sinister features are present. While the actual act of fundoscopy may be substituted with printed retinal photos due to time constraints, PACES candidates are expected to be proficient in direct fundoscopy and to be familiar with common abnormalities encountered in internal medicine.

---

[5] Quadrantanopias from branch retinal artery occlusion have been described in giant cell arteritis, although these are rare.

Table B4.6. Important causes of headache with visual disturbance for PACES.

Cause	Important clinical features
Giant cell arteritis	Age > 50, unilateral headache, jaw claudication, scalp tenderness, symptoms of polymyalgia rheumatica. May have optic disk swelling. Elevated erythrocyte sedimentation rate. Note: These patients present not with red eye or eye pain, but with visual blurring (arteritic anterior ischaemic optic neuropathy) or acute visual loss (central retinal artery occlusion).
Idiopathic intracranial hypertension	Typically overweight, female, childbearing age; bilateral headache worse when lying down or coughing. Fundoscopy is crucial and may reveal bilateral papilloedema.
Pituitary adenoma, apoplexy, etc.	Bitemporal hemianopia, systemic features of endocrinopathies (e.g., signs and symptoms of acromegaly)
Acute glaucoma	Red eye, fixed mid-dilated pupils
Uveitis	Red eye (absent in posterior uveitis), history of rheumatologic illness (e.g., rheumatoid arthritis, psoriasis)
Migraine with visual aura	Characteristic episodic headaches, positive visual phenomena (flashes of lights, zig-zag patterns, etc.)

As you move to address the patient's concerns, appreciate that acute giant cell arteritis is a sight-threatening emergency. Early initiation of steroid treatment is paramount and can prevent permanent visual loss.

Question and Answer

Suggested answer to the patient's concerns:

Mdm Grumps, this headache must be incredibly frustrating and worrying for you. I don't think a brain tumour is likely at this point, and we will need further tests to ensure that's not the case. However, the current headache appears different from your usual migraine headaches, especially when you also have visual problems, soreness when you chew, and muscle aches. I am worried that you may instead have an inflammatory condition called giant cell arteritis, in which your blood vessels, including those supplying your eyes, are inflamed. It is a serious condition as it can cause permanent blindness. I need to have you admitted urgently for further tests and treatment. If it truly turns out to be giant cell arteritis, the main treatment involves taking steroids, and the headache usually improves significantly.

Suggested presentation to the examiner:

Mdm Grumps presents with a new headache on a background of migraine. Her new headache is associated with transient visual disturbances, jaw claudication, lethargy, and polymyalgia. Her neurologic examination was otherwise unremarkable for significant deficits, and the temporal arteries were non-tender when palpated. My primary diagnosis is giant cell arteritis. My differentials include medication-overuse headache. Intracranial tumour is less likely.

I will admit her. Investigations include:

- Confirming my diagnosis by:
  - Checking erythrocyte sedimentation rate.
  - Performing temporal artery ultrasound and biopsy.
- Referral to an ophthalmologist for slit lamp examination (looking for features of optic nerve or retinal ischaemia), intraocular pressure measurement by Goldmann tonometry, and visual field testing.
- CT brain.
- Other routine labs including a full blood count, renal and liver biochemistries, and preparation for immunosuppression such as hepatitis B/C/HIV serology.

A multidisciplinary team inclusive of an ophthalmologist and a rheumatologist will be required to advise on her current and future treatment. She will require high dose oral steroids to prevent permanent visual loss; this should be started urgently without waiting for temporal artery biopsy results[6]. Additionally, her pain control should be optimised in accordance to the WHO analgesic ladder.

---

[6] The temporal artery biopsy can also be falsely negative due to skip lesions.

Consultation Case 13

Ms Ache (Painful Hands)

Use this case as practice! The pull-out booklet contains the candidate's information.

Information for the Candidate

Patient Details: Ms Ache, 28 years old

Your Role: Neurology Clinic SHO

Referral Letter:
> Dear Colleague,
>
> Thank you for seeing this pleasant lady who is complaining of painful hands but there doesn't appear to be an orthopaedic issue. Perhaps it could be a nerve problem?
>
> Thank you.
>
> Dr Carpenter, Orthopaedic Surgeon

Vital Signs: BP 100/62 mmHg, HR 57/min, RR 14/min, SpO2 95% RA, T 37.0°C

Patient's Brief

Synopsis: *A young lady presents with painful hands and the Raynaud's syndrome on a background of occupational exposure to vibrating tools, drug history of ergots and contraceptive pills, and smoking.*

Open the consult with: My hands have been painful for the past 3 months. The bone doctors gave me some painkillers, but it doesn't seem to get better. They said it could be a nerve problem and asked me to see you. *Do not volunteer any other information unless asked.*

History of current problem:

- Pain is most noticeable over the fingertips. There is no joint pain, stiffness, or swelling.
- Pain is not worsened by any specific movements of the hand or by rest.
- You have not noticed any numbness. However, when you enter a cold room or pick up a cold drink, your fingers turn white and then blue and feel slightly 'odd'. When the fingers are re-warmed, they turn pink before going back to normal.
- No weakness of hand grip, loss of dexterity of the fingers, or tingling sensation.
- No trauma to the hands.

- No fever.
- No pain in the neck, back, lower limbs, or any other joints.
- No difficulty swallowing, constipation, dyspnoea, dry eyes, dry mouth, muscle pain, mouth ulcers, rashes, or haematuria.
- No decrease in effort tolerance, lightheadedness, or purpura.
- No weight loss, lymphadenopathy, or fatigue.

Past medical and surgical history:
- Migraine without aura. You get disabling attacks every 2–3 weeks and get by with cafergot.

Medication list:
- Cafergot (ergotamine 1 mg with caffeine 100 mg), 2 tablets PRN. This was given to you half a year ago for better control of your migraine, as NSAIDs did not work well.
- Oral contraceptive pill.
- Supplements and herbal remedies: nil
- Drug allergy: nil

Family history:
- Mother – systemic lupus erythematosus with kidney failure, required dialysis at 35 years old, passed away in her 40s.

Relevant personal, social, occupational, and travel history:
- You work for a boutique craft firm making bespoke furnishings. Your job scope includes the use of hand-held tools (e.g., saw, drill) to process wooden and metal furniture parts.
- You smoke 5 cigarettes a day and have done so for the last 10 years.
- You drink socially but not more than 7 units of alcohol per week.
- You are engaged to a steady boyfriend and are sexually active. You have no children.

Relevant physical examination findings:

Use of a surrogate is likely at this station.
- Hands – no colour change, joint deformities, joint swelling, muscle wasting.
- Fingertips – no clubbing, distal infarcts, pulp atrophy, telangiectasia, calcinosis, or sclerodactyly.
- Radial pulse well-felt bilaterally.
- Thumb abduction full power, Froment's sign negative, no finger numbness.
- No conjunctival pallor.
- No rashes (e.g., malar rash, livido reticularis, heliotrope rash, salt and pepper appearance); no microstomia.

You have some specific questions for the doctor at this consultation:

- My mother had lupus and was dialysis-dependent for 5 years before passing away in her 40s. Will the same happen to me?

Approach and Clinical Reasoning

The differential diagnosis of painful hands can be systemically considered by thinking through the five tissues of the hand (Table B4.7). Certain aetiologies (e.g., occult fractures) are unlikely in PACES, but you must still demonstrate a reasonable clinical approach. Begin with open-ended questions, asking the patient to describe the pain (whether this affects the joints, in particular or the whole fingers) and any associated symptoms (e.g., numbness, weakness, joint swelling, stiffness). This will allow you to narrow down to possible aetiologies relatively quickly. Inspect the limb early as the

Table B4.7. Differentials to painful hands.

Tissue	Differential	Important features
Bone and joint	• Inflammatory arthritis – rheumatoid, psoriatic • Gout	Inflammatory pain (worse on rest), prolonged early morning stiffness Joint deformity, swelling, tophi
	• Osteoarthritis	Long history of mechanical pain (worse on movement) Bouchard, Heberden nodes
	• Trauma including occult fractures (e.g., scaphoid)	History of trauma Anatomical snuffbox tenderness
Muscle and tendon	• Enthesitis (e.g., De Quervain's tenosynovitis)	Provocation tests (e.g., Finklestein)
Skin and soft tissue	• Infection (cellulitis, abscess, tenosynovitis) • Dactylitis	Erythema and swelling of soft tissues
Nerve	• Peripheral neuropathy – diabetes, vasculitis, etc. • Compression neuropathy – carpel tunnel syndrome • Cervical spondylotic radiculopathy with referred pain	Wasting, weakness of intrinsic hand muscles Numbness – glove and stocking or medial nerve distribution (see neurology physical exam)
Vessels	• Raynaud's syndrome • Takayasu arteritis	Colour changes, pulp atrophy Weak radial pulse, radial-radial or radial-femoral delay
	• Thromboarteritis obliterans (Buerger's syndrome)	Young smoker with digital extremity ischaemia/gangrene

physical examination might give you the answer (remember that you can take a history and examine in any order).

Ms Ache quite readily offers a history of colour changes triggered by cold exposure. Recognise the Raynaud's phenomenon and explore causes of a secondary Raynaud's syndrome (Table B4.8).

Table B4.8. Causes of Raynaud's syndrome.

Type	Category	Causes
Primary	Idiopathic Raynaud's syndrome (typical onset between 15–30 years old)	
Secondary	Rheumatologic disease	Systemic sclerosis
		Systemic lupus erythematosus
		Sjogren's syndrome
		Rheumatoid arthritis
		Dermatomyositis
		Mixed connective tissue disease
	Exposures	Smoking
		Use of vibrating tools
	Medications	Migraine analgesics (cafergot, triptans)
		Chemotherapy (cisplatin)
		Beta blockers
		Oral contraceptive pills
	Endocrine	Hypothyroidism
	Hyperviscosity	Paraprotein (myeloma, Waldenstrom macroglobulinemia)
		Cryoglobulinaemia

Possible causes of Ms Ache's Raynaud's syndrome are:
- Secondary to drugs – cafergot, contraceptive pill.
- Secondary to occupational vibrating tool exposure (hand-held drill and saw).
- Associated with underlying rheumatologic disease – it is important to exclude symptoms or signs of rheumatologic disease, particularly given her family history. Note that Raynaud's may precede the development of other symptoms/signs of disease.
- Idiopathic/primary (Raynaud's disease). Features in keeping with idiopathic Raynaud's syndrome, as opposed to a secondary cause, include (a) typical epidemiology (i.e., young female < 40 years old), (b) absence of ulceration or tissue loss, (c) symmetry, and (d) absence of signs or symptoms of underlying rheumatologic disease.

Examination of Ms Ache's hands proceeds along the time-tested 'look, feel, move' paradigm, but pay attention to each tissue in turn. Look for deformities and swellings of the bones, joints, and soft tissues, as well as signs of rheumatologic disease such as scleroderma (sclerodactyly, pulp atrophy, calcinosis) or rheumatoid arthritis. <u>Feel</u> the joints for swelling. <u>Move</u> the fingers and check their range of motion. Examine the median and ulnar nerves in motor and sensory domains, and check that the pulse is well felt. You may get a patient with instantly recognisable signs of rheumatologic disease, or you may get one with no signs at all.

Move to the face and body, checking for conjunctival pallor (haematologic disease), rashes associated with rheumatologic disease (e.g., malar rash, livido reticularis, heliotrope rash, salt and pepper appearance), and microstomia. If the patient has an identifiable rheumatologic disease, proceed to examine for disease manifestations in other organs (e.g., auscultate lungs for interstitial lung disease).

Question and Answer

Suggested answer to the patient's concerns:

Ms Ache, I am sorry to hear about your mother's passing. It must have been so difficult for you and your family. There is a possibility that the hand pain you have is due to lupus, but at this moment you do not exhibit other signs or symptoms of lupus, and there are many other causes of hand pain including the medications you are on, the vibrating tools you use at work, and smoking. Even if you do have lupus, you can be treated; we will do whatever we can to prevent you from needing dialysis.

I will need to arrange for some tests for you to check the other organs in your body before we can fully assess the likelihood of lupus. I do not need to admit you, but I will get the tests done today and see you in a week. In the meantime, please stop taking cafergot and contraceptive pills. I will give you something else for your migraine instead. Stopping smoking is also helpful; if you are agreeable, I will like to refer you to a smoking cessation counsellor and we can discuss whether nicotine replacement therapy will be suitable for you.

Pitfall: The hidden communications station

> The patient's concern (that she might have lupus like her mother, end up on dialysis, and pass away) is a tricky one. You must acknowledge the possibility of lupus, while calming her fears and expressing empathy and support for her. Use the toolkit from the communications station — but keep it brief.

Suggested presentation to the examiner:

Ms Ache presents with Raynaud's syndrome without other systemic manifestations of rheumatologic or hematologic disease. She has a significant occupational exposure to vibrating tools, drug history of ergots and contraceptive pills, and smoking. Examination is normal with no peripheral signs of systemic sclerosis or lupus, no evidence of arthritis, and no neuropathy. My differentials include idiopathic Raynaud's syndrome, Raynaud's syndrome secondary to vibrating tools or drugs, or early rheumatologic disease such as systemic sclerosis or lupus as the Raynaud's phenomenon may precede other signs of disease.

Investigations include:

- Nailfold capillary microscopy looking for enlarged or missing capillary loops that suggest underlying rheumatic disease.
- Screen autoantibodies beginning with antinuclear antibody, double-stranded DNA (lupus), anti-topoisomerase/anti-Scl70, anticentromere, and anti-RNA polymerase III (systemic sclerosis).
- Check a full blood count, as well as renal and liver biochemistries to rule out other organ involvement as might occur in a systemic autoimmune disease.

Principles of management include:

- Minimise exposure to secondary causes of Raynaud's (e.g., vibrating tools), switch ergots to other analgesia, using barrier contraception in place of oral contraceptive pills, and smoking cessation.
- General measures such as avoidance of cold exposure, keeping hands warm.
- If these are insufficient, the next step will be to consider pharmacologic treatment such as calcium channel blockers, topical nitrates, and other vasodilators.

Consultation Case 14

Mrs Potts (Back Pain)

Use this case as practice! The pull-out booklet contains the candidate's information.

Information for the Candidate

Patient Details: Mrs Potts, 60 years old

Your Role: Medical Outpatients SHO

Referral Letter:
> Dear Colleague,
>
> Thank you for seeing Mrs Potts. She has back pain that did not seem to improve with paracetamol. Will you please assist to manage her?
>
> Thank you.
>
> Dr Vivien Lee, GP

Vital Signs: BP 135/82 mmHg, HR 87/min, RR 14/min, SpO2 97% RA, T 37.0°C

Patient's Brief

Synopsis: *A 60-year-old lady presents with inflammatory back pain, renal impairment not in keeping with well-controlled diabetes, and anaemia. The diagnosis is multiple myeloma.*

Open the consult with: I just don't understand why my back is giving me so much trouble. I can't even sit in the office for a good hour of work without this unbearable ache. *Do not volunteer any other information unless asked.*

History of current problem:
- Back pain started quite suddenly 3 months ago, but this was not related to any trauma or injury. It has gotten steadily worse since then.
- Back pain can get severe (pain score 7/10) and tends to wake you up from sleep.
- Back pain does not radiate anywhere.
- Back pain is worst while resting and gets better with activity.
- Paracetamol does little to relieve the pain. Your GP said that he could not give you NSAIDs because of your kidney problem. A friend has recommended some herbal remedies which seem to help.
- You have also felt more tired recently, with decreased effort tolerance and a tendency to feel lightheaded. Your GP told you that your blood count was low but also said that it was probably related to your kidney disease.

- You have not had any other joint pains, rashes, or mouth ulcers.
- No fever or night sweats.
- No lower limb weakness, numbness, difficulty passing motion/urine, or incontinence.
- Weight loss of 6 kg in 3 months.
- No blood in urine, frothy urine, post-menopausal bleeding, or blood in the stools. Your bowels are moving normally.

Past medical and surgical history:
- Type 2 diabetes, diagnosed 10 years ago. This is well controlled with a latest HbA1c of 7.2%. You have gone for yearly eye and foot screens, which are normal. You have not had any complications due to diabetes.
- You have been told that your kidneys are deteriorating rapidly due to diabetes, which you feel puzzled about as your diabetes had always been well-controlled.

Medication list:
- Metformin 500 mg TDS, Empagliflozin 10 mg OM, Losartan 50 mg OM, Paracetamol 1 g QDS PRN.
- You have been taking some herbal remedies (tablets) for the past 2 years. You purchased these online at the recommendation of a friend.
- No known drug allergy.

Family history:
- Your 85-year-old father (who migrated from South Africa) was diagnosed with tuberculosis 2 years ago. He has since been treated and is well.
- No other relevant family history.

Relevant personal, social, occupational, and travel history:
- Occupation: human resource manager, deskbound.
- You used to jog regularly but have since stopped due to your back pain.
- Non-smoker, non-drinker.
- Not married, no children.

Relevant physical examination findings:

A surrogate patient is likely at this encounter.
- Back – no midline tenderness, no step deformity, no paravertebral muscle spasm. Range of motion full and painless.
- Range of movement of the spine is normal. Able to reach forward and touch toes.
- Straight leg raise negative.
- Lower limb neurology normal, gait normal.
- Digital rectal examination (if offered) – normal anal tone, normal perianal sensation, no masses.

- Mild conjunctival pallor.
- No lymphadenopathy.

You have some specific questions for the doctor at this consultation:
- What is wrong with me? I used to be fit and healthy, but now I'm tired and my back is such a bother.

Approach and Clinical Reasoning

Back pain in PACES is usually a sinister systemic cause rather than a straightforward orthopaedic issue (i.e., degenerative spondylosis, or trauma). Begin by excluding trauma, cauda equina syndrome, or neurological deficits (sciatica, weakness, numbness, bladder or bowel disturbances). Determine if pain is acute or chronic, and mechanical (better at rest) or inflammatory (better on movement). Consider the dangerous causes of back pain (Table B4.9).

Table B4.9. Dangerous causes of back pain.

Category	Cause	Important clinical features
Acute onset	Cauda equina syndrome – various underlying causes	Bladder/bowel dysfunction Severe bilateral pain and weakness
	Trauma, hematoma formation	History of trauma or procedure
Chronic mechanical pain	Compression fracture Pathologic fracture – e.g., metastases, osteoporotic fractures	Pain worse on movement Onset with minor trauma, predisposition for osteoporosis, underlying cancer
Chronic inflammatory pain	Axial spondyloarthritis - Ankylosing spondylitis - Psoriatic arthropathy - IBD related arthritis - Reactive arthritis	Decreased range of motion Rash, other joint pains Chronic bloody diarrhoea
	Infective - Epidural abscess - Vertebral osteomyelitis - TB (Pott's disease)	Fever, night sweats Predisposition (e.g., IV drug use, immunocompromised)
	Neoplastic - Metastatic cancer - Multiple myeloma - Primary spinal tumour	Weight loss, other features of systemic malignancy (e.g., anaemia, hypercalcaemia, renal impairment in myeloma)
Referred pain	e.g., pancreatitis, aortic aneurysm, nephrolithiasis	Other features (e.g., abdominal pain, radiation to groin)

IBD: inflammatory bowel disease; TB: tuberculosis

Mrs Potts has chronic inflammatory back pain associated with weight loss. A careful history will also reveal unexplained anaemia and rapidly progressive renal impairment that is not in keeping with well-controlled diabetes without microvascular complications. The likely unifying diagnosis is multiple myeloma — Mrs Potts has three of the four classic 'CRAB' symptoms of myeloma (hyperCalcaemia, Renal impairment, Anaemia, and Bone pain).

Important differentials include:
- Other forms of malignancy, especially given her weight loss.
- Infection, such as spinal tuberculosis (i.e., Pott's disease), given the positive family history.
- Compression fracture given the possibility of steroid-induced osteoporosis should the herbal remedies that she is on contain steroids.

Don't forget: Always rule out an emergency

> For the complaint of back pain, you must demonstrate that you have considered and excluded the cauda equina syndrome.

Physical examination should focus on the presenting complaint (i.e., her back), look for any step deformity, nerve root irritation (straight leg raise), or restricted spinal motion, and perform a targeted lower limb neurological examination to ensure that this is normal. Do offer a digital rectal examination, although having to perform one in PACES is unheard of. Next, confirm conjunctival pallor; if time permits, examine for features of malignancy (for instance screening for abdominal masses), although this would be of lower priority.

Question and Answer

Suggested answer to the patient's concerns:

Mrs Potts, thank you for sharing all this with me. I can't imagine how frustrating this unexplained back pain and fatigue must have been. I am concerned that your back pain may be more than a run-of-the-mill muscle ache. I am wondering if you have a condition called myeloma, which is an abnormal overproduction of immune cells in your body that causes bone pain, low blood counts, and kidney problems. At this stage I'm not certain if this is the case, and I am also considering other possibilities such as a fracture, infection, or inflammation of your back. I will like to admit you and do some tests, such as a scan and blood and urine tests, so that we can give you an answer to what's causing your back pain. In the meantime, let me give you some stronger painkillers to help with the pain.

Suggested presentation to the examiner:

Mrs Potts has inflammatory back pain, renal impairment not in keeping with well-controlled diabetes, and anaemia. The unifying diagnosis is multiple myeloma. My differentials include other spinal tumours, infection such as tuberculosis given the contact history, and a compression fracture especially if the herbal remedies that she has been taking contains steroids.

I will like to admit her. In terms of investigations:

- I will like to confirm my diagnosis of myeloma by performing:
  - Full blood count for anaemia.
  - Serum creatinine and electrolytes, especially calcium.
  - Serum and urine protein electrophoresis, serum free light chains.
  - Bone marrow aspiration and trephine.
  - Skeletal survey.
- To evaluate for differentials/complications:
  - Imaging studies including a spinal MRI.
  - Anaemia work-up including iron studies, folate, and B12.
  - Consider urine microscopy, protein/creatinine ratio, and ultrasound kidneys, looking into other causes of renal impairment.

I will involve a multidisciplinary management team comprising the haematologist, nephrologist, allied healthcare professionals, and other specialists as necessary.

- The primary treatment of myeloma is multi-agent chemotherapy or haematopoietic stem cell transplant.
- I will also need to manage complications including:
  - Management of bone lesions with analgesia, bisphosphonates; orthopaedic consult should there be a pathologic fracture.
  - Hydration, bisphopshonates, and calcitonin if there is severe hypercalcaemia.
  - Management of anaemia including transfusion and iron supplementation.
- Adjuncts include patient education, physiotherapy to maximise function, and appropriate vaccinations.

Consultation Case 15

Mr Pop (Chest Pain)

Use this case as practice! The pull-out booklet contains the candidate's information.

Information for the Candidate

Patient Details: Mr Pop, 23 years old

Your Role: Respiratory Medicine SHO

Referral Letter:
> Dear Colleague,
>
> Thank you for following up on Mr Pop. I saw him today for a non-traumatic pneumothorax, which resolved with supplemental oxygen. A chest X-ray prior to discharge was normal.
>
> Dr Darius Pan, A&E Physician

Vital Signs: BP 115/85 mmHg, HR 67/min, RR 11/min, SpO2 97% RA, T 36.9°C

Patient's Brief

Synopsis: *This young gentleman with underlying Marfan's syndrome and a recent pneumothorax now presents with chest pain and breathlessness, which is worrisome for recurrent pneumothorax or aortic dissection.*

Open the consult with: My chest is starting to hurt again, and the breathlessness is back. *Do not volunteer any other information unless asked.*

History of current problem:
- While playing basketball with friends 2 weeks back, you experienced sudden-onset chest pain and breathlessness. This chest pain was left-sided, poking in nature, worse on taking a deep breath, and did not radiate anywhere. You were also feeling breathless. There was no wheeze and you could speak in full sentences.
- You were brought to the A&E. The A&E doctor told you that your lung had 'popped'. You felt better after having some oxygen, and was sent home. You did not require any procedure, needle drainage, or chest tube.
- Your chest pain recurred last night while you were doing static weights in the gym. You will describe the pain as 'pulling' in character, centrally located, radiating to the back, and worse on inspiration. The pain was sudden-onset and severe at its onset

(pain score of 8/10 initially), but it subsided to 2/10 after resting for 5 minutes. You think that the chest pain occurred because you pulled a muscle while doing weights.
- This chest pain is associated with mild breathlessness. The breathlessness is worse on exertion. It is not worse lying down.
- You have no palpitations, diaphoresis, cough, fever, wheeze, or leg swelling.
- You have no abdominal pain, foot pain, discolouration of the foot, or difficulty walking.
- You have no vomiting.
- You have no blurred vision or back pain.

Past medical and surgical history:
- Childhood asthma, no longer on follow up.
- You frequently dislocate both shoulders. In fact, you dislocate them so often that you have learnt how to 'pop' them back in yourself.

Medication list:
- Nil
- Supplements and herbal remedies: nil
- Drug allergy: nil

Family history:
- Your father is just as tall as you are. He required a heart valve replacement in his 50s and is on long-term blood thinners.
- You have a younger sister, who is far shorter than you are.

Relevant personal, social, occupational, and travel history:
- You are a university student who plays on the varsity basketball team. You enjoy basketball and are rather good at it — your height is an advantage.
- You have smoked 1 pack a day for the past two years.
- No relevant travel history.

Relevant physical examination findings:
- Comfortable, not in respiratory distress.
- Respiratory system – tracheal central, good chest expansion, no hyper-resonant percussion note, bilaterally clear to auscultation.
- Cardiac system – collapsing pulse, early diastolic murmur best heard in full expiration in the lower left sternal edge.
- Systemic features (see Photo 10) – arachnodactyly, tall with large arm span, elbow hyperextension (A and B) positive thumb and wrist sign (C), pes planus (D).
- Visual acuity normal, no iridodonesis. Myopic with thick spectacles.
- No leg swelling.

Photos to be shown to candidate upon request (use colour plates for full-colour photos).

Photo 10

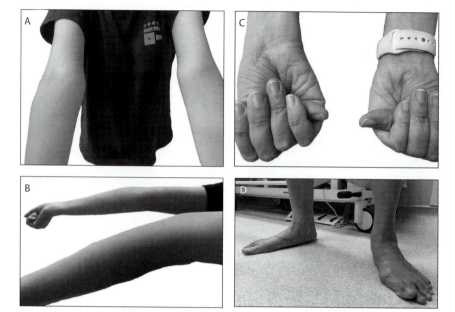

Clinical photo generously provided by Assoc Prof Tan Ju Le, National Heart Centre Singapore.

You have some specific questions for the doctor at this consultation:

- Can I go home?

- Why does this keep happening to me?

Approach and Clinical Reasoning

Most candidates will find the spot diagnosis of Marfan's syndrome relatively obvious. Think through the causes of secondary pneumothorax (Table B4.10).

Mr Pop presents with acute-onset chest pain and dyspnoea on a background of Marfan's syndrome. Complications of Marfan's must be specifically considered, in addition to general causes of chest pain and dyspnoea. Key differentials are:

- Recurrent pneumothorax, given the history of pneumothorax and pain worse on inspiration. You must rule out tension pneumothorax.

- Aortic dissection. His pain was maximal at onset and radiates to the back, and patients with Marfan's are at risk of dissection.

- Other causes of chest pain in a young man – pulmonary embolism, asthma, pericarditis, musculoskeletal chest pain.

Physical examination should aim to elicit:

- Features of pneumothorax – hyper-resonant percussion note, decreased air entry, tracheal deviation (obviously you will not get a tension pneumothorax in PACES, but you must demonstrate an effort to rule this out)
- Features of aortic dissection – checking lower limb pulses, as well as radial-radial and radial-femoral delay
- Other differentials – auscultate chest for wheeze, check calves for swelling
- Other features of Marfan's:
  - Aortic regurgitation (collapsing pulse, early diastolic murmur).
  - Mitral valve prolapse (pansystolic murmur).
  - Systemic features (increased arm span:height ratio, thumb sign, wrist sign, pectus carinatum, scoliosis, elbow hyperextension, pes planus).
  - Ocular features – iridodonesis suggesting ectopia lentis, myopia > 3 diopters.

Practice makes perfect: Marfan's syndrome

> Create an examination routine that you would use to demonstrate the signs of Marfan's syndrome. Do revise these features and the diagnostic criteria of Marfan's syndrome — they should be at your fingertips for the exam!

Table B4.10. Causes of secondary pneumothorax.

Cause	Important clinical features
Chronic obstructive pulmonary disease	Smoking, longstanding dyspnoea and productive cough, hyperinflated lungs
Marfan's syndrome	Arachnodactyly, systemic features of Marfan's
Cystic fibrosis	Recurrent lung infections, persistent productive cough, extra-pulmonary disease, coarse inspiratory crepitations
Infections – pneumocystis pneumonia, necrotising pneumonia	Exercise desaturation, acute fever and cough. Underlying immunocompromise, HIV, or risk factors
Lymphangioleiomyomatosis	Primary or with underlying tuberous sclerosis: facial angiofibromas, shagreen patch, ash-leaf spots, seizures
Lung malignancy	Weight loss, chronic cough
Trauma	Trauma, thoracic procedures, positive-pressure ventilation

Question and Answer

Suggested answer to the patient's concerns:

Mr Pop, I'm afraid that I'm not comfortable with letting you go home. You are not well and I need to admit you for treatment. You may indeed have popped your lung again, although I am also thinking about other causes of chest pain such as an abnormal tear in the large blood vessel that leads out of your heart. We need an X-ray, a CT scan of the blood vessel, and an ECG. It's important that we do this as some of these conditions can be life threatening if not acted on in a timely manner.

As to why this keeps occurring, I suspect that you have a genetic condition called Marfan's syndrome. This makes you more likely to pop a lung, have problems with your heart valve and vessels, and dislocate your shoulder. It's not entirely a bad thing — it may be why you are so tall, which is a huge advantage in basketball. However, the potential complications must be managed.

Suggested presentation to the examiner:

Mr Pop presents with acute-onset chest pain and dyspnoea. He has Marfan's syndrome with a history of pneumothorax, recurrent atraumatic shoulder dislocations, and a family history of valve replacement. Physical examination is significant for a collapsing pulse and early diastolic murmur suggestive of aortic regurgitation, as well as systemic features of Marfan's syndrome such as arachnodactyly, positive thumb sign and wrist sign, increased arm span to height ratio, and a high arched palate. There is no tracheal deviation or hyper-resonant percussion note of the chest. Air entry in the chest is good and peripheral pulses are well felt. My differentials for his chest pain include aortic dissection and pneumothorax. Other differentials such as pulmonary embolism, asthma, and musculoskeletal chest pain are less likely.

Mr Pop will require admission and urgent investigation, including a chest X-ray to look for pneumothorax or widened mediastinum, ECG, and a CT aortogram to confirm the diagnosis. Adjunctive tests include a blood count, renal biochemistry, coagulation studies, and a cross-match in the event that surgery is required. He will also need an echocardiogram to confirm aortic regurgitation and assess severity.

Management requires a multidisciplinary team including the cardiologist, respiratory physician, and cardiothoracic surgeon.

- If he has an aortic dissection, management includes beta-blockade, analgesia, and consideration of aortic repair.
- If he has a pneumothorax, supplemental oxygen and a chest tube is indicated. He may benefit from pleurodesis.
- Subsequent follow up includes:
  - Yearly monitoring of aortic root diameter and surgical replacement if criteria are met.
  - Ophthalmology referral for evaluation of ectopia lentis.
  - Orthopaedic input for recurrent shoulder dislocation and shoulder strengthening exercises.
  - Patient education, smoking cessation.
  - Genetic counselling and screening of family members.

Consultation Case 16
Ms Slim (Weight Loss)

Use this case as practice! The pull-out booklet contains the candidate's information.

Information for the Candidate

Patient Details: Ms Slim, 60 years old

Your Role: Internal Medicine Clinic SHO

Referral Letter:
> Dear Colleague,
>
> Thank you for seeing Ms Slim, who complains of a 2-month history of weight loss.
>
> Thank you.
>
> Dr Atkins, GP

Vital Signs: BP 102/64 mmHg, HR 70/min, RR 12/min, SpO2 99% RA, T 36.2°C

Patient's Brief

Synopsis: *This 60-year-old lady presents with weight loss, proximal myopathy, and cutaneous features of dermatomyositis. She also has a chronic cough and post-menopausal bleeding that raises concerns of underlying malignancy.*

Open the consult with: I don't know what's wrong. I feel so weak and everyone says I've lost weight. *Do not volunteer any other information unless asked.*

History of current problem:

- You have lost 10 kg (22 lb) in the last two months without trying to lose weight. You currently weigh 50 kg (110 lb). Your appetite has been poor.

- This has been accompanied by weakness. If asked, you find it particularly challenging to climb up the stairs, get up from a chair, or lift up heavy objects. You are no longer able to take your morning jog. You have no weakness of your fingers or difficulty writing. This weakness does not vary during the course of the day.

- You have no muscle pain, numbness, imbalance, slurred speech, blurring of vision, or facial droop.

- You have noticed a rash over the back of your fingers and around your eyes. It appeared a few months ago and is not itchy or painful. It does not bother you very much.

- You have an occasional dry cough for many years. Previous doctors have told you it is a smoker's cough. There is no blood in your sputum.
- You have also had some vaginal spotting for the past 3 months. You find this quite odd because you have had your menopause many years ago, but because you last had a pap smear 6 months ago which was normal, you did not think too much of this.
- You have no giddiness, chest pain, or breathlessness. You have no change in bowel habit or rectal bleed.
- You have no tremors or heat/cold intolerance.

Past medical and surgical history:
- Nil

Medication list:
- Nil
- No supplements or traditional medicine.
- No known drug allergy.

Family history:
- Your sister had Graves' disease.
- No family history of malignancy.

Relevant personal, social, occupational, and travel history:
- You work as an office secretary.
- You are married with two adult children.
- You do not drink. You smoke half a pack a day since you were 20.
- You have no relevant travel history.

Relevant physical examination findings:

The patient will have real physical signs, but the history is likely to be simulated to mimic an acute presentation.

- Gottron's papules (erythematous violaceous plaques over the extensor bony prominences of the metacarpophalangeal and proximal interphalangeal joints; Photo 11).
- Mechanics' hands (this is new – appearing 2 months ago. Your hands do not come into contact with industrial or household chemicals; Photo 12). You arrange for a part time cleaner to come in and do the bulk of the housework, and you routinely wear rubber gloves when washing the dishes.
- No overt rash over the face, chest, or neck.
- Neurology: symmetrical proximal muscle weakness without fatigability; normal tone, reflexes, and sensation.

Consultation Case 16

- Lungs clear, no crepitations.
- Abdomen – examiner will provide information that this is normal.
- Rectal examination – examiner will provide information that this is normal.

Photos to be shown to candidate upon request (use colour plates for full-colour photos).

Photo 11

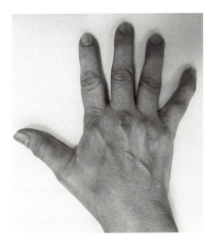

Photo 12

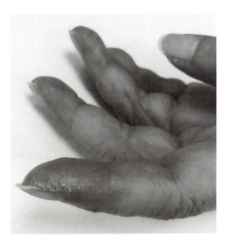

You have some specific questions for the doctor at this consultation:

- Do I have cancer? Is that why I'm losing so much weight?

Approach and Clinical Reasoning

Unintentional weight loss is a broad presenting complaint with many causes (Table B4.11).

Tip: Begin with open ended questions

> The fastest way to narrow down your differentials is to use open-ended questions. Two particularly helpful questions are:
> - "Tell me more about your weight loss" – most patients in the exam will have a prepared script that they will begin on.
> - "Apart from weight loss, is there anything else bothering you at the moment?" – eliciting the symptom complex is very helpful to focus further questioning, particularly for a nonspecific symptom like weight loss.

Table B4.11. Causes of unintentional weight loss.

Category	Important causes	Important clinical features
Malignancy	Gastrointestinal, lung, others	Rectal bleeding, chronic cough, early satiety; other associated symptoms
Infective	Tuberculosis HIV	Cough, haemoptysis, contact history Positive sexual history, diarrhoea
Malabsorption	Parasitic infection Inflammatory bowel disease Chronic pancreatitis Celiac disease	Chronic diarrhoea Bloody diarrhoea, abdominal pain Diarrhoea, history of alcohol use Chronic diarrhoea, abdominal bloating
Endocrine	Hyperthyroidism Diabetes Adrenal insufficiency	Tremor, heat intolerance Polyuria, polydipsia Postural giddiness, dehydration
Advanced chronic illness	Active autoimmune disease including new-onset myositis Major organ failure (e.g., cardiac cachexia, renal failure)	Joint pain, rashes, haematuria, proximal weakness Symptoms of organ failure
Reduced food intake	Psychiatric – depression, eating disorders Neurologic – dysphagia or cortical factors (e.g., dementia)	Mood symptoms, fixed delusions about food, etc. Weakness, speech difficulty, dysphagia
Social factors	Chronic vigorous exercise Poor access to food	Professional athletes, fads Poverty, social isolation, etc.

The history of weakness should not be dismissed as 'generalised lethargy'. Attempt to characterise this weakness as proximal or distal, symmetrical or asymmetrical, and associated with numbness or otherwise. Symmetrical proximal weakness without numbness localises to the anterior horn cell, muscle, or neuromuscular junction (refer to the neurology physical examination). Asking about fatigability is critical; upon finding proximal weakness (worse on getting up from a chair) without fatigability, consider acquired causes of a new-onset myopathy — thyroid disease, Cushing's disease, drug and alcohol, dermatomyositis (see Physical Exam, Syndrome 2.4).

Weight loss is an important clue to the diagnosis of dermatomyositis. Its characteristic skin findings can be obvious (full-fledged Gottron's papules and a heliotrope rash) or subtle (e.g., mechanics' hands alone). Some candidates may find it challenging to tie in the history of weakness with the weight loss so as to achieve a *complete* diagnosis of malignancy-associated dermatomyositis.

Dermatomyositis is strongly associated with malignancy, which you must search for. Note, however, that a clinically apparent malignancy can present before or after the cutaneous features of dermatomyositis appear. The clinical concern for Ms Slim is the post-menopausal bleeding (suggestive of uterine or cervical cancer) and her chronic cough (possible lung cancer).

Don't forget: Paraneoplastic disorders

> Dermatomyositis is highly associated with malignancy. A thorough evaluation for underlying malignancy must be sought.

Examination should focus on:
- Demonstrating the cutaneous features of dermatomyositis.
- Examining neurology to confirm the presence of a proximal symmetrical weakness with lower motor neuron signs and intact sensation, and the absence of fatigability or prominent fasciculations.
- If time permits, search for the source of the malignancy (e.g., auscultating the chest, but note that physical examination is poorly sensitive for lung nodules).

Question and Answer

Suggested answer to the patient's concerns:

You sound worried, Ms Slim. You are right that losing this much weight is not quite normal. I am worried about your cough and your vaginal bleeding — it's too early to say, but sometimes these may be symptoms that something is not quite right. We will get to the bottom of this, and if we find something, we will do our best to treat it as soon as possible.

Let's begin with some simple blood tests and a chest X-ray. I will speak to the gynaecologist, who will need to a full gynaecological examination and ultrasound for you. I will also get the neurologist to do a nerve and muscle study to check out the weakness, and the rheumatologist to give an opinion.

Suggested presentation to the examiner:

Ms Slim presents with proximal weakness, weight loss, post-menopausal bleeding, and a chronic cough. Physical examination reveals significant Gottron's papules, mechanics' hands, as well as symmetrical proximal weakness with lower motor neuron signs. She has dermatomyositis, and I am concerned about an underlying gynaecological or lung malignancy.

Tip: Physical signs in dermatomyositis

> The classic heliotrope rash, a photosensitive 'salt and pepper' rash in a shawl-like distribution, and Gottron's papules are unmistakable. More subtle signs of dermatomyositis include the mechanics' hands (often just an unexplained 'finger eczema'), periungual erythema, and the Holster sign (poikiloderma on the lateral thighs) — these need to be specifically sought, or they may be missed.

Investigations – I will like to confirm my diagnosis of dermatomyositis with:
- Blood tests, particularly looking for elevation in muscle enzymes (creatinine kinase, aldolase) and myositis-specific antibodies (e.g., anti-Jo-1, anti-SRP, anti-Mi-2, anti-MDA-5, etc.), as well as general studies such as a blood count and renal and liver biochemistries.
- Nerve conduction study and electromyography.
- Consideration of muscle biopsy.

I will like to search for an underlying malignancy beginning with a chest X-ray and subsequently CT chest, as well as referral to the gynaecologist for a speculum examination, pelvic ultrasound, and endometrial sampling.

Management will involve a multidisciplinary team including the rheumatologist, neurologist, gynaecologist, and pulmonary physician. The first aim of management is to treat any underlying malignancy. Therapeutic options for the dermatomyositis alone include glucocorticoids and steroid-sparing agents. Non-pharmacological adjuncts include physiotherapy, patient education, and rehabilitation.

Consultation Case 17

Mr Bocelli (Difficulty Seeing)

Co-authored with Dr Nicole Chan, Ophthalmology, National University Hospital

Use this case as practice! The pull-out booklet contains the candidate's information.

Information for the Candidate

Patient Details: Mr A. Bocelli, 40 years old

Your Role: Medical Outpatients SHO

Scenario: Mr Bocelli complains of difficulty seeing.

Vital Signs: BP 120/78 mmHg, HR 50/min, RR 10/min, SpO2 98% RA, T 36.3°C

Patient's Brief

Synopsis: *This gentleman has chronic progressive bilateral visual field loss, tunnel vision, family history of blindness, and classic fundoscopic findings of retinitis pigmentosa.*

Open the consult with: I have been having problems seeing. *Do not volunteer any other information unless asked.*

History of current problem:
- Both eyes appear to be equally affected.
- You have found it difficult to drive at night for many years. However, each time your optician checks your vision, he tells you that your visual acuity is normal and that your current spectacles do not need to be changed. You have not seen him for the past 5 years.
- You have been in 5 car accidents in the past two years. Interestingly, the accidents all involve another car filtering into your lane from the side.
- You have also been bumping into objects and people on your sides.
- You do notice that your eyesight is not as sharp as it used to be. However, this does not bother you too much as you are still able to work on a computer.
- There is no eye pain or redness.
- You have no history of diabetes. You just went for a company-sponsored health screening last year and was told that your blood sugar is normal.

- No headaches, nausea, or vomiting.
- No cold intolerance, constipation, weight gain, decrease in libido, change in facial appearance, or increase in shoe or ring size.
- No weakness or numbness elsewhere in your body.
- You are not aware of any congenital/childhood infections.

Past medical and surgical history:

- Tuberculosis – You were treated for tuberculosis 10 years ago. You recall having to take multiple pills daily for 6 months. You do not recall ever having seen an eye doctor.

Medication list:

- Nil. In particular, you have never taken malaria prophylaxis or medications for joint pains or psychiatric problems.
- Supplements and herbal remedies: nil
- Drug allergy: penicillin.

Family history:

- Your maternal grandmother was blind but you do not remember why.

Relevant personal, social, occupational, and travel history:

- You are a professional singer.
- You are married with 2 children.
- You do not smoke or drink.

Relevant physical examination findings:

- Fundoscopy – peripheral bone spicules, attenuated arterioles, and waxy disc pallor (similar finding in both eyes) (Photo 13).
- Visual fields – bilateral symmetrically constricted visual fields.
- Visual acuity – able to read newspaper headlines but difficulty reading the fine print, 6/18 for both eyes.
- No RAPD.
- No hearing loss or hearing aid.
- No polydactyly.
- No cerebellar signs.
- No other cranial neuropathy.

You have some specific questions for the doctor at this consultation:

- Can I drive?

Photos to be shown to candidate upon request (use colour plates for full-colour photos).

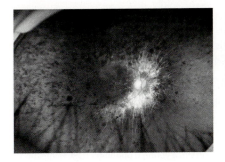 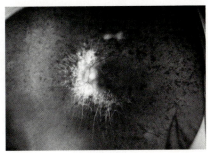

Photo 13 (Right eye) **Photo 14 (Left eye)**

Clinical photos generously provided by Dr Nicole Chan, National University Hospital

Approach and Clinical Reasoning

Clarify what the patient means by 'difficulty seeing'. Remember that visual function encompasses much more than visual acuity. 'Difficulty seeing' or 'blurring of vision' may mean a reduced visual acuity, visual field defect or scotoma, diplopia, red eye/eye pain, reduced colour vision, night blindness, and so on. Beware of the patient who complains of blurring of vision but has good visual acuity — always remember to check the visual fields! In blurring of vision, it is key to establish the following:

- Whether it is unilateral or bilateral.
- Time course – acute (hours to days), subacute (weeks), or chronic (months to years).
- Progression – non-progressive, slowly or rapidly progressive, or intermittent/episodic.

Pitfall: Use the correct differential list

> Do not bark up the wrong tree! First ascertain which is the correct differential list to use:
> 1. Acute blurring of vision with eye pain or red eye (Table B4.15)
> 2. Acute-subacute blurring of vision, without eye pain/red eye (Table B4.14)
> 3. Chronic progressive painless blurring of vision (Table B4.12)
> 4. Visual field defect (Table B4.13)
> 5. Diplopia (see Physical Exam, Syndrome 3.2)

Mr Bocelli has chronic progressive bilateral visual loss (Table B4.12) with an additional history of bumping into things on the sides, suggesting a visual field defect (Table B4.13).

Table B4.12. Causes of chronic painless progressive blurring of vision in PACES.

Localisation	Cause	Important clinical features
Retina *Abnormal fundoscopy* *May have peripheral visual field defect*	Retinitis pigmentosa (RP)	Family history of blindness may or may not be present (RP is most commonly sporadic) Tunnel vision/constricted visual fields Fundoscopy: diffuse bone spicules
	Diabetic retinopathy	Longstanding, poorly controlled diabetes May have previous panretinal photocoagulation or intravitreal anti-VEGF injections
	Chorioretinitis	Poor vision since young (congenital TORCH infection) Immunocompromised (e.g., CMV, HIV) Fundoscopy: patchy scarring
Optic neuropathy (ON) *Reduced visual acuity* *Reduced colour vision* *RAPD* *Optic atrophy (disk pallor)**	Compressive	Graves' ophthalmopathy: proptosis, goitre, hyperthyroidism Orbital apex syndrome (eg., tumour): may have CN III, IV, VI involvement
	Toxic/metabolic	Drug history: ethambutol, hydroxychloroquine, methanol poisoning, ethambutol Nutritional: B12 deficiency (gastric surgery, celiac disease), alcoholism
	Raised intracranial pressure	History of idiopathic intracranial hypertension Intracranial tumours
	Glaucoma	Often asymptomatic (red painful eye is only seen in acute intraocular pressure rise, and not in chronic cases)
Intracranial	Optic glioma	Neurofibromatosis type 1
	Pituitary adenoma and other intracranial lesions	Often causes visual field defect – always check visual fields See Table B4.13 on next page
Lens (cataract) **Macula**	Less likely in PACES but must be considered in clinical practice.	

CMV: cytomegalovirus; ICP: intracranial pressure; RAPD: relative afferent pupillary defect; TORCH: congenital toxoplasmosis, rubella, cytomegalovirus, herpes simplex

*An initially swollen optic disc loses its ability to swell after 6 weeks following axonal death.

Table B4.13. Visual field defects in PACES.

Defect	Localisation	Important causes
Bitemporal hemianopia	Optic chiasm	• Pituitary adenoma – look for features of acromegaly, Cushing's syndrome, suppression of thyroid, adrenal, and sex hormone axes • Craniopharyngioma and other tumours
Homonymous hemianopia	Contralateral brain involving occipital lobe (visual cortex) or parietal + temporal lobe (optic tract)	• Vascular: infarct, haemorrhage • Inflammatory/demyelinating (multiple sclerosis) • Neoplastic • Infective • Iatrogenic (radiation)
Tunnel vision	Retinal disease	• Retinitis pigmentosa • Extensive panretinal photocoagulation (most commonly for proliferative diabetic retinopathy)
	Optic neuropathy	• Glaucoma • Compressive optic neuropathy
Altitudinal defect	Retinal disease	• Branch retinal artery or vein occlusion • Retinal detachment
	Optic neuropathy	• Non-arteritic ischaemic optic neuropathy • Compressive optic neuropathy • Glaucoma

While Mr Bocelli's history of night blindness, tunnel vision, and slowly progressive visual loss is classical for retinitis pigmentosa, always consider differentials — especially treatable ones.

- As you enter the room, look out for spot diagnoses (i.e., thyroid eye disease and acromegaly).
- History is key. In most cases, the diagnosis can be made with careful history taking. Fundoscopy is challenging for most medicine trainees and simply serves to confirm the diagnoses and exclude differential diagnoses. In this scenario, particular note should be made of:
  - Any history of diabetes.
  - Drug history – Mr Bocelli has had multidrug treatment of tuberculosis — he is likely to have had ethambutol, which can cause visual loss.
  - The symmetry of the symptoms between the two eyes. Retinitis pigmentosa is typically bilateral and symmetrical. If unilateral or significantly asymmetrical, consider other pathologies (e.g., compressive, ischaemic, infective, inflammatory).

Leave sufficient time for physical examination. This should include:

- Visual acuity. Carry a mini Snellen chart in your kit and have the patient read from it. If the patient is unable to read, use the semiquantitative scale of 'counting fingers', 'hand movement', 'light perception', and 'no light perception' to grade the severity of visual impairment.

- Fundoscopy. Find the disc first, which provides you a clear landmark to orientate yourself. With the suspected diagnosis of retinitis pigmentosa in mind, go for the peripheries and look for peripheral bone spicules[7]. Most patients with retinitis pigmentosa listed for PACES have florid signs and reduced light perception. Waxy disc pallor and arteriolar attenuation (arterioles look thinner than usual) are subtle if you are not familiar with the normal calibre of retinal vessels. However, they may be appreciable once you have a high index of suspicion for retinitis pigmentosa.
- Confrontational visual fields, looking for bilateral symmetrically constricted visual fields.

The fundoscopic appearance of diffuse bony spicules and disc pallor can appear similar to that of extensive panretinal photocoagulation or chorioretinal atrophy from previous chorioretinitis. Again, the history will help you to differentiate these vastly different causes. The latter two diagnoses should not have gradually progressive visual field loss.

If time permits, look out for syndromic forms of retinitis pigmentosa (RP) by asking for any other medical history, checking hearing, and looking for visible dysmorphisms. Syndromic retinitis pigmentosa include:

- Usher syndrome – RP + deafness, ataxia.
- Bardet-Biedl syndrome – RP + polydactyly, obesity, renal disease, and reduced IQ.
- Kearns-Sayre syndrome – RP + chronic progressive external ophthalmoplegia, ptosis, heart block.
- Refsum disease – RP + peripheral neuropathy, cardiomyopathy, deafness, ataxia.

Finally, recognise that there is a safety issue that must be addressed in this station. The patient is getting into accidents, so he should be counselled to stop driving. Patients with occupations in which poor peripheral vision also poses a safety concern, such as those working with heavy machinery or working from heights, should be advised to consider other less hazardous work environments.

---

[7] In retinitis pigmentosa, there is degeneration of the photoreceptors, atrophy of the outer retina, and retinal pigment epithelium. Migration of the retinal pigment epithelium cells into the retina gives rise to the peripheral bone spicule appearance.

Practice makes perfect: Fundoscopy

Fundoscopy can be challenging, but do not be afraid — think of the fundoscope as merely a magnifier to help you directly visualise the retina and optic disc.

Tips to improve your fundoscopy:

- Turn off the lights and have the patient look into the distance. This optimises pupil dilation for you to examine the fundus more easily.
- Starting from about an arm's length away from the patient, compare the red reflex of both eyes. Causes of reduced red reflex include media opacity (cataracts, vitreous haemorrhage) and diseases that affect reflection of light from the retina (e.g., retinal detachment).
- Begin with a clear landmark — the optic disc. Find the optic disc easily by standing 15° lateral to the patient's line of sight, gradually moving closer while keeping your eye on the red reflex. Look for optic disc, atrophy, swelling, and cupping.
- Trace the vascular arcades. Pay attention to the calibre and appearance of the blood vessels (e.g., attenuation, tortuousity).
- Look at the retina beyond the vascular arcades for haemorrhages, cotton wool spots, laser scars (panretinal photocoagulation), bony spicules, etc.
- Examine the macula by moving temporally from the optic disc.
- As with any physical examination, examine with differential diagnoses in mind. Knowing what to expect and looking out for specific signs is the first step to making fundoscopy meaningful and effective.
- Practice makes perfect — contact your local medical retina clinic and ask if you can sit in to practice. Build up your confidence by practicing on dilated eyes in the 'right' patients. Examine cooperative patients with relatively clear media, such as younger patients (or your colleagues). Examining elderly patients with cataracts, poorly dilating pupils, or patients who are particularly photosensitive will be more challenging.

Question and Answer

Suggested answer to the patient's concerns:

Mr Bocelli, I am worried to hear that you have been driving and getting into accidents. I do not have good news for you. Is this a good time to talk about this? Is there anyone you will like with you as we discuss this? *(Use the breaking bad news framework but keep it short).*

The most likely cause of your blurred vision is retinitis pigmentosa, a condition affecting the retina, which is a layer of cells in your eye that detect light. This condition will continue to progress slowly over the years and your vision will slowly worsen. Although you are still able to read, your side vision is affected. As you cannot see things on the sides very well and your current vision is reduced, you should stop driving and stop handling heavy machinery at work, as this concerns your safety and the safety of others. We will refer you to the eye doctor for further assessment and monitoring, and to our low vision colleagues who can help to optimise your current vision with aids and teach you techniques to navigate safely.

Suggested presentation to the examiner:

Mr Bocelli is a 40-year-old gentleman with chronic progressive bilateral visual field loss, tunnel vision, and a positive family history of blindness. Examination findings of bilateral symmetrical bony spicule pigmentations, attenuated arterioles, waxy disc pallor on fundoscopy, and constricted visual fields are consistent with the diagnosis of retinitis pigmentosa. I do not note any deafness, polydactyly, or ptosis which might suggest syndromic retinitis pigmentosa.

Differentials are optic neuropathy secondary to ethambutol, but the temporal sequence does not fit and the fundoscopic findings cannot be explained by this.

I would like to refer him to the ophthalmologist for slit lamp examination, formal visual field assessment, retinal photography, follow up, and genetic testing.

Management is supportive and includes patient education, low vision aids, registration in support groups[8], family screening, and genetic counselling[9].

---

[8] Support groups include — Singapore: Singapore Association for the Visually Handicapped (SAVH); UK: Royal National Institute of Blind People.

[9] Retinitis pigmentosa can be inherited in an autosomal dominant, autosomal recessive, or X-linked recessive pattern. 50% are sporadic mutations. In Mr Bocelli's case, only his grandmother is affected and the disease 'skips a generation'. Therefore, it is likely autosomal recessive. His child is unlikely to be affected unless his partner has a spontaneous mutation.

Consultation Case 18

Mdm Kant Xi (Difficulty Seeing)

Co-authored with Dr Nicole Chan, Ophthalmology, National University Hospital

Use this case as practice! The pull-out booklet contains the candidate's information.

Information for the Candidate

Patient Details: Mdm Kant Xi, 50 years old

Your Role: Early Access Clinic SHO

Referral Letter:

> Dear Colleague,
>
> Mdm Xi is in follow-up with this clinic for diabetes, which has been quite difficult to control. She has a new complaint of difficulty seeing. Will appreciate if you could see her.
>
> Thank you,
>
> Dr David Ng, GP

Vital Signs: BP 130/89 mmHg, HR 60/min, RR 11/min, SpO2 99% RA, T 36.5°C

Patient's Brief

Synopsis: *This patient with poorly controlled diabetes presents with acute painless unilateral visual loss.*

Open the consult with: The vision in my left eye has been blurred for the past week. *Do not volunteer any other information unless asked.*

History of current problem:

- Current vision – left eye: can barely make out text on a handphone; right eye: no complaints, able to read newspaper.
- You were sitting down just reading something on your handphone when there was a sudden shower of floaters, followed quickly by sudden severe blurring of vision which has persisted.
- No eye pain, redness, discharge.
- No flashes of light or floaters.
- No headache.

- No weakness, numbness, or slurring of speech.
- You do not use contact lenses.
- You have no foot pain, ulcers, or numbness.
- You have no chest pain, difficulty breathing, or decreased effort tolerance. You are able to walk a distance of at least 3 bus stops.
- You have no increased thirst or frequent passing of large amounts of urine, although your urine has been frothy.
- No falls or injuries due to the visual loss.

Past medical and surgical history:
- Diabetes – you were diagnosed 10 years ago and were initially on follow up with the GP. You attend appointments inconsistently – you are busy with work and you do not see why you need to attend them so frequently because you feel well. Your latest HbA1c 1 year ago is 9.0%.
- You have never had any eye screen/retinal photographs, laser eye treatment or injections into the eyes.
- No history of tuberculosis, joint pains, or toxic alcohol ingestion.

Medication list:
- Atorvastatin 20 mg ON
- Losartan 50 mg OM
- Metformin 500 mg BD
- Insulin mixtard 40 units pre-breakfast, 28 units pre-dinner. You have frequently missed doses in the last 3 months.
- Supplements and herbal remedies: nil
- Drug allergy: nil

Family history:
- Both your parents had diabetes.
- Your father passed away in his 60s after 10 years on dialysis.
- There is no family history of blindness.

Relevant personal, social, occupational, and travel history:
- You are divorced and no longer in contact with your ex-spouse and children.
- You stay alone in a small rental flat.
- You have been working in odd jobs.
- Finances are challenging and you often have to scrimp on food.
- You smoke 5 cigarettes a day for the past 30 years.
- You do not drink alcohol.
- You do not drive.

Consultation Case 18

Relevant physical examination findings:

- Visual acuity – left eye hand movements, right eye 6/12
- Fundoscopy (or retinal photograph)
    o Left eye: large area of vitreous hemorrhage, obscuring the disc and macula, widespread dot/blot haemorrhages, neovascularisation elsewhere inferonasally and superonasally.
    o Right eye: no vitreous haemorrhage, findings of diabetic retinopathy as per left eye.
- Visual fields – normal.
- No relative afferent pupillary defect.
- No focal weakness in limbs, no cranial nerve palsy.
- Hydration status fair.

Photos to be shown to candidate upon request (use colour plates for full-colour photos).

Photo 15 (Left eye)

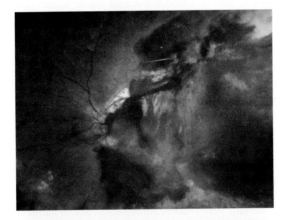

Photo 16 (Right eye)

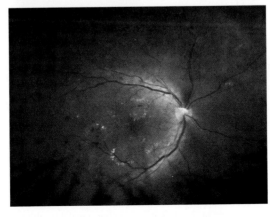

Clinical photos generously provided by Dr Nicole Chan, National University Hospital

You have some specific questions for the doctor at this consultation:

- The GP told me that I am going to go blind if I do not seek treatment. He is bluffing me, isn't he?

Approach and Clinical Reasoning

Mdm Xi has acute unilateral severe painless visual loss on a background of long-standing, poorly controlled diabetes mellitus. The absence of eye pain, which would suggest anterior segment pathology (Table B4.15), is a significant negative. Therefore, the pathology is most likely located in the posterior segment, optic nerve, or brain.

The clues in this case are the floaters preceding the sudden onset of blurring of vision. The floaters suggest vitreous opacities which, when severe and dense enough, result in media opacity obscuring the vision. Given the rapid onset and progression, the most likely differential is a vitreous haemorrhage[10].

In a patient with painless blurring of vision, the time course (transient or persistent, acute vs. subacute vs. chronic onset) is helpful to narrow the differential diagnoses (Table B4.14). Diabetic patients are at higher risk of developing certain sight-threatening conditions that present with visual loss (marked * in Table B4.14). The other causes may co-exist in a patient with diabetes.

In every ophthalmology case with a diabetic patient, always ask about previous pan-retinal photocoagulation ('laser eye treatment') and intravitreal injections (of anti-vascular endothelial growth factor agents or steroids). The patient may remember having several laser sessions (as pan-retinal photocoagulation is often fractionated) and seeing bright lights and feeling some pain during the laser treatment.

Background diabetic retinopathy, even when severe or proliferative, is often asymptomatic in the absence of concomitant diabetic macular oedema. Unfortunately, untreated retinal ischaemia predisposes to retinal neovascularisation that can present acutely with sight-threatening complications, including vitreous haemorrhage and neovascular glaucoma. Macula-involving tractional retinal detachment has a more subacute or chronic presentation. Additionally, vasculopaths are predisposed to other causes of visual loss:

- Retinal vascular disease – retinal artery or vein occlusion.
- Ocular ischaemic syndrome (secondary to carotid stenosis).
- Ischaemic optic neuropathy.
- Ischaemic or hemorrhagic stroke with homonymous visual field defects.
- Cataracts – diabetes is also a risk factor, which presents with chronic progressive blurring of vision.

---

[10] Vitritis (inflammation of the vitreous) is another possibility, although the onset is slightly less rapid (e.g., within hours, instead of seconds to minutes).

Table B4.14. Causes of acute-subacute painless blurring of vision.

Course	Differentials	RAPD^	Important features
Transient (recovers)/ episodic	Amaurosis fugax*	No	Vascular risk factors
	Migraine with aura	No	Typical migraine history: positive visual phenomena (bright lights, zigzag lines) preceding onset of throbbing headache
	Hypoglycaemia*	No	Associated with palpitations, diaphoresis, relieved by glucose intake
	Idiopathic intracranial hypertension	No	Headache Transient visual loss (lasting seconds) often following changes in posture or Valsalva manoeuvre Pulsatile tinnitus exacerbated by positional changes ± Horizontal diplopia (sixth nerve palsy from raised intracranial pressure)
Sudden, persistent *Typically vascular causes*	Vitreous haemorrhage*	No	Sudden-onset floaters, followed by blurring of vision which progresses within minutes Diminished red reflex Fundoscopy: view may be poor
	Retinal artery occlusion (RAO)*	Yes	Sudden onset of severe visual loss that persists (not progressive) Central RAO: pale fundus, cherry red spot Branch RAO: monocular superior or inferior visual field defect Risk factor (e.g., atrial fibrillation, giant cell arteritis)
	Retinal vein occlusion	Possible	'Blood and thunder' fundus, macular oedema, may have disc swelling Underlying risk factor, hyperviscosity, hypercoagulable state, contraceptive pill use
	Ischaemic optic neuropathy (ION)	Yes	Features of optic neuropathy: loss of colour vision, visual field defect, ± disk swelling Non-arteritic anterior ION classically causes an inferior altitudinal visual field defect Giant cell arteritis: headache, scalp tenderness, jaw claudication, polyrheumatica myalgia, systemic symptoms
	Intracranial infarct/ haemorrhage involving optic tracts, optic radiation or visual cortex*	No	Visual field defect: homonymous hemianopia (optic nerve lesion), quadrantanopia (parietal or temporal lobe lesion), or hemianopia (occipital lobe lesion) Have a high index of suspicion for visual field defects if the patient complains of blurring of vision but has relatively good visual acuity May have other neurological deficit depending on the location of the pathology

(Cont'd)

Course	Differentials	RAPD^	Important features
	Neovascular glaucoma*	Yes#	Acute eye pain, ipsilateral headache, nausea, vomiting Mid-dilated unreactive pupil, hazy cornea
Subacute, persistent (hours to days)	Retinal detachment (RD)	If large	Progressive visual field loss (a shadow or curtain obscuring the peripheral vision) May be preceded by floaters or flashes of light Fundoscopy: bullous retinal detachment Rhegmatogenous RD (from retinal tears, often in patients with high myopia) presents over hours Tractional RD* (when proliferative diabetic retinopathy pulls on the retina) presents with subacute or chronic visual loss if the macula is involved
	Optic neuritis, as in multiple sclerosis and neuromyelitis optica	Yes	Features of optic neuropathy: reduced visual acuity and colour vision, visual field defect May have pain on eye movement May have disc swelling May have other neurologic deficits

^Relative afferent pupillary defect.
*Causes particularly associated with diabetes and/or diabetic retinopathy.
#RAPD is present because neovascular glaucoma usually arises from posterior segment ischaemia.

Examination should include fundoscopy and a screen for focal neurologic deficits. The following features may be found:

- Vitreous haemorrhage. There may be a poor view of the fundus due to vitreous haemorrhage.
- Features of diabetic retinopathy (it may be easier to examine this in the contralateral eye without vitreous haemorrhage). Mild or moderate diabetic retinopathy may be subtle on direct fundoscopy, but you should not miss frank proliferative diabetic retinopathy.
  - Proliferative: neovascularisation, traction bands, vitreous haemorrhage.
  - Severe non-proliferative: > 20 intraretinal haemorrhages in 4 quadrants, venous beading in ≥ 2 quadrants, or intraretinal microvascular abnormality in ≥ 1 quadrant (the '4-2-1' rule)
  - Moderate: more than microaneurysms but not meeting criteria for 'severe'.
  - Mild: only microaneurysms.
- Previous laser photocoagulation scars in the peripheral regions of the retina.
- RAPD. The presence of RAPD and reduced colour vision in the affected eye points towards an optic neuropathy. RAPD can also arise from severe retinal disease.
- Do a quick screen of visual fields to exclude homonymous hemianopia.

Tip: Fundoscopy signs in diabetic retinopathy

The signs of diabetic retinopathy shown in the photos include:

- Neovascularisation elsewhere (marked NVE)
- Hard exudates (marked HE)
- Venous beading (marked VB)
- Vitreous hemorrhage (marked VH)
- Blot hemorrhages (scattered in image)

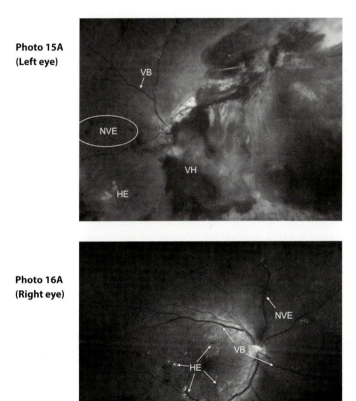

Photo 15A (Left eye)

Photo 16A (Right eye)

The additional issue in this station is Mdm Xi's poorly controlled diabetes. If time permits, it will be good to explore whether she has systemic complications of diabetes, her disease understanding, and the factors behind her non-compliance. Ensure that she is not having frank osmotic symptoms or a hyperglycaemic crisis.

Question and Answer

Suggested answer to the patient's concerns:

Mdm Xi, your vision has become blurred suddenly because of bleeding in your left eye. This bleeding is due to abnormal blood vessels that are a result of advanced diabetes changes affecting your eye. Your GP is right — this is a blinding condition if not urgently treated. I will refer you to the eye doctor today for a more thorough eye examination. They will speak to you about the required treatment. They will also need to treat your other eye to reduce the risk of a similar event occurring.

The bleeding in your eye is an indicator that your diabetes is causing severe damage. We need to take steps immediately to improve your diabetic control to prevent similar or more serious problems from happening, as poorly controlled diabetes affects other organs as well, such as the kidney.

Suggested presentation to the examiner:

Mdm Xi is a poorly controlled diabetic who presents with acute painless unilateral visual loss. She has markedly reduced left visual acuity, vitreous hemorrhage, and features of underlying proliferative diabetic retinopathy including neovascularisation and widespread dot/blot haemorrhages.

The immediate step is an urgent ophthalmology consult. She will require treatment for both eyes, which may include pan-retinal laser photocoagulation or intravitreal vascular endothelial growth factor inhibitors. Some patients may require vitrectomy if there is non-resolving vitreous hemorrhage. Visual prognosis is guarded.

Subsequent follow up will need to address her poor diabetic control, for example:

- Establishing HbA1c, screening for other organ complications (creatinine, urine protein/creatinine ratio, foot screen), and checking for comorbids (lipids, blood pressure).
- Addressing barriers to compliance. A diabetic nurse educator consult may be helpful.
- Intensifying treatment if suboptimal HbA1c despite compliance.
- Dietician consult.
- Improve the patient's understanding of her disease.

Consultation Case 19

Ms See (Difficulty Seeing)

Co-authored with Dr Nicole Chan, Ophthalmology, National University Hospital

Use this case as practice! The pull-out booklet contains the candidate's information.

Information for the Candidate

Patient Details: Ms See, 30 years old

Your Role: Medical Walk-In Clinic SHO

Referral Letter:
> Dear Colleague,
>
> Thank you for seeing Ms See for difficulty seeing.
>
> Dr Benjy, GP

Vital Signs: BP 120/88 mmHg, HR 70/min, RR 14/min, SpO2 98% RA, T 36.0°C

Patient's Brief

Synopsis: *This young lady has right optic neuritis and symptoms suggestive of a previous transverse myelitis. The differentials are relapsing-remitting multiple sclerosis or neuromyelitis optica.*

Open the consult with: I've found the vision in my right eye somewhat blurry in the past 5 days. *Volunteer the history of reduced colour vision and numbness.*

History of current problem:

- You first noticed a mild ache behind the right eye that is worse on eye movement, which started around 7 days ago.
- Next, you found that bright colours seem less 'intense' in your right eye than before, when compared to your left eye.
- Vision was sharp initially but has started to become blurry in the last 2–3 days. You can still make out the road signs, but not read a newspaper.
- You have tried using dry eye eyedrops with no improvement in symptoms.
- You do recall having a flu one week before all these symptoms started.
- There is no red eye, discharge, floaters, flashes of light, or double vision.
- No headache or nausea/vomiting.

- No weakness or numbness at present. However, after running a marathon last month, you experienced some numbness in both feet which lasted for 3–4 days and resolved thereafter. You think that this was because of over-exertion.
- No incoordination, slurring of speech, facial droop, difficulty passing urine or passing motion.
- No rashes, oral ulcers, dry eyes or mouth, joint pains, abnormal bleeding, fatigue, reduced effort tolerance, difficulty breathing, or frothy urine.

Past medical and surgical history:
- Graves' disease. You had your thyroid removed 3 years ago and are on thyroid hormone replacement.
- No diabetes.

Medication list:
- Thyroxine, 100 mcg OM
- Supplements and herbal remedies: nil
- Drug allergy: nil

Family history:
- No family history of blindness, stroke, or other neurological disease.

Relevant personal, social, occupational, and travel history:
- You are newly married to your childhood sweetheart.
- Your last menstrual period was 1 week ago.
- You do not smoke or drink.
- You work as an interior designer.

Relevant physical examination findings:
This station can be run with a real patient or a surrogate. Even if a real patient is used, signs may disappear if the patient is listed for exam in advance.
- Visual acuity: grossly normal.
- Right relative afferent pupillary defect.
- Fundoscopy: right optic disc swollen (Photo 17).
- Extraocular eye movements normal.
- Ocular motility normal.
- Offer to check colour vision (Ishihara chart or comparison of intensity of a red object between both eyes) – colour vision is reduced in the right eye.
- Other neurology: cranial nerves normal, no cerebellar signs, limb power and reflexes full, gait normal, sensation grossly intact.
- No malar rash.

Consultation Case 19

Photo to be shown to candidate upon request (use colour plates for full-colour photos).

Photo 17

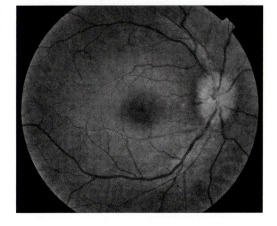

Clinical photo generously provided by Clin Assoc Prof Sharon Tow, Singapore National Eye Centre

You have some specific questions for the doctor at this consultation:

- Do you think I could be having a stroke? The GP did say that he was worried about a stroke.
- Will my colour vision be permanently affected? I'm an interior designer and I find it increasingly difficult to differentiate between the different colour shades.

Approach and Clinical Reasoning

This is a young female with acute onset of unilateral blurring of vision and reduced colour vision. Initial differentials to this complaint are broad (see complete differentials list, Table B4.14). The absence of eye pain or red eye is a significant negative which makes the pathology most likely located in the posterior segment, optic nerve, or brain. The prominence of reduced colour vision narrows the differentials to optic nerve[11] or macular disease. An obvious RAPD makes optic nerve disease the likely localisation[12]. In essence, reduced colour vision, blurring of vision, and an RAPD are typical features of optic neuropathy.

Differentials to an optic neuropathy include:

- Optic neuritis: Ms See's presentation is classical. Her retroorbital pain, worse on eye movement, is a consequence of inflammation of the extraocular recti muscles that surround the optic nerve. Causes of optic neuritis include multiple sclerosis (more common in Caucasian populations) and neuromyelitis optica (more common in Asian populations).

---

[11] Pain on eye movements (which is different from eye pain), is another clinical feature that would be strongly supportive of optic neuritis had it been present in this case.

[12] Large retinal pathology (e.g., severe retinal detachment) can also cause a relative afferent pupillary defect.

- Compressive optic neuropathy (e.g., orbital apex neoplasm and thyroid eye disease), which must be considered with Ms See's history of Graves' disease. Thyroid eye disease can occur even in patients without obvious proptosis or who are euthyroid (as thyroidectomy or anti-thyroid drugs do not remove the autoantibodies).
- Ischaemic optic neuropathy (ION): arteritic ION (giant cell arteritis) is unlikely in a young female, and non-arteritic ION is unlikely in a young patient without vascular risk factors.
- Metabolic: toxic alcohols (methanol, ethylene glycol), B12 deficiency.
- Infectious and reactive: TB, syphilis, HIV, lyme disease, post-infectious, acute disseminated encephalomyelitis (ADEM).

Additionally, Ms See has not only subacute visual blurring but also an episode of transient bilateral lower limb numbness (suggestive of a spinal cord lesion). These are multiple lesions disseminated in space and time which is classic for multiple sclerosis. Neuromyelitis optica spectrum disorder remains a differential.

Physical examination should focus on:

- Ocular signs
  - Inspect for proptosis in thyroid eye disease.
  - Pupils: check for relative afferent pupillary defect (RAPD). This is an important sign.
  - Fundoscopy: for any disc swelling.
  - Extra-ocular eye movements: internuclear ophthalmoplegia, cranial nerve palsies, restrictive myopathy in thyroid eye disease.
- Screen for other neurology, particularly lower limb reflexes, sensation, and cerebellar signs.

Question and Answer

Suggested answer to the patient's concerns:

Ms See, thank you for sharing this concern with me. Your symptoms are not suggestive of a stroke. Rather, it is likely to be caused by inflammation affecting the nerve that transmits signals from your eye to your brain. The episode of numbness in your legs is likely to be caused by similar inflammation affecting your spinal cord. The most likely diagnosis is a condition known as multiple sclerosis. We will need to do some blood tests and an MRI scan of your optic nerves, brain, and spinal cord to confirm this.

This inflammation is treatable. The good news is that most patients recover their vision, including colour vision which is important to you. While multiple sclerosis can have long-term problems from episodes of inflammation, together with the neurologist and the ophthalmologist, we will start you on treatment to ensure the best possible recovery.

Suggested presentation to the examiner:

Ms See is a young lady with multiple central nervous lesions disseminated in space and in time, including right optic neuritis and bilateral lower limb numbness which localise to the spinal cord. She has a right RAPD and optic disc swelling. Ocular motility and other aspects of the neurological examination are normal. My principal diagnosis is relapsing-remitting multiple sclerosis. A differential is neuromyelitis optica spectrum disorder.

My investigations will include:

- Confirming my diagnosis by performing contrasted MRI orbits, brain and spine, and looking for lesions disseminated in space and time.
- Lumbar puncture to look for oligoclonal bands.
- Looking for differentials by checking autoantibodies and aquaporin 4 (for neuromyelitis optica).
- Blood tests including full blood count and renal and liver biochemistries.
- Referral to the ophthalmologist for slit-lamp examination and visual field assessment, and to exclude other causes of blurring of vision.

In terms of management, I will involve a multidisciplinary team involving a neurologist, ophthalmologist, and allied healthcare professionals such as the physiotherapist and occupational therapist. Principles of management include:

- Treatment of disease with a course of IV methylprednisolone and subsequently discussing disease modifying therapy.
- Supportive management to prevent complications and maximise function, especially if she becomes more symptomatic with time. This includes physiotherapy, adjuncts to address spasticity, and management of bladder, bowel, and sexual function.

Consultation Case 20

Mr Hong Yan (Red Eye)

Co-authored with Dr Nicole Chan, Ophthalmology, National University Hospital

Use this case as practice! The pull-out booklet contains the candidate's information.

Information for the Candidate

Patient Details: Mr Hong Yan, 32 years old

Your Role: Emergency Department SHO

Referral Letter:
> Dear Colleague,
>
> Thank you for seeing Mr Hong Yan. He complains of redness and discomfort of the left eye, which did not respond to levofloxacin eyedrops.
>
> Warm regards,
>
> Dr Andrew Tan, GP

Vital Signs: BP 107/63 mmHg, HR 74/min, RR 11/min, SpO2 98% RA, T 36.2°C

Patient's Brief

Synopsis: *This young gentleman presents with unilateral red eye, inflammatory back pain, and dactylitis. The diagnosis is ankylosing spondylitis.*

Open the consult with: My left eye is still red, doc. The GP gave me some eyedrops but they don't work. *Do not volunteer any other information unless asked.*

History of current problem:
- You have been experiencing redness and pain of the left eye for 6 days. The pain is quite bothersome and you find it uncomfortable to look at bright lights. Pain is not worse on looking around.
- There is mild blurring of vision and tearing, but no discharge, gritty sensation, or itch.
- Your right eye is unaffected.
- You have had no similar episodes in the past.
- You have no floaters or double vision, and you do not bump into things on the sides.

Consultation Case 20   329

- There is no one else around you who has red eyes/conjunctivitis.
- You do not use contact lenses. There is no injury to the eye. You do not have any recent eye surgeries or procedures.
- You have no headache, giddiness, weakness, numbness, or facial droop.
- You have been well with no fever, cough, flu, or muscle aches.
- You have noticed mild back pain for the past 6 months. This is most noticeable at the start of the day and is associated with stiffness, but it gets much better after an hour or two once you 'get moving'. You are not too bothered by the back pain and have not taken any painkillers.
- There is no pain in any other joints.
- Incidentally, you also had an episode 3 months ago where the entire left ring finger became swollen. This got better on its own after 2–3 weeks.
- You have no pain in the ankles or any tendons.
- You have no diarrhoea or blood in your stools.
- You have no rashes, mouth ulcers, hair loss, change in colour of the hands upon going into a cold room, or dry eyes/mouth.

Past medical and surgical history:
- Nil
- No history of diabetes or joint problems.

Medication list:
- Levofloxacin eyedrops, given by the GP on the first day of your symptoms.
- No drug allergy.

Family history:
- Nil. In particular, no history of autoimmune disease, joint problems, or eye problems.

Relevant personal, social, occupational, and travel history:
- You work as a nurse.
- You have a steady girlfriend.
- You do not smoke or drink.

Relevant physical examination findings:
This encounter will use a real patient who will have been treated. As ophthalmic signs (i.e., red eye) may no longer be present, photographs may be shown.
- Left eye conjunctival injection, hypopyon (Photo 18).
- No proptosis. Able to close eyes fully.
- No relative afferent pupillary defect (if present, this would suggest that the posterior chamber is affected in addition to the anterior chamber – this would be worrisome for an endophthalmitis which is immediately sight-threatening).

- Question mark posture with loss of lumbar lordosis and thoracic kyphosis, occiput to wall distance 4 cm (Photo 19).
- Restricted spinal movements: reduced forward flexion (Schober's test 3 cm).
- Sacroiliac tenderness (positive FABER test)
- Chest expansion not significantly reduced.
- No dactylitis or enthesitis.
- No rash or psoriatic nail changes (e.g., nail pitting, onycholysis).
- Heart S1S2, no collapsing pulse, no murmur.
- Lungs clear.

Photos to be shown to candidate upon request (use colour plates for full-colour photos).

Photo 18

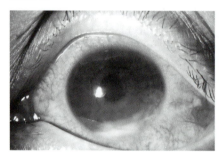

Photo 19

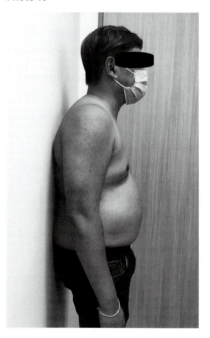

Clinical photos generously provided by
Dr Jay Siak, Singapore National Eye Centre, and
Dr Stanley Angkodjojo, Sengkang General Hospital

You have some specific questions for the doctor at this consultation:

- Is there anything to help with the eye pain?

Approach and Clinical Reasoning

A painful red eye suggests pathology of the anterior segment (cornea, conjunctiva, iris) or the sclera. Quickly rule out common causes of red/painful eyes, such as trauma, contact lens overwear syndrome, and corneal erosion, which are unlikely in PACES (but you should still do due diligence to exclude them). The PACES patient complaining of a painful red eye almost always has an underlying systemic cause (Table B4.15). Begin by looking for spot diagnoses (Graves' ophthalmopathy) and asking for symptoms of rheumatologic disease (Sjogren's syndrome, spondyloarthritis, rheumatoid arthritis, and granulomatosis with polyangiitis).

Table B4.15. Important and systemic causes of red/painful eyes.

Cause	Key ocular features	Underlying causes
Dry eyes	Dry, gritty sensation	Sjogren's syndrome
Exposure keratopathy	Inability to close eyes fully (lagophthalmos)	Thyroid eye disease Lower motor neuron CN VII palsy
Anterior uveitis (iritis)	Circumciliary (perilimbal) injection (erythema) Pupil may be smaller and/or irregular shaped (due to ciliary spasm and/or posterior synechiae) Hypopyon (if significant inflammation) Note: Isolated posterior uveitis does not cause eye redness	Spondyloarthritis: ankylosing spondylitis, psoriatic arthropathy, IBD-arthritis Lupus, Sjogren's syndrome Sarcoidosis Infective: HSV, VZV, CMV, Toxoplasmosis, syphilis, TB
Anterior scleritis	Diffuse redness and vascular engorgement	Rheumatoid arthritis, lupus, other vasculitis Infectious: VZV, HSV, HIV
Infective keratitis	Corneal opacity Epithelial defect on fluorescein staining	Bacterial, often associated with improper contact lens use
Herpetic keratitis	Dendritic lesion on fluorescein staining Corneal haze and oedema	HSV (history of periocular vesicles) VZV (zoster involving V1 dermatome)
Endophthalmitis	Acute severe visual loss. Hypopyon Relative afferent pupillary defect	Endogenous (e.g., Klebsiella bacteraemia) Exogenous (intraocular procedures or ocular trauma/foreign body)
Acute ↑ intraocular pressure (e.g., acute glaucoma)	Fixed mid-dilated pupil Conjunctival injection Hazy cornea Ipsilateral headache	Ocular causes: neovascular glaucoma, intumescent or subluxed cataract, narrow angles (in hyperopic eyes) Drug history: topiramate

Note: A painful eye (anterior segment pathology) should be differentiated from pain behind the eye that is worse with eye movement (retrobulbar optic neuritis).

CMV: cytomegalovirus; HSV: herpes simplex virus; IBD: inflammatory bowel disease; TB: tuberculosis; VZV: varicella zoster virus

In addition to a red and painful left eye, Mr Hong Yan has a 6-month history of inflammatory back pain, as well as a history of 'swelling of the entire left ring finger' consistent with dactylitis. This cluster of symptoms suggests spondyloarthritis; in the absence of bloody diarrhoea (inflammatory bowel disease associated arthritis), rash (psoriatic arthropathy), or antecedent gastrointestinal or genitourinary infection (reactive arthritis/Reiter syndrome), the unifying diagnosis is ankylosing spondylitis. It is not uncommon for acute anterior uveitis to be the first problem requiring medical evaluation.

Pertinent points in history to cover in a patient with suspected spondyloarthritis will include:

- Excluding red flags in the back pain history (see Case 14 for an approach to back pain)
- Asking about other musculoskeletal manifestations of ankylosing spondylitis:
  - Back and neck pain, reduced mobility, and postural abnormalities.
  - Sacroiliitis – patients will describe having buttock pain rather than leg/hip pain.
  - Peripheral arthritis.
  - Enthesitis.
  - Dactylitis (sausage digits).
- Asking about extra-articular manifestations, such as:
  - Anterior uveitis (as in this case).
  - Aortic regurgitation and apical pulmonary fibrosis – ask for breathlessness.

Examination has the dual aims of (1) confirming ocular pathology and (2) eliciting the features of ankylosing spondylitis. Remember that fulminant signs of uveitis are unlikely as the patient would have been treated. Similarly, textbook presentations of a 'question-mark posture' are increasingly rare, with aggressive and early treatment to prevent deformities.

Appropriate examination steps include:

- Checking visual acuity
- Examining the eye with a pen torch – look for a circumciliary injection, an irregular pupil, and hypopion. Exclude differentials (particularly thyroid eye disease by checking for proptosis).
  - Fundoscopy is of less value in this case (unless you are looking for disc swelling, macular exudates, retinitis or vasculitis that would suggest concomitant posterior uveitis).
  - In a patient with acute eye redness, pain, and a hypopyon, it is imperative to exclude endophthalmitis which is sight-threatening.
- Checking spinal mobility including the occiput to wall distance, and performing Schober's test to assess lumbar flexion.
- Assessing for sacroiliitis by checking the FABER test.
- Screening for rash, enthesitis, dactylitis, and peripheral arthritis.

- If time permits, auscultating the heart (for aortic regurgitation) and apex of the lung (for apical fibrosis).

Question and Answer

Suggested answer to the patient's concerns:

Mr Hong Yan, yes we can help you with the eye pain. This is a condition known as ankylosing spondylitis, which is a condition in which inflammation affects your eyes, joints, and back. I will refer you to see the eye specialist today for a more detailed evaluation. They may give you some eyedrops to reduce inflammation and help with the eye pain.

Suggested presentation to the examiner:

This young gentleman presents with acute unilateral eye redness and pain, photophobia, and blurring of vision associated with inflammatory back pain and dactylitis. Physical examination is significant for left eye conjunctival injection and hypopyon. He has a question-mark posture, reduced spinal flexion with forward excursion of 3 cm on Schober's test, thoracic kyphosis with occiput to wall distance of 4 cm, and sacroiliac tenderness with a positive FABER test. The unifying diagnosis is acute anterior uveitis secondary to ankylosing spondylitis.

Investigations:

- I will refer him to the ophthalmologist for detailed examination and to exclude differentials, particularly infection.
- Imaging: I will perform an X-ray followed by MRI of the spine and sacroiliac joints looking for sacroiliitis (the 'bamboo spine' appearance i.e., extensive syndesmophytes is unlikely in early ankylosing spondylitis).
- Laboratory: I will check an erythrocyte sedimentation rate, HLA-B27, and baseline blood count, as well as renal and liver biochemistries.

Management: He will benefit from a multidisciplinary team including a rheumatologist, ophthalmologist, and allied healthcare professionals such as the physiotherapist. Principles of management include:

- The anterior uveitis will require treatment with topical steroids and cycloplegic eyedrops.
- Initial treatment of back symptoms includes physiotherapy and NSAIDs.
- If response to NSAIDs is inadequate, then a TNF-alpha inhibitor (e.g., infliximab, adalimumab, golimumab) or interleukin-17 inhibitor (secukinumab) will be indicated.

Consultation Case 21

Mr Pei (Haematuria)

Use this case as practice! The pull-out booklet contains the candidate's information.

Information for the Candidate

Patient Details: Mr Pei, 45 years old

Your Role: Medicine Clinic SHO

Referral Letter:
> Dear Colleague,
>
> A pre-employment screening done for this patient 1 week ago identified blood 3+ and protein 2+ on urine dipstick. A repeat dipstick today showed persistence of these abnormalities. Please kindly assist with further investigation and management.
>
> Thank you.
>
> Dr Smily Lock, GP

Vital Signs: BP 145/92 mmHg, HR 70/min, RR 14/min, SpO2 97% RA, T 36.5°C

Patient's Brief

Synopsis: *A 45-year-old gentleman presents with haematuria, bilateral ballotable kidneys, and a family history of kidney failure. The likely diagnosis is polycystic kidney disease.*

Open the consult with: I have been having blood in my urine, I don't know why. *Do not volunteer any other information unless asked.*

History of current problem:
- Over the past months, you have noticed several episodes in which your urine turns red for several days, then resolves.
- You have not sought medical attention so far as you have felt well with no flank pain, groin pain, pain on passing urine, frequent passage of urine, or frequent urge to pass urine.
- You are unsure whether the blood in urine occurs in early, mid, or late stream.
- You do not have any symptoms of cough, runny nose, fever, or sore throat.
- You have not noticed any bubbles or froth in your urine. Your urine is not foul smelling.

- There is no change/decrease in your urine output. You do not have any incontinence, poor urine stream, hesitancy when starting to pass urine, or sensation of incomplete voiding.
- You have no joint pain, rashes, abnormal bruising, breathlessness, or leg swelling.
- There is no loss of weight or appetite.
- You have no headache, weakness, numbness, or double vision.
- You have no hearing problems.

Past medical and surgical history:
- Nil
- You think that your blood pressure was last checked a year ago and was normal.

Medication list:
- Nil
- No supplements or traditional medicine.
- No drug allergy.

Family history:
- Your mother had kidney failure in her 50s and is currently on peritoneal dialysis. You do not know the cause of her kidney failure.
- Your late aunt was also on dialysis and passed away from a dialysis catheter infection.
- There is no family history of bleeding in the brain or sudden death.

Relevant personal, social, occupational, and travel history:
- You are a never-smoker.
- You are an engineer. Your area of expertise is silicon wafer production; you mainly do design work and have no exposure to industrial chemicals.
- You are not married and do not have children.
- Your hobby is playing golf with friends.

Relevant physical examination findings:

This encounter will use a real patient.
- Patient is well.
- No abdominal scars.
- No peripheral findings, no dialysis fistula, no vascular catheter scars.
- Abdomen is soft and non-tender with bilateral ballotable kidneys ± hepatomegaly.
- Renal punch negative.
- No pedal oedema or basal lung crepitations.
- Cardiac and neurological examinations are normal.

You have some specific questions for the doctor at this consultation:
- Will I need dialysis like my mum?

Approach and Clinical Reasoning

The approach to haematuria (Figure B4.2) begins by excluding urinary tract infection and confounders. The stem helpfully provides that haematuria is persistent. The next step is to distinguish between renal vs. urological aetiologies. This scenario does not provide enough information to make a definite conclusion either way — there is hypertension but no proteinuria or renal impairment, and no information on whether the haematuria is isomorphic or dysmorphic.

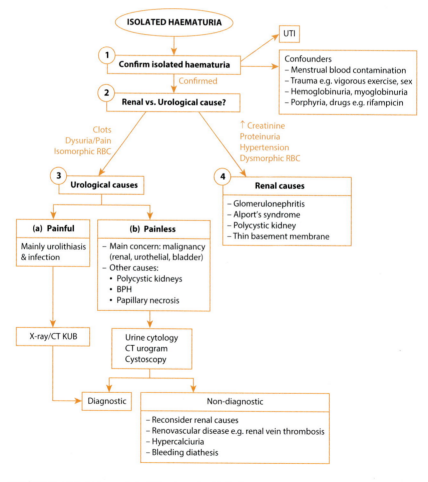

BPH: benign prostatic hyperplasia; UTI: urinary tract infection

Figure B4.2. Approach to isolated haematuria.

Key points in history include:

- The absence of pain makes infection and urolithiasis less likely.
- Look for features which should suggest glomerulonephritis (GN) – systemic rheumatic disease, relationship of haematuria with infections (IgA nephropathy, infection-associated GN), chronic viral hepatitis, etc.
- Explore the possibility of urological malignancy. Ask about loss of weight/appetite and risk factors (smoking, occupational chemical exposure, pelvic radiation, exposure to schistosomiasis).
- Ask for a family history.

The diagnosis of polycystic kidney disease (PKD) reveals itself in the physical examination when bilateral kidneys are balloted. Even before examination, this diagnosis should be suspected with Mr Pei's strong family history of kidney failure — it is quite easy to miss polycystic kidneys if one is not looking for them.

Think this through: Suspecting polycystic kidneys

> This station hinges on the identification of a critical physical sign (i.e., bilateral ballotable kidneys). If not carefully felt for, this sign is easy to miss. What are the presenting stems that will prompt you to examine the abdomen carefully for renal masses?

Haematuria is common in PKD and can often be the presenting symptom. Consider whether there is any complication of PKD that contributed to haematuria (Table B4.16).

Table B4.16. Causes of haematuria in polycystic kidney disease.

Differential	Important features
Cyst rupture, haemorrhage into cyst	Haematuria usually resolves within a week (occasionally can persist) There may be brisk haematuria
Nephrolithiasis	Classically with loin to groin pain
Malignant change	May be asymptomatic or present with persistent haematuria (Note: PKD increases risk of renal tract malignancies)
Infection	Fever, flank pain, dysuria, foul-smelling urine more common than haematuria

Apart from eliciting bilateral ballotable kidneys, the physical examination should also cover:

- Renal punch for possible pyelonephritis.
- Examine for suggestions of renal insufficiency – fluid status, dialysis fistulae, parathyroidectomy scar.

It will be a bonus to consider the other manifestations of polycystic kidney disease:
- Anaemia (due to chronic kidney disease).
- Cerebral aneurysm with subarachnoid haemorrhage – asking for episodes of thunderclap headache, screening pronator drift.
- Hepatic cyst: examining for hepatomegaly (this would have been a part of the abdominal examination).
- Cardiac valvular disease: auscultating for mitral valve prolapse, aortic regurgitation (if time permits).

Question and Answer

Suggested answer to the patient's concerns:

Mr Pei, thank you for sharing this worry with me. The possibility of being on dialysis must scare you especially after seeing your loved ones go through it. I am concerned that you and your family members may have an inherited condition known as polycystic kidney disease, which can cause blood in the urine as in your case. Some patients with this condition do end up on dialysis; however, the decline in kidney function is quite gradual, over many years. I will need to do a blood test to know how well your kidneys are functioning at this moment.

Suggested presentation to the examiner:

Mr Pei presents with painless microscopic haematuria. I suspect that he has polycystic kidney disease as evidenced by bilateral ballotable kidneys and a strong family history. He is hypertensive, but there is no other suggestion of fluid overload or renal insufficiency at the moment. There is no hepatomegaly to suggest large hepatic cysts, or pronator drift to suggest subarachnoid haemorrhage.

Investigations:

- Confirm the diagnosis of polycystic kidney disease by doing ultrasound kidneys or CT kidneys.
- Characterise urinary abnormality: urine microscopy, phase contrast, and protein/creatinine ratio.
- Evaluate for the cause of haematuria, ideally with a CT urogram if renal function allows.
- Assess renal function and electrolytes.
- Look for complications of chronic kidney disease: electrolytes, blood count, and evaluation for mineral bone disease (calcium/phosphate/vitamin D/parathyroid hormone).
- Discuss MRI screening for intracranial aneurysm (especially if there is a family history of intracranial haemorrhage or high-risk occupation or hobby).

Management:

- Treatment of haemorrhagic cysts in PKD is generally conservative (nephrectomy indicated only if there is unusually severe and persistent bleeding or malignant change).
- Longer-term management of polycystic kidney disease:
  - Regular follow up to monitor progression of renal disease
  - Standard care of chronic kidney disease including blood pressure control, antiproteinuric therapy, dietary advice, and managing anaemia
  - Managing complications of PKD

Note: Tailor the management to this patient. As there is no fluid overload at this moment, diuretics should not be part of the management plan.

Consultation Case 22

Mrs Childless (Amenorrhoea)

Use this case as practice! The pull-out booklet contains the candidate's information.

Information for the Candidate

Patient Details: Mrs Childless, 34 years old

Your Role: General Medicine Clinic SHO

Referral Letter:
> Dear Colleague,
>
> Thank you for seeing Mrs Childless. She has missed her menstrual period for 3 months and is complaining of fatigue. A urine pregnancy test is negative.
>
> Thank you.
>
> Dr Stork, GP

Vital Signs: BP 90/52 mmHg, HR 57/min, RR 11/min, SpO2 98% RA, T 37.0°C

Patient's Brief

Synopsis: *This lady has a pituitary macroadenoma, presenting with bitemporal hemianopia, oligomenorrhoea, weight gain, symptoms of hypothyroidism, adrenal insufficiency, and hyperprolactinemia.*

Open the consult with: My husband and I have been trying for a child for the past 3 years, but we have not been successful. My periods are infrequent and scanty. I have also been feeling tired. *Do not volunteer any other information unless asked.*

History of current problem:
- Last menstrual period 3 months ago. Periods have been irregular (every 2–3 months) and light (1–2 pads/day at the heaviest) for the past year. You had your first period at 14 years old and have always had 'normal periods' (every 30 days, lasting 5 days each time, 5 pads/day at the heaviest).
- You do not have painful periods, vaginal discharge, or intermenstrual bleed.
- No previous pregnancies, miscarriages, abortions, or uterine instrumentation.
- You have been feeling unusually tired and cold for the last 4 months. No constipation or diarrhoea.

- Occasional giddy spells particularly when getting up from a seated position.
- No tummy swelling or stretch marks over your abdomen.
- Decreased sex drive for the past 3 months – you desire a child and there are no marital issues; however, you have found it difficult to become sufficiently aroused to allow penetrative vaginal intercourse. You do not have any history of pain during sexual intercourse (vaginismus).
- No hot flushes or unusual mood swings.
- No increase in shoe/ring size and no sweaty palms.
- No breast pain. You occasionally do have small amounts of milky discharge from both breasts.
- You do not notice any appreciable change in your vision. However, you have recently gotten into 2 car accidents in the past year — both times with a car that was attempting to filter into your lane from the side. You had always been a very careful driver.
- No previous brain tumour, surgery, or radiation. No headaches or vomiting.
- You have been otherwise well with no loss of appetite or major stressors.
- You have persistent concerns about being overweight (BMI 34). You recently started a rather extreme diet (one meal a day) and exercise regime (running 10 km a day). This has been spectacularly unsuccessful; you have in fact gained 5 kg in the last 2 months.
- You have always had bothersome acne since teenage years.

Past medical and surgical history:
- Obesity
- Impaired fasting glucose, on yearly glucose checks

Medication list:
- Nil
- No herbal remedies
- Drug allergy: nil

Family history:
- Nil

Relevant personal, social, occupational, and travel history:
- Married. Yet to successfully conceive despite 3 years of regular unprotected sexual intercourse.
- You work as a real estate agent and drive around for work.
- You do not smoke or drink.
- No relevant travel history.

Relevant physical examination findings:

This station can be run with either a real patient, or with a surrogate who has been trained to simulate the visual field findings.

- Large body habitus
- Visual acuity grossly normal
- Bitemporal hemianopia on confrontation visual field testing
- Extraocular eye movements normal
- No goitre, no peaches and cream skin
- No spade-like hands/feet, increase in shoe/ring size, macroglossia, or coarse facial features
- No cushingoid features
- Neurological examination normal, no delayed relaxation of reflexes
- If postural blood pressure is offered – 90/52 mmHg supine, 68/40 mmHg standing

You have some specific questions for the doctor at this consultation:

- My husband and I have been longing for a child. Do you think I will ever be able to get pregnant?

Approach and Clinical Reasoning

Mrs Childless has oligomenorrhoea. Pregnancy is, of course, the most common cause of amenorrhoea, but the stem has helpfully ruled this out. Although a gynaecological cause of oligomenorrhoea is unlikely in MRCP PACES, you will still need to demonstrate a reasonable approach to oligomenorrhoea including consideration of gynaecological causes. The causes of oligomenorrhoea are easily remembered by considering structural and functional disease along each part of the hypothalamic-pituitary-gonadal axis (Table B4.17).

Always begin history-taking with open-ended questions; in particular, explore if Mrs Childless has additional symptoms that may suggest an aetiology of oligomenorrhoea. The stem provides information that the patient is fatigued. In addition, Mrs Childless readily offers information that she has symptoms of hypothyroidism (cold intolerance, weight gain), hypogonadism (decreased libido), and hypocortisolism (postural hypotension). This is panhypopituitarism and the history of car accidents suggest bitemporal hemianopia from a pituitary adenoma. Further, Mrs Childless' history of galactorrhoea points to hyperprolactinemia; she may have a prolactinoma or a non-functioning macroadenoma (which compresses the pituitary stalk, preventing dopamine transport from the hypothalamus to the pituitary, and therefore removing the inhibition of dopamine on prolactin secretion).

Table B4.17. Causes of oligomenorrhoea.

	Structural	**Functional**
Hypothalamus	Tumour (rare) Infiltration (e.g., sarcoidosis, Langerhans cell histiocytosis (rare))	Major illness, stressors Anorexia, intense exercise
Pituitary	Adenoma (screen hormone axes and symptoms of mass effect) - Prolactinoma - Cushing's disease - Acromegaly - Non-functioning tumour Surgery, haemorrhage, infiltration	Drugs – hyperprolactinaemia from dopamine antagonists (drug history especially antipsychotics)
Ovary	Oophorectomy	Hyperthyroidism Polycystic ovary syndrome (mild hyperandrogenism, metabolic syndrome) Premature ovarian failure (menopausal symptoms)
Adrenal	Androgen-producing adrenal tumour Adrenal Cushing's disease	
Uterus	Hysterectomy Asherman's syndrome (prior uterine instrumentation)	Pregnancy

Practice makes perfect: Screening the pituitary hormone axes

> Asking about each pituitary hormone axis is not straightforward and thus time-consuming. Prepare and practice a set of 10–15 questions that you can use to quickly screen through the pituitary hormonal axes (thyroid, adrenal, growth hormone, prolactin, sex hormones, antidiuretic hormone) and mass symptoms (bitemporal hemianopia, headache, giddiness). This can come in useful in many presenting complaints.

Differentials to consider:

- Polycystic ovarian syndrome (PCOS) is an important differential given that Mrs Childless has mild hyperandrogenism (acne), impaired fasting glucose, and obesity (although hypothyroidism can also explain weight gain).
- Functional hypothalamic oligomenorrhoea is possible given her extreme diet and exercise regime. However, this is less likely given her weight gain and the associated symptoms.

- Ensure that you take an adequate menstrual history and ask about gynaecological causes of oligomenorrhoea and use of dopamine antagonists (which can cause hyperprolactinemia) such as metoclopramide.

Physical examination should focus on demonstrating mass effect of the pituitary adenoma (test visual fields) and features of hypothyroidism (peaches and cream skin, bradycardia, slow-relaxing reflexes, etc.). It is important to request a postural blood pressure (you will rarely be asked to do it).

The safety issues that need to be addressed in a pituitary disorder scenario are:
- Mrs Childless has hypocortisolism with borderline blood pressure; this is worrying and warrants admission.
- Ensure that Mrs Childless has no acute headache, vomiting, or hypotension to suggest pituitary apoplexy.
- Mrs Childless is driving despite bitemporal hemianopia. She must be advised otherwise.

Question and Answer

Suggested answer to the patient's concerns:

Mrs Childless, it must have been really difficult to desire a child this much and yet not be able to have one. I suspect that you have not been able to get pregnant because of a problem with a hormone gland in your brain called the pituitary. What you have told me suggests a benign growth of this gland, which has caused your hormone levels to be low. This is why you have been tired, feeling cold, gaining weight, and struggling with your sex drive. We need to confirm this through a brain scan and blood tests, but if you have what I suspect, it is something that we can treat. You may also need hormone replacement but with treatment, there is a reasonable chance that you can get pregnant some time in the future.

For the time being, please do not drive until your vision is normal.

Suggested presentation to the examiner:

Mrs Childless presents with longstanding oligomenorrhoea and a 3- to 4-month history of weight gain, hypothyroidism, postural hypotension, decreased libido, and hyperprolactinemia. My examination is significant for bitemporal hemianopia and large body habitus. I suspect that she has panhypopituitarism due to a pituitary adenoma, which may be a prolactinoma or another adenoma with pituitary stalk compression. My differentials include polycystic ovarian syndrome in view of metabolic syndrome and mild hyperandrogenism, as well as functional hypothalamic disease due to extreme diet and exercise, although this is less likely. There is no suggestion of pituitary apoplexy.

I am inclined to admit her in view of adrenal insufficiency and borderline blood pressure.

My investigations will include:
- MRI pituitary fossa looking for a pituitary adenoma.
- Blood tests for the pituitary hormonal axes including:
  - ACTH levels and ACTH stimulation (short synacthen) test; renal panel looking for hyponatraemia and hyperkalaemia.
  - T4 and thyroid stimulating hormone levels.
  - Follicle stimulating hormone, luteinising hormone, estradiol.
  - Prolactin.
  - Insulin-like growth factor 1.
- Referral to ophthalmology for formal visual field assessment.

Should these investigations confirm the diagnosis of a pituitary adenoma, management involves a multidisciplinary team including an endocrinologist, neurosurgeon, ophthalmologist, and allied healthcare professionals. This includes:

- Replacement of hormone deficiencies. especially physiologic cortisol replacement.
- Prolactinoma: dopamine agonists (i.e., cabergoline; bromocriptine is rarely used now).
- Other pituitary tumours: definitive management involves transphenoidal resection of the pituitary.
- She must stop driving for now.

Consultation Case 23

Ms Liu B. Xue (Epistaxis)

Use this case as practice! The pull-out booklet contains the candidate's information.

Information for the Candidate

Patient Details: Ms Liu B. Xue, 30 years old

Your Role: Internal Medicine Clinic SHO

Referral Letter:
> Dear Colleague,
>
> Thank you for seeing Ms Liu. She has been seeing me for repeated episodes of nosebleeds. I have tried silver nitrate cautery, but this was only of limited effectiveness.
>
> Dr Sherilyn Liew, ENT Surgeon

Vital Signs: BP 115/60 mmHg, HR 60/min, RR 12/min, SpO2 99% RA, T 36.2°C

Patient's Brief

Synopsis: *This young lady has recurrent epistaxis, gastrointestinal bleeding, symptomatic anaemia, mucocutaneous telangiectasia, and a positive family history. The diagnosis is hereditary haemorrhagic telangiectasia.*

Open the consult with: I've always had on and off nosebleeds all my life, but they never bothered me too much. I feel well otherwise. *Do not volunteer any other information unless asked.*

History of current problem:

- You have nosebleeds every 1–2 weeks. This usually stops after you pinch your nose for 10–15 minutes. You have never needed to visit the emergency department, undergo surgery, or receive transfusions as a result of nosebleeds.
- You occasionally notice small amounts of fresh red blood in your stools, which you attribute to haemorrhoids — you are chronically constipated because you dislike fruits and vegetables.
- You do notice that you have been slightly more lightheaded and more tired recently. You used to run 10 km every weekend but are no longer able to.
- Your periods are not unusually heavy (3–4 pads/day for 5 days).

- You have no gum bleeding.
- You have not noticed any easy bruising or joint swelling after minor trauma.
- You have had an uneventful wisdom tooth extraction 2 years ago. You do not recall having prolonged bleeding after this.
- No weight loss or night sweats.
- No jaundice or change in urine colour.
- No blood or froth in urine, decrease in urine volume, or leg swelling.
- No fever, joint pain, or rashes.
- No blood-stained nasal discharge, cough, blood in sputum, or breathlessness.
- No headache, weakness, numbness, seizures, or double vision.

Past medical and surgical history:
- Nil

Medication list:
- Nil; specifically, no blood thinners
- Supplements and herbal remedies: nil
- Drug allergy: penicillin

Family history:
- Your father passed away suddenly in his 30s while you were an infant. You recall that he had a sudden bleed in the brain in his sleep.
- Your older sister has also always had frequent nosebleeds.
- Your younger brother is unaffected.
- No family history of nose cancer.

Relevant personal, social, occupational, and travel history:
- You are practicing as a lawyer.
- You are engaged to be married next year. You do not have any children.
- You are sexually active with your fiancé. You use condoms 100% of the time.
- You do not smoke, drink, or use recreational drugs.

Relevant physical examination findings:
- Telangiectasia over oral mucosa and the lips (Photo 20), as well as the fingertips; none over the face/chest/back.
- No sclerodactyly, pseudoclubbing, acroosteolysis, microstomia.
- No conjunctival pallor or scleral icterus.
- No liver or lung bruit, and no chest scars.
- No focal neurological deficit.

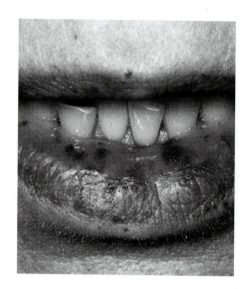

Photo 20

Photo by Raimo Suhonen. Reproduced with permission from DermNet NZ www.dermnetnz.org

You have some specific questions for the doctor at this consultation:

- If I have children, will my children also have this condition?

Approach and Clinical Reasoning

This case can be a spot diagnosis if you recognise the oral and finger telangiectasia of hereditary haemorrhagic telangiectasia (HHT, Osler-Weber-Rendu syndrome). HHT is a PACES staple and epistaxis is its most common stem.

Pitfall: Jumping to a spot diagnosis

Do not jump to the spot diagnosis. Examiners want to see a sound clinical approach to the presenting complaint.

Additionally, remember that not every patient with telangiectasia has HHT. Differentials for telangiectasia/mucosal hyperpigmentation include:

- Telangiectasia in HHT (specifically over oral and buccal mucosa, as well as the fingertips)
- Telangiectasia in systemic sclerosis (may be more generalised in distribution)
- Spider naevi in chronic liver disease
- Hyperpigmented macules in Peutz-Jegher's syndrome
- Hyperpigmentation in Addison's disease
- Benign oral naevi

Begin by taking a bleeding history, which should cover:
- Site of bleeding: mucocutaneous (platelet disorder), intramuscular/intra-articular (clotting factor disorder), or palpable purpura (vasculitis)
- Frequency and severity of bleeding
- Spontaneous vs. provoked bleeding
- Menstrual history
- Previous haemostatic challenges (e.g., childbirth, surgeries, dental procedures)
- Onset – congenital vs. acquired disorder

Next, consider the consider the causes of epistaxis (Table B4.18).

Table B4.18. Differentials to epistaxis in PACES.

	Aetiology	Important features
Systemic causes	Bleeding diathesis (e.g., immune thrombocytopenia, Von Willebrand disease, liver and renal disease)	Other bleeding manifestations apart from epistaxis (e.g., bruising, menorrhagia)
	Drugs (antiplatelets, anticoagulants)	Drug history
	Granulomatosis with polyangiitis (Wegener's)	Systemic manifestations (e.g., cough, dyspnoea, nephritis, neuropathies)
Local causes	Hereditary haemorrhagic telangiectasia	Oral and finger telangiectasia, visceral arteriovenous malformations (e.g., rectal bleeding), family history
	Nasopharyngeal carcinoma and other nasal cancers	Blood tinged nasal discharge, cranial neuropathy; more common in patients of southern Chinese ancestry
	Carotid blowout	Previous carotid surgery or radiation therapy
	Chronic intranasal drug use	History of sniffing drugs (e.g., cocaine)
	Idiopathic	Exacerbated by nose picking, cold and dry air

Ms Liu has a longstanding history of epistaxis, rectal bleeding complicated with symptomatic anaemia, and a positive family history with her father having had a fatal intracranial bleed. Apart from HHT, a bleeding diathesis such as Von Willebrand disease is a differential. Quickly exclude liver disease, renal disease, drugs, and myeloproliferative and autoimmune disease.

Finally, it is important to screen for complications of HHT, in particular that of visceral arteriovenous malformations (AVM):
- Anaemia
- Gastrointestinal AVM: rectal bleeding, hepatomegaly, hepatic encephalopathy (from porto-systemic AVMs)
- Cerebral AVM: intracranial haemorrhage, seizures

- Pulmonary AVM: haemoptysis, high output heart failure, paradoxical embolism/stroke

Note: Dyspnoea in HHT can be multifactorial, due to anaemia, high output cardiac failure, and venous thromboembolism

Examination should:

- Demonstrate the characteristic features of HHT (i.e., telangiectasia over oral and buccal mucosa and fingertips). Telangiectasia can be subtle — you must look hard inside the mouth.
- Check for complications of HHT, such as:
  - Anaemia – conjunctival pallor, offer digital rectal examination
  - CNS – screen pronator drift and cranial nerves
  - Lungs – chest scars, auscultate for lung bruit
  - Abdomen – examine for hepatomegaly, auscultate for liver bruit
  - Cardiac – check for pedal oedema and raised jugular venous pressure (high output cardiac failure)
- Exclude differentials (e.g., check for other stigmata of chronic liver disease)

Question and Answer

Suggested answer to the patient's concerns:

Ms Liu, thank you for sharing this worry with me. I suspect that you may have an inherited condition known as 'hereditary haemorrhagic telangiectasia', although I do need to do some tests to look for other conditions. This condition makes you bleed more easily, and you are right to point out the possibility that you can pass it to your children. This is an inherited condition and your children do have a 50% chance[13] of inheriting it, assuming that your partner is normal.

Suggested presentation to the examiner:

Ms Liu has recurrent epistaxis, gastrointestinal bleeding, symptomatic anaemia, and a significant family history of epistaxis and fatal intracranial bleed. Physical examination is significant for telangiectasia over oral and buccal mucosa and over the fingertips. She has symptoms of anaemia but is not pale. My primary diagnosis is hereditary haemorrhagic telangiectasia. Differentials include a bleeding diathesis such as Von Willebrand disease. I do not note any focal neurology to suggest complications of a cerebral arteriovenous malformation or paradoxical embolism through a pulmonary arteriovenous malformation, and no evidence of heart failure. I will like to complete my examination by performing a rectal examination.

---

[13] This is an autosomal dominant disorder.

The diagnosis of HHT is clinical (Curaçao criteria). My investigations will include:

- Checking haemoglobin and iron studies.
- Check platelets and coagulation studies to look for differentials to HHT.
- Consider sending Von Willebrand factor antigen, ristocetin cofactor activity, and factor VIII to screen for Von Willebrand disease.
- Check liver and renal biochemistries.
- Genetic testing to confirm the diagnosis is possible but may not be necessary if the diagnosis can be made on clinical criteria.

Management:

- She may require admission for blood transfusion if significantly anaemic.
- Advice on epistaxis first aid; obtain ENT input on cautery and packing for persistent or unresolving bleeds.
- Iron supplementation.
- Discuss screening for pulmonary and cerebral arteriovenous malformations[14].
- Do genetic counselling and screen family members.

---

[14] Embolisation or resection of pulmonary AVMs may be indicated. Screening for cerebral AVMs is controversial in an asymptomatic patient with HHT as it is unclear whether the risk of intervention outweighs the risk of resection.

Consultation Case 24

Mr A. M. Indra (Hyperlipidaemia)

Use this case as practice! The pull-out booklet contains the candidate's information.

Information for the Candidate

Patient Details: Mr A. M. Indra, 40 years old

Your Role: Cardiology Outpatients SHO

Referral Letter:
> Dear Colleague,
>
> Mr A. M. Indra was diagnosed with hyperlipidaemia on health screening 6 months ago. Despite Atorvastatin 40 mg ON, his low-density lipoprotein (LDL) levels remain at 5.6 mmol/L, from 5.7 mmol/L previously (normal < 4.1 mmol/L; optimal < 2.6 mmol/L). He is concerned about the risk of a heart attack and wishes to see you.
>
> Thank you.
>
> Dr Cheryl Lie, GP

Vital Signs: BP 125/82 mmHg, HR 57/min, RR 12/min, SpO2 99% RA, T 37.0°C

Patient's Brief

Synopsis: *This 40-year-old gentleman has nephrotic syndrome with hyperlipidaemia, pedal oedema, and frothy urine.*

Open the consult with: *The GP told me that my cholesterol levels are still high and I'm going to get a heart attack if I don't do anything about it.* Do not volunteer any other information unless asked.

History of current problem:

- You saw the GP 6 months ago for company-sponsored health screening and were diagnosed with hyperlipidaemia.
- Since then, you have consistently taken atorvastatin 40 mg every night at bedtime. You set a reminder on your phone and never miss a dose.
- You have cut down on high-cholesterol foods in your diet and started exercising at least 2–3 times a week (from none previously).
- You have no muscle aches or liver problems due to atorvastatin.

Consultation Case 24

- You have noted mild bilateral leg swelling in the past year, but you think this is because of prolonged standing.
- You are not obese. However, you have gained 5 kg in the past year despite a decrease in your diet intake and an increase in exercise.
- Your urine has been frothy. There is no blood in your urine or difficulty passing urine.
- You do not have cold intolerance, constipation, menorrhagia, or lethargy.
- No jaundice, generalised itch, or change in urine colour.
- You have no joint pains, mouth ulcers, or rashes.
- No weight loss, change in bowel habit, chronic cough, or rectal bleeding.
- No prior kidney disease, kidney stones, or bladder problems.
- No chest pain or breathlessness.

Past medical and surgical history:
- Nil
- In particular, no history of HIV, hepatitis B or C.
- You have been screened for diabetes and high blood pressure during health screening and were told that you had neither.

Medication list:
- Atorvastatin 40 mg ON
- Supplements and herbal remedies: nil
- Drug allergy: nil

Family history:
- Father and grandfather had both passed away from myocardial infarctions in their early 40s.

Relevant personal, social, occupational, and travel history:
- You work in a sedentary office job.
- Married with a 10-year-old daughter and a 7-year-old son.
- No sexual activity apart from regular intercourse with your wife.
- No intravenous drug use.
- Smoker, half pack a day for 30 years.
- Social drinker, approximately 10 units of alcohol a week.

Relevant physical examination findings:

This station can be run with either a real patient or a surrogate.
- Not obese.
- Bilateral symmetrical mild pedal oedema, nontender, no erythema.

- No orbital xanthelasma or tendon xanthoma.
- No jaundice.
- No goitre, peaches and cream skin, loss of lateral third of eyebrows, or slow-relaxing reflexes.
- No rashes or joint swelling.
- No significant pleural effusion.

You have some specific questions for the doctor at this consultation:

- Am I going to get a heart attack? My father and grandfather both died in their early 40s and I have two young children.

Approach and Clinical Reasoning

Mr Indra has persistent hyperlipidaemia despite statin treatment. The most common causes of refractory hyperlipidaemia are non-compliance to medication or incorrect dosing (statins should be taken at bedtime, instead of in the morning) and dietary indiscretion. This is easy to rule out as Mr Indra is compliant to both medications and lifestyle changes.

Next, consider secondary causes of hyperlipidaemia (Table B4.19).

Table B4.19. Secondary causes of hyperlipidaemia.

Cause	Important clinical features
Familial hypercholesterolaemia	Family history, tendon xanthomas, orbital xanthelasmas
Nephrotic syndrome	Frothy urine (proteinuria), pedal oedema
Cholestatic liver disease, particularly primary biliary cholangitis	Jaundice, pruritus, and dark urine. Hepatosplenomegaly, xanthelasma
Hypothyroidism	Cold intolerance, menorrhagia, constipation, lethargy
Metabolic syndrome	Diabetes, obesity
Drugs	Drug history (e.g., atypical antipsychotics, antiretrovirals)

Further history will reveal clues for both familial hyperlipidaemia (family history of premature coronary disease) and nephrotic syndrome (frothy urine, pedal oedema) in Mr Indra.

Next, screen for secondary causes of the nephrotic syndrome, particularly ruling out features of autoimmune disease or malignancy (MN = membranous nephropathy, MCD = minimal change disease, FSGS = focal segmental glomerulosclerosis):

- Inflammatory: Lupus nephritis (class V)

- Malignancy: solid organ (MN), leukaemia/lymphoma (MCD), myeloma
- Amyloidosis – AL (light chain/myeloma) or AA (due to chronic inflammatory disease)
- Infection: HIV (collapsing FSGS), hepatitis B (MN), hepatitis C (membranoproliferative GN)
- Drugs: NSAIDs, penicillin, lithium, penicillamine, bisphosphonates, sulfasalazine, mercury (in whitening creams), heroin, interferon
- Causes of hyperfiltration: obesity, reflux nephropathy, reduced kidney mass (FSGS)

As always, ensure that there is no immediate emergency — that Mr Indra has no angina symptoms or breathlessness (from nephrotic syndrome).

Physical examination would aim to demonstrate features of nephrotic syndrome (pedal oedema, lung crepitations, ascites) and differentials to hyperlipidaemia (xanthelasma, tendon xanthoma, jaundice, goitre).

Question and Answer

Suggested answer to the patient's concerns:

Mr Indra, I hear your worry. You are right that uncontrolled cholesterol levels will increase the risk of a heart attack, so we must do everything we can to bring down your cholesterol levels. I need to investigate why your cholesterol is persistently high. In particular, I suspect that you may be having a condition called nephrotic syndrome, whereby your kidneys leak protein. This is probably why your urine is bubbly and your legs are swollen; it can also cause your cholesterol levels to be high. I will do some blood and urine tests and if it confirms what I suspect, I will refer you to the kidney doctor. Nephrotic syndrome is a treatable illness and the good news is that your cholesterol levels should come down with treatment. One more thing you can do to minimise the risk of a heart attack is to stop smoking — if you are keen to consider, please allow me to refer you to a smoking cessation counsellor and get you some nicotine patches.

Suggested presentation to the examiner:

Mr Indra has refractory hyperlipidaemia despite compliance with high-intensity statin, which is associated with frothy urine and pedal oedema. Physical examination is significant for pedal oedema; significant negatives include the absence of xanthelasma, jaundice, goitre, and obesity.

My principle diagnosis is nephrotic syndrome without any obvious secondary cause. I will also wish to consider familial hypercholesterolemia in view of the significant family history of premature coronary artery disease. Less likely causes of refractory hyperlipidaemia include hypothyroidism, cholestatic liver disease, or metabolic syndrome.

I will like to investigate by:

- Repeating the lipid panel.

- Confirming my diagnosis of nephrotic syndrome by doing:
  - Urinary microscopy and 24-hour urinary protein.
  - Urea, creatinine, and electrolytes.
  - Serum albumin.
- Investigating for a cause of nephrotic syndrome:
  - Ultrasound kidneys.
  - Fasting glucose and HbA1c.
  - Viral serology (e.g., HIV, hepatitis B and C).
  - Anti-phospholipase A2 receptor antibody (primary membranous nephropathy).
  - Autoimmune serology beginning with antinuclear antibody (ANA) and anti-double-stranded DNA (anti-dsDNA).
  - Myeloma study (serum and urine protein electrophoresis, serum free light chains).
  - Refer for renal biopsy.
- Considering differentials:
  - Thyroid function test.
  - Liver function test.
  - Consider genetic testing for familial hypercholesterolemia if clinical criteria (Simon-Broome criteria) are not met.

Mr Indra can be managed as an outpatient unless he is very symptomatic. I will enlist a multidisciplinary team including the GP, nephrologist, smoking cessation counsellor, and dietician. Key tenets of management include:

- Intensive statin therapy.
- Treatment of nephrotic syndrome including:
  - Immunosuppression or treatment of secondary causes as appropriate.
  - Diuresis.
  - Angiotensin inhibition.
  - Fluid restriction, low-sodium diet.
  - Avoidance of nephrotoxins.
- Minimise cardiac risk by treating other coronary risk factors, diet, exercise, and smoking cessation.
- Patient education.

Consultation Case 25

Mdm Hashi (Fatigue)

Use this case as practice! The pull-out booklet contains the candidate's information.

Information for the Candidate

Patient Details: Mdm Hashi, 36 years old

Your Role: Endocrine Clinic SHO

Referral Letter:
> Dear Colleague,
>
> Mdm Hashi is on my follow up for hypothyroidism. She is complaining of persistent fatigue in spite of thyroxine replacement. Her latest free T4 is 12 pmol/L (normal: 11 - 21 pmol/L), and thyroid stimulating hormone is 3.0 mIU/L (normal: 0.5 - 5.0 mIU/L). Could you please see her?
>
> Thank you.
>
> Dr Moto, GP

Vital Signs: BP 91/52 mmHg, HR 62/min, RR 10/min, SpO2 100% RA, T 35.8°C

Patient's Brief

Synopsis: *This patient with a previous history of Hashimoto thyroiditis now presents with adrenal insufficiency, difficulty lactating, and decreased libido following postpartum haemorrhage. Differentials include Sheehan's syndrome, autoimmune adrenalitis, and symptomatic anaemia.*

Open the consult with: I have been feeling very tired for the last 2 months, I don't really know why. *Do not volunteer any other information.*

History of current problem:
- Your fatigue started 2 months ago after the birth of your youngest daughter.
- You had undergone a normal vaginal delivery under epidural anaesthesia but suffered severe blood loss after delivery, had a low blood pressure, and needed transfusion of multiple packs of blood. You were told that this bleeding occurred because of retained placental tissue, which was removed.
- Apart from fatigue, you have also been having giddiness, especially when you stand up suddenly from a sitting or lying position. You recall almost passing out several times when you stood up on a crowded bus.

- There is no increase in fatigue throughout the day or with any activity.
- You have lost 5 kg in the last 2 months, and your appetite is poor.
- You have had difficulty breastfeeding due to minimal milk production; you have had to rely on formula milk.
- You have experienced a decrease in libido after delivery, but you think that this is expected. Prior to this pregnancy, you had typical periods (5 pads/day at the heaviest, lasting 5 days, every 25–30 days) and you conceived within 6 months of starting to try for a baby. Your period has not returned post-partum.
- You have no cold or heat intolerance, diarrhoea or constipation, mood symptoms, or leg swelling.
- You have no muscle stiffness/aches, fever, night sweats, loud snoring, or daytime sleepiness. Your mood has been good.
- You do not have any easy bruising, heavy periods, further vaginal or gastrointestinal bleeding, or history of bleeding tendencies.
- You have no headaches or change in your vision. You did not have any episode of severe headache in the past few months.
- There is no darkening of your skin.
- You have had no major infection, recent trauma, or chronic cough.

Past medical and surgical history:
- You have Hashimoto thyroiditis, diagnosed in your late 20s. You are on thyroxine replacement, which you take first thing in the morning with a glass of water, separated from other food by at least 2 hours. You have never missed a dose of thyroxine.
- No other medical or surgical history.

Medication list:
- Thyroxine 75 mcg OM. You take this first thing every morning, at least 2 h before breakfast. There were a number of dose changes during and after pregnancy, but you have been told that your thyroid hormone levels (last checked 1 week ago) were within acceptable limits.
- Ferrous fumarate 200 mg with lunch.
- Supplements and herbal remedies: nil.
- Drug allergy: nil.

Family history:
- No relevant family history.

Relevant personal, social, occupational, and travel history:
- You are married with two children aged 4 years and 3 months. You are currently a home maker.

- No travel history and no personal or contact history of tuberculosis.
- You do not smoke or drink.

Relevant physical examination findings:

- No pallor.
- No cutaneous hyperpigmentation.
- Small, smooth goitre which ascends on swallowing, no bruit or retrosternal extension.
- Visual fields normal.
- No pedal oedema.
- Offer postural blood pressure – 91/52 mmHg falls to 65/37 mmHg on standing.

You have some specific questions for the doctor at this consultation:

- Why am I feeling so tired? Can I be treated?

Approach and Clinical Reasoning

The most obvious cause of fatigue in a patient with Hashimoto thyroiditis is, of course, hypothyroidism. This can occur due to (i) non-compliance to thyroxine replacement, (ii) dose reduction or significant changes in weight, or (iii) concomitant intake of calcium supplements, calcium-rich food, or ciprofloxacin causing interference with thyroxine absorption. However, the stem makes clear that Mdm Hashi is biochemically euthyroid. Therefore, quickly verify compliance and move on to look for other causes of fatigue.

Fatigue is a difficult complaint to approach cold because its differentials are incredibly broad (Table B4.20). Always use open-ended questions to prod for more clues (e.g., "apart from fatigue, is there anything else troubling you recently?") rather than diving into specific questions. Look out for any spot diagnoses as fatigue commonly complicates known conditions.

Table B4.20. Common differentials for fatigue in PACES*.

Category	Differential	Important features
Endocrine	Adrenal insufficiency	Postural hypotension/giddiness, hyperpigmentation (primary adrenal insufficiency), hyponatraemia; some patients complain of diffuse muscle aches
	Hypothyroidism	Cold intolerance, weight gain, constipation, menorrhagia
Rheumatologic	Myositis	Myalgia, proximal myopathy, rash (Gottron papules, heliotrope rash), underlying malignancy

(Cont'd)

Category	Differential	Important features
	Polymyalgia rheumatica	Aching and morning stiffness over the neck, shoulder, and hip girdle; may have features of giant cell arteritis
	Fibromyalgia	Chronic widespread muscle pain
Hematologic and oncologic	Anaemia	Blood loss, conjunctival pallor
	Malignancy	Night sweats, B symptoms, other specific features
Respiratory	Obstructive sleep apnoea	Loud snoring, witnessed apnoea, excessive daytime sleepiness
		Look for a secondary cause (e.g., acromegaly, hypothyroidism[15])
Psychiatric	Depression	Low mood, loss of interest
Nonspecific	Any chronic organ failure (e.g., heart failure, uraemia, liver disease)	
	Any cause of systemic inflammation (e.g., lupus)	
	Drugs (e.g., benzodiazepines, opioids, antihistamines, substance use)	

* This table summarises common differentials for fatigue in PACES, but the complete approach to fatigue is much broader.

Important differentials for Mdm Hashi are:

- Adrenal insufficiency – postural giddiness is prominent.
- Anaemia – given recent obstetric blood loss.

The next step is to search for an aetiology of adrenal insufficiency (Table B4.21). Note the key differences between primary adrenal insufficiency and secondary adrenal insufficiency (ACTH deficiency):

- Cutaneous hyperpigmentation arises from ACTH excess and is specific to primary adrenal insufficiency.
- Salt wasting, volume contraction, and hyperkalaemia are more prominent in primary adrenal insufficiency as aldosterone deficiency is more pronounced in primary adrenal insufficiency.
- Deficiencies of other pituitary hormones may be present in secondary adrenal insufficiency.

---

[15] Note: Excessive daytime sleepiness is a feature of myotonic dystrophy. However, this is thought to be a consequence of disordered central sleep regulation, rather than obstructive sleep apnoea.

Table B4.21. Causes of adrenal insufficiency.

Category	Differential	Important features
Primary (Addison's disease)	Autoimmune	Isolated or as part of an autoimmune polyendocrine syndrome (APS): • APS type 1: Addison's + hypoparathyroidism + candidiasis • APS type 2: Addison's + autoimmune thyroiditis + type 1 diabetes
	Infection	Most commonly tuberculosis; ask for night sweats, weight loss, contact and personal history
	Haemorrhage	Classically associated with meningococcaemia
	Metastatic	Adrenal metastases in lung, breast, stomach, or colon cancer, and melanoma
Secondary	Pituitary tumour, trauma, or infiltration	Bitemporal hemianopia; derangements in other pituitary endocrine axes Haemorrhage may also occur into a pituitary tumour (pituitary apoplexy)
	Pituitary infarction	Characteristically due to postpartum haemorrhage (Sheehan's syndrome)
Exogenous	Drugs	Adrenal suppression due to steroid use – sudden cessation leads to adrenal insufficiency Others: etomidate, ketoconazole, etc.

Don't forget: Exogenous steroid use

> Sudden cessation of exogenous steroids is a common cause of adrenal insufficiency. Probe hard for exogenous steroid use, including supplements and traditional medicine.

The two key differentials in Mdm Hashi are:

1. **Sheehan's syndrome.** She gives a history of postpartum haemorrhage preceding the onset of symptoms. She also has decreased libido and lactation difficulties which suggest derangements in the other pituitary hormone axes. Sheehan's syndrome occurs because the pituitary gland enlarges during pregnancy and is vulnerable to infarction from hypovolemic shock. It can present in the immediate postpartum period with hypotension, or up to years later with any manifestation of hypopituitarism (e.g., failure to lactate post-delivery, amenorrhoea, adrenal insufficiency, or hypothyroidism).

2. **Autoimmune adrenalitis**, particularly autoimmune polyendocrine syndrome type 2 as Mdm Hashi also has thyroiditis.

Additionally, pay attention to the temporal relationship between pregnancy and the onset of symptoms. If Mdm Hashi has a history of menstrual irregularities and subfertility preceding this pregnancy, then she may well have an existing pituitary tumour. On the other hand, if symptoms are new-onset, then the diagnosis of Sheehan's syndrome may be more likely.

Physical examination should focus on:

- Looking for features of primary and secondary adrenal insufficiency (i.e., cutaneous hyperpigmentation (primary adrenal insufficiency), visual fields (for bitemporal hemianopia from a pituitary tumour)).
- Checking for differentials (i.e., anaemia).
- Assessing thyroid status and examining goitre. While this is not diagnostically high-yielding, it is still a 'physical sign' that examiners may expect you to identify.

Finally, look out for frank Addison's crisis (hypotension, hypoglycaemia, abdominal pain) which will require you to admit the patient.

Question and Answer

Suggested answer to the patient's concerns:

Mdm Hashi, you are feeling so tired because your body is not producing enough steroid hormone. I also suspect that your body is not producing enough of other hormones, which is why you have difficulty breastfeeding. I will do some blood tests right now to confirm my diagnosis. I think it's best if we admit you to do these tests and make sure you are alright.

This is a very treatable condition, but you must take steroid replacements every day. If you are unwell, you may need to double the dose of your steroids. We will teach you how to give yourself injections in case you are vomiting and can't take tablets. Everyone worries about steroid side effects, but they do not apply to you because we are just replacing what you don't have, not giving you extra steroids. There are some very good patient support groups and an expert nurse whom I will like you to speak to.

Suggested presentation to the examiner:

Mdm Hashi presents with fatigue, weight loss, difficulty lactating, and decreased libido following postpartum haemorrhage. Clinical examination is significant for postural hypotension and a diffuse goitre. There is no cutaneous hyperpigmentation, visual field abnormality, or conjunctival pallor. My principal diagnosis is Sheehan's syndrome presenting with derangements of adrenal, prolactin, and sex hormone axes. My differentials include anaemia and autoimmune adrenalitis.

Investigations:

- I will like to confirm my diagnosis by performing:
  - ACTH stimulation test (short synacthen test).
  - ACTH levels to distinguish primary vs. secondary adrenal insufficiency.
  - Checking the pituitary hormone axes including T4, TSH, LH, prolactin, IGF-1.

- ○ Renal panel looking for hyponatraemia and hyperkalaemia.
- ○ MRI pituitary fossa looking for empty sella.
- I will like to assess for Addisonian crisis by checking glucose.
- I will like to look for differentials, in particular by checking her haemoglobin. I may also consider doing adrenal autoantibodies if autoimmune adrenalitis remains on the cards.

Management: I will admit Mdm Hashi for stabilisation as her blood pressure is borderline low. She will require a multidisciplinary team including the endocrinologist, obstetrician, and allied healthcare professionals such a nurse counsellor and lactation nurse. Principles of management include:

- Physiologic hormone replacement including hydrocortisone[16], estradiol, and any other deficient hormones.
- Patient education, particularly counselling on sick day protocols.
- Assistance with lactation.

---

[16] Fludrocortisone replacement is usually required in Addison's disease, but typically not required in central hypocortisolism.

Consultation Case 26

Mr Rachmaninoff (Numbness)

Use this case as practice! The pull-out booklet contains the candidate's information.

Information for the Candidate

Patient Details: Mr Rachmaninoff, 50 years old

Your Role: Neurology Clinic SHO

Referral Letter:
> Dear Neurology Colleague,
>
> Mr Rachmaninoff is on my follow up for diabetes. He has been complaining of hand numbness. I wonder if you could have a look at him?
>
> Thank you and warmest regards.
>
> Dr Tung Lin, GP

Vital Signs: BP 155/92 mmHg, HR 77/min, RR 11/min, SpO2 99% RA, T 36.0°C

Patient's Brief

Synopsis: *This professional pianist has carpal tunnel syndrome and underlying acromegaly.*

Open the consult with: I don't know what's going on; both of my hands are numb and tingling. I can't play the piano. *Do not volunteer any other information unless asked.*

History of current problem:

- This hand numbness and tingling started 3 months ago and has gotten worse since.
- Both the thumbs, index, middle, and ring fingers are numb. You are not sure about your little fingers.
- The numbness is worse when you bend your wrists, and especially if you sleep in the 'wrong position' at night.
- There is no numbness affecting your toes or elsewhere. You have no feet ulcers.
- You have no weakness; you are able to use your hands well.
- You have not injured your hands, wrists, elbows, or neck.
- You have no neck pain.

- You notice that your wedding ring no longer fits, and your shoe size has increased in the past year.
- You also notice that your palms are quite sweaty even in a cold room and this affects your work.
- Your wife complains that you snore loudly at night and you do wake up feeling unrefreshed. You have even fallen asleep while listening to piano recitals.
- You have occasional mild to moderate headaches. These are squeezing in nature and tend to affect the back part of the head. You do not note any specific triggers other than fatigue or lack of sleep. The headaches get better with rest and paracetamol.
- You have no nausea/vomiting, difficulty seeing, bumping into things on the sides, car accidents, rectal bleeding, skin tags, or joint pains.
- You have not been unusually thirsty or passing large quantities of dilute urine. You have no blood or bubbles in your urine.
- You have no cold/heat intolerance, constipation or diarrhoea, anxiety or lethargy, weight loss or weight gain, nipple discharge, or reduction in sexual drive.
- You have no joint pains, rashes, or mouth ulcers.

Past medical and surgical history:
- Diabetes, diagnosed 6 months ago. Your last HbA1c 3 months ago was 7% (53 mmol/mol).
- You are not known to have hypertension, thyroid, or kidney problems.
- No recent surgeries.

Medication list:
- Metformin 850 mg BD
- Linagliptin 5 mg OM
- Supplements and herbal remedies: nil
- Drug allergy: nil

Family history:
- Nil

Relevant personal, social, occupational, and travel history:
- You are a professional pianist and have always noted that your rather large hands give you an advantage[17]. You do not use any vibrating tools.
- You are married without children.
- You do not smoke. You drink socially, approximately 1–2 pints of beer a week and the occasional glass of wine.
- No relevant travel history.

---

[17] Ramachandran M, Aronson JK. The diagnosis of art: Rachmaninov's hand span. *J R Soc Med* 2006 99(10):529–30.

Relevant physical examination findings:

This station will feature a real patient. Neurologic findings may be simulated.

- Spade-like hands (Photo 21), no wasting or deformities.
- Numbness to pinprick on medial 3.5 fingers with split ring finger. Proprioception and vibration sense normal. Tinel's positive over carpal tunnel. There is sparing of sensation over both thenar eminences.
- Power 5/5 in thumb abduction and finger flexion/abduction. Froment's sign negative.
- Sensation normal in feet.
- Coarse facial features, macroglossia with indentation of teeth (Photo 22), and widened interdental spaces (Photo 23).
- Visual fields normal; no bitemporal hemianopia.
- No neck scar, skin tags, or goitre.

Photos to be shown to candidate upon request (use colour plates for full-colour photos).

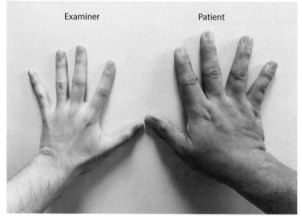

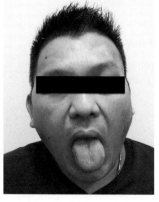

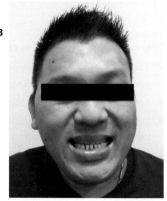

Clinical photos generously provided by Dr Loh Lih Ming, Singapore General Hospital

Consultation Case 26

You have some specific questions for the doctor at this consultation:

- What is happening to me? Is it diabetes causing my hand numbness?
- Will I be able to continue playing the piano?

Approach and Clinical Reasoning

Mr Rachmaninoff presents with hand numbness on a background of diabetes. The first step is to distinguish between carpal tunnel syndrome, peripheral neuropathy, mononeuritis multiplex, and radiculopathy. It may be advantageous to leave more time for yourself to examine him.

Careful examination will identify a pattern of numbness affecting the medial 3.5 fingers, with a split ring finger suggestive of median nerve palsy. Sparing of sensation over the thenar eminences localizes the issue to the carpel tunnels. Perform provocation testing (i.e., Tinel's or Phalen's signs; note that his numbness is also worse with wrist flexion and extension, which is consistent). Look for weakness or wasting in the hands, which is a marker of severity and chronicity. Examine the feet — the absence of sensory loss here again favours carpal tunnel syndrome over peripheral neuropathy.

The next step is to search for a cause as to *why* he has carpal tunnel syndrome (Table B4.22) — idiopathic carpal tunnel syndrome is unlikely to appear as a consultation station.

Pitfall: Anchoring and premature closure

> Just because Mr Rachmaninoff has diabetes does not necessarily mean that his hand numbness is a consequence of diabetic peripheral neuropathy. It is easy to lock on to this diagnosis too early without exploring appropriate differentials.

Table B4.22. Differentials to hand numbness and paraesthesia.

Cause	Key features	Important secondary causes
Carpal tunnel syndrome	Numbness over lateral 3.5 digits, worse on wrist flexion & extension, positive Tinel's sign. If severe, also thenar wasting, weak thumb abduction.	Autoimmune: rheumatoid arthritis, others Endocrine: acromegaly, hypothyroid Metabolic: diabetes, chronic kidney disease, amyloidosis Repetitive use/occupational Pregnancy
Peripheral neuropathy	Glove and stocking numbness: symmetrical numbness in all fingers, toes typically more severely affected than fingers	Metabolic: diabetes, B12 deficiency (e.g., gastrectomy, ileal resection) Toxic: alcohol, isoniazid, phenytoin, platinum chemotherapy drugs Endocrine: hypo/hyperthyroidism, acromegaly

(Cont'd)

Cause	Key features	Important secondary causes
		Autoimmune: GBS, CIDP, systemic vasculitides
Paraneoplastic
Hereditary: Charcot-Marie-Tooth disease
Infective: leprosy, HIV
Critical illness
Infiltrative: amyloidosis, sarcoidosis
Mononeuritis multiplex	Asymmetrical patchy numbness affecting distribution of multiple peripheral nerves (in upper and lower limbs)	Endocrine: diabetes, acromegaly
Autoimmune: RA, SLE, ANCA vasculitis, Sjogren's syndrome
Infective: HIV, lyme disease, leprosy
Infiltrative: amyloid, sarcoid
Paraneoplastic
Radiculopathy from cervical spine disease	Affects one dermatome/myotome; neck pain; UMN signs in lower limb if concomitant cervical myelopathy	Degenerative disk disease (can affect exiting nerve roots, i.e., radiculopathy or descending cord, i.e., myelopathy)
Others: abscess, tumour, etc.

CIDP: chronic inflammatory demyelinating polyneuropathy; GBS: Guillain-Barré syndrome; RA: rheumatoid arthritis; SLE: systemic lupus erythematosus; UMN: upper motor neuron

Recognise that he has a history of coarsening of facial appearance and increase in ring and shoe size suggestive of acromegaly. The next tasks are to (1) demonstrate the physical signs of acromegaly, (2) assess disease activity, (3) look for complications, and (4) search for an aetiology.

1. Demonstrate the physical signs of acromegaly:
   - In the hands: spade-like hands, absence of ring (outgrown).
   - In the face: coarse features, macroglossia, widened interdental space, proganthism.
   - It is helpful to ask for old photos, such as on a driving license or identity card.
2. Assess disease activity. Clinically active disease in acromegaly is indicated by the presence of sweaty palms (which Mr Rachmaninoff has) and skin tags (which you should look for). In contrast, features of soft-tissue overgrowth (e.g., macroglossia, spade-like hands) may persist even after acromegaly is treated.
3. Search for an aetiology — particularly a pituitary adenoma. Check for bitemporal hemianopia and ask for symptoms of mass effect (headache, bitemporal hemianopia) and suppression of other pituitary hormone axes.
4. Look for complications:
   - Cardiac – hypertension, left ventricular hypertrophy, cardiomyopathy.
   - Respiratory – sleep apnoea.

- Endocrine – diabetes (glucose check marks), goitre, thyroid nodule.
- Gastrointestinal – colonic polyps/cancer (conjunctival pallor, offer rectal examination).
- Neurologic – entrapment neuropathy (e.g., carpal tunnel syndrome).
- Musculoskeletal – joints for arthritis.

In addition to carpal tunnel syndrome, Mr Rachmaninoff has new-onset diabetes and hypertension (note the vitals given in the stem) complicating his acromegaly.

Question and Answer

Suggested answer to the patient's concerns:
Mr Rachmaninoff, this numbness must be very distressing for you. I will do what I can to get to the bottom of this and get you better. It is true that diabetes is one of the causes of hand and feet numbness. In your case, however, I am concerned about another condition called acromegaly which may be causing your hand numbness. Acromegaly is a condition of hormone overproduction, which can cause high blood pressure and growth of soft tissue, leading to a change in appearance, increase in shoe and ring size, and compression of nerves which has led to hand numbness. We will need to do some tests to confirm this diagnosis and get you started on treatment right away.

Suggested presentation to the examiner:
Mr Rachmaninoff has acromegaly complicated by carpal tunnel syndrome, new-onset diabetes, and hypertension. Physical examination is significant for spade-like hands, coarse facial features, macroglossia with dental malocclusion, and increase in shoe and ring size. There is decreased pinprick sensation in the medial three and a half fingers, with a split ring finger, and a positive Tinel's sign over carpal tunnel. There is no weakness of the abductor pollicis brevis or wasting of the thenar eminence, and no lower limb numbness. I looked for but did not find any bitemporal hemianopia. Other causes of carpal tunnel syndrome include diabetes, hypothyroidism, renal insufficiency, or idiopathic factors.

I will like to investigate by:

- Performing a nerve conduction study to confirm carpal tunnel syndrome.
- Confirm diagnosis of acromegaly by checking insulin-like growth factor 1 (IGF-1), growth hormone suppression with oral glucose tolerance test, formal visual field testing, and MRI pituitary fossa.
- Screening the rest of the pituitary hormones.
- Checking for differentials of numbness including checking thyroid and B12 levels and assessing his HbA1c.

Management should be taken by a multidisciplinary team including the endocrinologist, neurosurgeon, and allied healthcare professionals. This will entail:
- Transphenoidal resection of pituitary tumour (gold standard).
- Treatment of metabolic complications (i.e., diabetes and hypertension).
- Adjunctive treatment for carpel tunnel syndrome which may include wrist splint, glucocorticoid injections, and consideration of surgical decompression.
- Screening for colonic neoplasia.

Consultation Case 27

Ms Kat (Hypertension)

Use this case as practice! The pull-out booklet contains the candidate's information.

Information for the Candidate

Patient Details: Ms Kat, 30 years old

Your Role: Medical Outpatients Clinic SHO

Scenario:
> Dear Colleague,
>
> Ms Kat seems to be hypertensive at a rather young age, and her hypertension is difficult to control. Would you please see and manage her?
>
> Warm regards,
>
> Dr April Toh, GP

Vital Signs: BP 175/91 mmHg, HR 80/min, RR 18/min, SpO2 98% RA, T 37.0°C

Patient's Brief

Synopsis: *This young lady with previously undiagnosed neurofibromatosis now presents with difficult-to-control hypertension and episodic headaches and palpitations, which are concerning for phaeochromocytoma.*

Open the consult with: The GP says that my blood pressure isn't well controlled. But I take my medicine all the time and I feel just fine! *Do not volunteer any other information unless asked.*

History of current problem:

- The GP started you on some blood pressure medicines which you have been taking diligently with no missed doses.
- You have been monitoring your home blood pressure, which remains around 160s systolic despite the medications.
- You notice that you develop occasional bouts of giddiness, palpitations, and headache. Each episode lasts 5–10 minutes and resolves spontaneously. You attribute this to your anxious personality, but interestingly, these episodes occur even while you are relaxing or watching TV.
- You have not gained weight or noticed any skin thinning.

- You have no decrease in urine output, blood in the urine, frothy urine, or leg swelling.
- You have no change in appearance, sweaty palms, or increase in shoe or ring size
- You have no visual problems, and you do not bump into things on the sides.
- You have no tiredness, constipation, abnormally light or heavy menses, and you do not feel unusually cold.
- You have no skin tightening over the fingers and no pain or colour change when going into a cold environment.
- You do not snore at night; you are alert on waking up in the morning.

Past medical and surgical history:
- You have had 'skin lumps' all over your body for as long as you can remember. You do not know what they are, but they have never bothered you. You usually wear long sleeved tops and long pants to hide them. You did well in school and had no learning difficulty. You do not have any seizures.

Medication list:
- Losartan 100 mg OM
- Amlodipine 10 mg OM
- No supplements or traditional medicine
- Drug allergy: diclofenac

Family history:
- Your older sister and mother both have the 'skin lumps' that you have.
- There is no significant family history of hypertension, heart disease, or stroke.

Relevant personal, social, occupational, and travel history:
- You work as a teacher.
- You do not take any recreational drugs.
- You have a fiancé to whom you are getting married next month. You use barrier contraception and are certain that you are not pregnant. You are having your period now.

Relevant physical examination findings:
- Cutaneous: café-au-lait macules (Photo 24) and multiple neurofibromas (Photo 25).
- No supraclavicular or dorsocervical adiposities, and no abdominal striae or thin skin.
- No macroglossia or spade-like hands.
- No sclerodactyly or microstomia.
- No finger or toe clubbing, radial-radial delay, or radio-femoral delay.

- 4-limb blood pressure – no discrepancy between limbs (information provided on request, candidates are not expected to perform 4-limb blood pressure).
- No palpable or ballotable renal masses. No renal bruit.
- No goitre.
- No pedal oedema.

Photos to be shown to candidate upon request (use colour plates for full-colour photos).

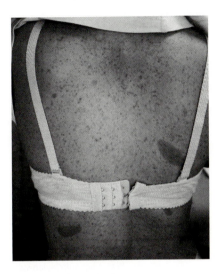

Photo 24. Patient's back

Photo generously provided by Assoc Prof Mark Koh and Dr Cheryl Lie, KK Women's and Children's Hospital

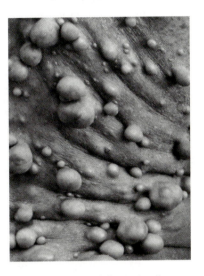

Photo 25. Anterior abdominal wall, close up.

Reproduced with permission from DermNet NZ www.dermnetnz.org

You have some specific questions for the doctor at this consultation:

- Can I get pregnant?
- Will my child have these skin lumps too?

Approach and Clinical Reasoning

Young hypertension (< 35 years old) and resistant hypertension (uncontrolled despite optimal doses of three antihypertensives from different classes, including a diuretic) are common presenting complaints. Apart from excluding non-compliance to treatment, look hard for a secondary cause (Table B4.23) — 'essential hypertension' is unlikely in PACES!

A typical strategy for a hypertension station will include:

- Inspection for spot diagnoses (i.e., acromegaly, Cushing's syndrome, scleroderma).

Table B4.23. Causes of secondary hypertension.

Category	Cause	Important clinical features
Renal	Renal insufficiency	Oliguria, pedal oedema, decreased urine output
	Nephritic syndrome	Haematuria, oliguria
	Polycystic kidney	Family history, ballotable renal masses
	Renal artery stenosis	Abdominal bruit, disproportionate (> 30%) creatinine rise with renin-aldosterone blockade.
Endocrine	Hyperaldosteronism	↑ Na^+, ↓ K^+
	Cushing's syndrome/disease	Weight gain, central obesity, supraclavicular adiposity, thin skin, abdominal striae; may have bitemporal hemianopia, history of steroid use
	Acromegaly	Sweaty palms, macroglossia, spade-like hands, change in ring/shoe size; may have bitemporal hemianopia
	Phaeochromocytoma	Paroxysmal headache, tachycardia, diaphoresis
	Hypothyroidism	Weight gain, lethargy, cold intolerance, menorrhagia
Vascular	Coarctation of aorta	Unequal 4-limb blood pressure, radial-femoral pulse delay, differential finger/toe clubbing
Rheumatologic	Scleroderma renal crisis	Sclerodactyly, microstomia, Raynaud's syndrome
	Takayasu arteritis	Poorly felt pulses. May have claudication or subclavian steal syndrome (giddiness or syncope with upper limb activity)
Others	Pre-eclampsia	Pregnancy, missed periods
	Obstructive sleep apnoea	Loud snoring, witnessed apnoea, excessive daytime sleepiness
	Drugs	Stimulants, recreational drug use

- Asking for any other associated symptoms. Be sure to pursue any clue volunteered by the patient, such as sweaty palms (acromegaly), fatigue (sleep apnoea, hypothyroidism) and so on.
- Screen through the specific causes. As the list is long, you may only be able to ask 1 to 2 'screening questions' for each of the causes above.
- Examine for any causes suggested during screening questions. In particular, it would be important to check pulses and ask for a 4-limb blood pressure.

As you enter the consult room, the patient's underlying neurofibromatosis will be immediately obvious. As you consider the causes of secondary hypertension, look particularly hard for causes related to neurofibromatosis — phaeochromocytoma, renal artery stenosis, and aortic coarctation are more common in patients with neurofibromatosis.

For Ms Kat, important differentials include:
- Phaeochromocytoma, given her history of episodic headaches and palpitations.
- Renal artery stenosis, which you will not be able to exclude on history and examination alone (renal artery bruit is rare).

The safety point in this station is to exclude a hypertensive emergency (aortic dissection, cerebrovascular accident, acute kidney injury, etc.) given that her blood pressure is quite high.

Physical examination should focus on:
- Demonstrating the features of neurofibromatosis:
  - Cutaneous: neurofibromas, café au lait spots, axillary freckling.
  - Offering slit lamp examination for lisch nodules.
  - Screening vision for optic gliomas.
  - Looking for scoliosis.
- Checking pulses and offering 4-limb blood pressure.
- Examining for renal bruit.

Question and Answer

Suggested answer to the patient's concerns:

Ms Kat, I would advise not getting pregnant right now. Firstly, your blood pressure is not controlled, which puts you at risk of dangerous complications for pregnancy. Secondly, one of your blood pressure medicines can potentially harm your baby, so we do need to change it to something else if you are trying for a baby. Thirdly, it is quite unusual to have such high blood pressure at such a young age. I am concerned that your hypertension may not be so straightforward; for instance, there may be a hormone overproduction causing this high blood pressure. I will do some blood tests, urine tests, and scans for you.

As for whether your baby will get the skin lumps, these lumps are due to a condition known as neurofibromatosis, which you and probably your mother and older sister have. It is a genetic condition; assuming that your husband is not affected, there is a 50% chance[18] that your baby may get the gene. Of those who have the gene, some may only be mildly affected, while some have more skin lumps.

Suggested presentation to the examiner:

Ms Kat presents with young hypertension and stigmata of neurofibromatosis. The history of intermittent headaches and palpitations is concerning for a phaeochromocytoma. I will also like to exclude renal artery stenosis which neurofibromatosis predisposes to.

---

[18] Neurofibromatosis has an autosomal dominant pattern of inheritance. Therefore, there is a 50% chance that her child will have neurofibromatosis (assuming her husband is unaffected). Penetrance is complete but expression is variable. Therefore, her daughter may be only mildly (or severely) affected.

My investigation will include:

1. Working up the cause of secondary hypertension, in particular:
   - Checking urinary catecholamines and metanephrines for phaeochromocytoma.
   - Ultrasound doppler renal artery.
   - Low dose dexamethasone suppression and 24 h urinary cortisol.
   - Checking bloods for renal function, electrolytes, thyroid function for hypothyroidism, and urine for pregnancy test and microscopy.
   - If these are negative, I may consider renin/aldosterone testing as well.
2. Screening for other cardiovascular risk factors including fasting glucose and lipid panel.
3. Screening for other complications of neurofibromatosis, in particular, slit lamp examination for lisch nodules.

For management:

- If she does have phaeochromocytoma, I will control her blood pressure using alpha blockade before beta blockade and localise the tumour by performing imaging such as CT adrenals. I will refer her to an endocrinologist as well as an experienced surgeon for adrenalectomy.
- Management of neurofibromatosis is tailored to its manifestations. The aim is to detect and treat complications as they occur. She will also require patient education, management of psychosocial issues, genetic counselling, and family screening.

Consultation Case 28

Mr Kay (Blackout)

Use this case as practice! The pull-out booklet contains the candidate's information.

Information for the Candidate

Patient Details: Mr Kay, 30 years old

Your Role: Medical Admissions Unit SHO

Scenario: Mr Kay was brought to A&E after passing out at a charity fun run.

Vital Signs: BP 120/80 mmHg, HR 70/min, RR 10/min, SpO2 100% RA, T 36.5°C

Patient's Brief

Synopsis: *This young man presents with exertional syncope, and a pansystolic murmur over the apex plus an ejection systolic murmur over the upper right sternal edge. The likely diagnosis is hypertrophic obstructive cardiomyopathy.*

Open the consult with: I don't know what happened. I was 1 km into my run when I suddenly lost consciousness. *Do not volunteer any other information unless asked.*

History of current problem:

- You were at a fund-raising 'fun run' today. You felt well before commencing the run and do not have any ongoing flu/illnesses.
- You did not experience any symptoms before passing out, such as lightheadedness, giddiness, darkening of vision, cold sweats, nausea, a rising sensation in your tummy, chest pain, palpitations, or breathlessness.
- You do not remember the episode of passing out.
- You did not bite your tongue or lose control of your bladder.
- You do not recall how long it took for you to regain consciousness. You woke up under a tree right next to the running route. You were alert immediately when awake, and you remember bystanders helping you up and offering you water.
- You had no weakness or numbness after getting up. After a cold drink, you walked away and left the race site.
- You did not suffer any injuries except some minor scratches over your elbow.

- You have had faints as a teenage boy, particularly when standing at attention under the hot sun (you were a military band member in school) — you do not recall any recent episodes.
- You have no palpitations, chest pain, shortness of breath, or leg swelling.
- You have no fever, headache, vomiting, or rash.

Past medical and surgical history:
- Depression, diagnosed 2 years ago.

Medication list:
- Fluoxetine 20 mg OM
- Supplements and herbal remedies: nil
- Drug allergy: nil
- You do not use intravenous drugs

Family history:
- No family history of heart problems, seizures, or sudden death.

Relevant personal, social, occupational, and travel history:
- You work as a lawyer.
- You are a fitness enthusiast and cycle 20 km to work every morning.
- You are planning to marry your fiancée in a year's time.
- You do not smoke.
- You drink relatively heavily (up to 10 shots of hard liquor a day), but have not done so for the past 48 hours.
- You do not use recreational drugs.
- No relevant travel history.

Relevant physical examination findings:
- General condition well.
- Regular pulse, normal volume.
- Undisplaced, heaving apex.
- Normal first and second heart sound. Grade 3/6 pansystolic murmur best heard at the apex, radiating to the axilla. Grade 2/6 ejection systolic murmur at the upper right sternal edge, without radiation. This gets louder with the Valsalva manoeuvre or squatting to standing.
- Neurologic examination normal.

You have some specific questions for the doctor at this consultation:
- This was just a faint from the heat and dehydration, like what I used to have in school right?

Consultation Case 28 379

Approach and Clinical Reasoning

Mr Kay presents with a sudden loss of consciousness. Begin by distinguishing between syncope and seizure by eliciting elicit pre-, intra-, and post-event features (Table B4.24).

Table B4.24. Clinical features to distinguish syncope vs. seizure.

	Syncope	Seizure
Context	Prolonged standing, heat, emotion, crowds Postural change Exertion, palpitations, chest pain Known heart disease	Head injury, structural brain disease Infection, metabolic disturbances Sleep deprivation, alcohol, bright lights (triggers) Prior seizures
Pre-event	Usually with a prodrome of light-headedness, fading of vision, pallor, diaphoresis Except cardiac syncope, which is without warning	May have aura*: déjà vu feeling, rising epigastric sensation, familiar smell or taste May be sudden, without warning
During event	Sudden loss of tone Hypotension or bradycardia (if observed) Brief motor activity, including clonic jerks	Features more specific for seizure include: – Sustained tonic–clonic or myoclonic movements – Automatisms* or blank staring – Lateral tongue biting* – Forceful head turn to one side (version)*
Post-event	Pallor, diaphoresis, flushing. Rapid, complete recovery to full alertness	Post-ictal drowsiness* (especially generalised seizure) May have transient weakness (Todd's paralysis) Nose wiping (in focal seizure)

*Features particularly specific to seizures. On the other hand, other features may not differentiate between syncope and seizure, for example, incontinence occurs in both conditions, and unsustained twitches can occur in syncope, potentially leading to misdiagnosis as seizure.

The features in Mr Kay's history (no aura, no tongue biting, alert immediately when awake) favour syncope over seizure. Recognise that his syncope occurred while running, suggesting an arrhythmia precipitated by exertion or an inability of cardiac output to meet the demands of physical exertion — this would be worrisome for cardiogenic syncope. Ask for a family history and look for a cause of cardiogenic syncope (Table B4.25).

Table B4.25. Important causes of cardiogenic syncope.

Mechanism	Conditions	Clinical features
Outflow tract obstruction	Critical aortic stenosis Hypertrophic obstructive cardiomyopathy	Chest pain, dyspnoea, murmur
Poor cardiac output	Heart failure Cardiomyopathy	Dyspnoea, oedema, raised jugular venous pressure
Arrhythmias	Ventricular tachycardia High grade atrioventricular block Sick sinus syndrome Pacemaker malfunction	Palpitations Irregular pulse Abnormal ECG
Channelopathy	Long QT – congenital or acquired (e.g., fluoroquinolones, antipsychotics) Brugada syndrome Wolff-Parkinson-White syndrome	Drug history Family history

Think through and exclude other forms of syncope:

- Postural hypotension-related: any history of postural giddiness or syncope triggered by standing up suddenly. Screen for important underlying causes, in particular:
  - Adrenal insufficiency.
  - Drugs (e.g., diuretics, beta blockers).
  - Autonomic failure (e.g., diabetes, other neuropathies, multiple system atrophy, late Parkinson's disease).
- Situational syncope: syncope triggered by coughing, swallowing, urinating, etc.
- Vasovagal syncope: his previous episodes of passing out after prolonging standing in the hot sun would be classic.

Pitfall: Look out for spot diagnoses

> An uncharitable question setter might list a patient with myotonic dystrophy for this syncope scenario and have the patient deny having any past medical conditions. The candidate would be required to recognise the spot diagnosis of myotonic dystrophy and identify its association with cardiomyopathy, which can present as syncope. Always begin the station with careful inspection for spot diagnoses!

In this encounter, history alone is unable to distinguish between the causes of cardiogenic syncope — there is no suggestion of fluid overload, no palpitation, and no relevant drug or family history. Examine the patient with your ears primed to pick up the murmurs of outflow tract obstruction or the displaced apex of a cardiomyopathy, and look carefully for any implanted cardiac device. Look for stigmata of neurocutaneous syndromes. If time permits, also briefly screen neurology for any focal deficits.

The unifying diagnosis is hypertrophic obstructive cardiomyopathy, and this is clinched on examination. Recognise that his daily 20 km cycle is a safety point that must be addressed.

Question and Answer

Suggested answer to the patient's concerns:

Mr Kay, I am worried that what you have experienced may not be 'just a faint'. It is quite different from your previous faints in that this happened suddenly while running. I am concerned that you may have a heart condition which blocks blood flow out of the heart and could have caused you to faint. This is something we need to act on.

I need to send you for some tests. Let's do an ECG now and check your blood tests. I will send you for a heart scan and ask you to wear something that measures your ECG for 24 hours. I will arrange for you to see the cardiologist immediately once these are done. As it does take quite a while to get these organised outpatient, I think it's best if we admit you as you are having symptoms.

Until you are fully evaluated, I think it's best that you do not participate in strenuous exercise, including your daily cycle to work, and avoid driving.

Suggested presentation to the examiner:

Mr Kay presents with exertional syncope. Examination is remarkable for a pansystolic murmur best heard over the apex as well as an ejection systolic murmur best heard over the upper right sternal edge, which gets louder with the Valsalva manoeuvre. My presumptive diagnosis is hypertrophic obstructive cardiomyopathy.

Investigations:

- To confirm the diagnosis:
  - ECG looking for left ventricular hypertrophy.
  - Echocardiogram to confirm hypertrophy, left ventricular outflow tract obstruction, and systolic anterior motion of the mitral valve.
- To look for differentials – bloods including glucose and electrolytes (particularly sodium) and 24 h ECG monitoring looking for arrhythmias.

I will refer him to the cardiologist for further management. Principles of management include:

- Prevention of sudden cardiac death: avoidance of extreme/competitive sports, consideration of an automated implantable cardioverter-defibrillator.
- Treatment of left ventricular outflow tract obstruction: options include pharmacologic therapy such as a beta blocker or calcium channel blocker, and interventions such as alcohol or surgical septal ablation.
- Treatment of heart failure, if any.
- Adjuncts: patient education, family screening, genetic counselling (autosomal dominant transmission), and appropriate vaccinations.

Consultation Case 29

Ms Oh (Blackout)

Use this case as practice! The pull-out booklet contains the candidate's information.

Information for the Candidate

Patient Details: Ms Oh, 30 years old

Your Role: Medical Admissions Unit SHO

Scenario: Ms Oh has been admitted after losing consciousness in public.

Vital Signs: BP 105/62 mmHg, HR 111/min, RR 11/min, SpO2 99% RA, T 36.2°C

Patient's Brief

Synopsis: *This young lady presents with a first-onset seizure, physical findings suggestive of tuberous sclerosis, and a history of recent abstention from heavy alcohol use. Key considerations include tuberous sclerosis and alcohol withdrawal seizures.*

Open the consult with: I was on my way home in the train from a job interview. I don't know what happened. Somehow I woke up in the emergency room. *Also volunteer how difficult finding a job has been, and the history of renal tumour.*

History of current problem:

- You were sitting in a train reading a newspaper. You do not recall experiencing unusual sensations, giddiness, chest pain, diaphoresis, lightheadedness, or blurring of vision prior to passing out.
- You were unaware that you lost consciousness. You regained awareness only after reaching the hospital's emergency room. You remember feeling sleepy when you woke up.
- The right side of your tongue is bruised and painful, but there were no other noticeable injuries.
- You did not lose control of your bladder or bowel during the episode of unconsciousness.
- You have no prior history of seizures or any previous episodes of loss of consciousness, unexplained tongue injuries, unexplained bony injuries, blood stains on pillows or within the mouth when waking from sleep, or unexplained loss of bladder control at night.

- You feel anxious and fidgety, and this is because you haven't had an alcoholic drink for a while.
- You do not have fever, headache, neck stiffness, giddiness, nausea, vomiting, weakness, numbness, slurred speech, or blurred or double vision.
- You do not have a recent history of head injury.
- There is no change in your urine output, and your urine is neither bloody, dark, nor frothy.

Past medical and surgical history:
- You have a benign tumour in the right kidney (the exact scientific name is unknown to you), which you were told can be left alone. It was incidentally discovered when you underwent an ultrasound of your abdomen for suspected gallstones several years ago — no gallstones were found.

Medication list:
- Nil (including supplements, contraceptive pills, and traditional medicines).
- No recreational drug use.
- No drug allergy.

Family history:
- No family history of seizures, stroke, brain problems, or kidney problems.
- No family history of tuberous sclerosis or neurofibromatosis.

Relevant personal, social, occupational, and travel history:
- You are currently unemployed and have been between odd jobs for the past 3 years. Your previous employer had to sack you because you were too slow while working as a supermarket cashier.
- You have always struggled in school and at work, taking far longer than others to complete simple tasks, and you were unable to complete your GCE 'O' levels.
- You drink heavily especially when unemployed, averaging 1 bottle of wine per day for the past year. However, you stopped drinking alcohol for the past 2 days because you have a job interview today, hoping to be employed as a packer at a warehouse. You have been feeling somewhat more jittery these few days as you have not had a drink.
- You are single and not sexually active.
- Your last menstrual period was 6 days ago.
- You do not have a driving license.
- You have no history of recent travel.

Relevant physical examination findings:
This encounter will use a real patient who has been treated.
- Alert, but somewhat anxious and fidgety.

384 A STRATEGY TO AND WORKED PRACTICE FOR THE MRCP PACES

- Facial angiofibromas (adenoma sebaceum; Photo 26).
- Shagreen patch (Photo 27).
- Periungual fibroma (Photo 28).
- Pupils equal and reactive.
- No cranial nerve deficits.
- Normal power, sensation, and cerebellar function in the limbs.

Photos to be shown to candidate upon request (use colour plates for full-colour photos).

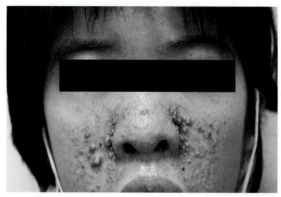

Photo 26

Photo 27

Photo 28

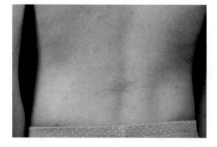

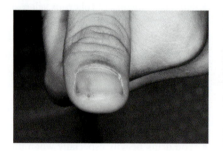

Clinical photos generously provided by Assoc Prof Mark Koh and Dr Cheryl Lie, KK Women's and Children's Hospital

You have some specific questions for the doctor at this consultation:

- Why did I lose consciousness?
- Do I have epilepsy?

Approach and Clinical Reasoning

Ms Oh presents with an unwitnessed episode of loss of consciousness. Distinguish seizure from syncope by eliciting pre-, intra-, and post-event features (see Table B4.24).

Features in favour of seizure in Ms Oh's case include tongue injuries and a prolonged duration before full awareness was regained. The absence of typical vasovagal complaints, postural triggers, and cardiac symptoms render vasovagal syncope and cardiogenic syncope less likely.

Next, distinguish between (a) a first seizure, (b) recurrent seizures, and (c) breakthrough seizures in a patient with known epilepsy. This distinction is important as it affects subsequent management (i.e., whether to start anti-epileptic drug therapy). Note that seizures due to non-compliance, sub-therapeutic levels of anti-epileptic medications, or inappropriate use of anti-epileptic medications are not considered breakthrough seizures.

In Ms Oh's case, it is likely that this was her first seizure. It is therefore imperative to search for an underlying cause or provocative factor to gauge the long-term risk of seizure recurrence (Table B4.26).

Table B4.26. Important provoking factors and causes of seizures.

Mechanism	Conditions	Clinical features
Structural brain lesion	Traumatic brain injury Acute vascular event (e.g., haemorrhage), cerebral venous thrombosis (CVT) Old cerebral insult (e.g., infarct) Mass lesions: abscess, tumour Congenital malformations Neurocutaneous syndromes (neurofibromatosis, Sturge-Weber syndrome, tuberous sclerosis)	History of trauma, stroke Worst-ever headache Chronic progressive headache Raised intracranial pressure (e.g., vomiting, headache worse lying down) Neurocutaneous stigmata Hypercoagulable state (CVT)
Metabolic	Hypo- or hyperglycaemia Electrolytes: low Na^+, Ca^{2+}, Mg^{2+} Uraemia	Diabetes, insulin use Causes of electrolyte derangements
Drugs	Alcohol or benzodiazepine withdrawal Drugs of abuse (cocaine, amphetamine) Medications: cefepime, ertapenem	Drug and alcohol history
Infective	Meningitis, encephalitis	Fever, headache, drowsiness, neck stiffness, purpuric rash
Autoimmune	Autoimmune encephalitis (e.g., anti-NMDA receptor encephalitis)	Short-term memory loss Behaviour change

It becomes apparent that Ms Oh has two possible underlying causes of seizures:

1. Her history of chronic heavy alcohol use with recent abstention from alcohol (as she was going for a job interview), as well as her being anxious and fidgety, raise concern for seizures due to alcohol withdrawal. The absence of tremors and sympathetic symptoms, though, are less in keeping.

2. The neurocutaneous stigmata of facial angiofibromas (adenoma sebaceum) and ash-leaf spots, along with a history of 'benign renal tumour' at a young age (angiomyolipoma) and poor academic achievement (possible cognitive deficit), are suggestive of underlying tuberous sclerosis. Note that a family history is often absent as up to 80% of cases are de novo mutations.

Other causes of seizures (e.g., electrolyte disturbances, cerebral insults) are difficult to elicit without laboratory investigations or imaging, and you should mention these differentials and the necessary work-up.

Question and Answer

Suggested answer to the patient's concerns:

Thank you for sharing your concern with me. I can't imagine how frightening it is for patients to be told that they have epilepsy. However, epilepsy is a disorder in which someone is at long-term risk recurrent seizures. As you have only had one seizure at the moment, we will need to find out what caused your seizure to occur. Although suddenly stopping alcohol intake can cause seizures, your history of benign kidney tumours and difficulty in school and at work make it likely that you have another condition which itself can predispose to you having seizures. I will need to admit you for further investigations, including a scan of the brain and a study of your brainwaves, so that we can better assess the risk of recurrence and whether you have epilepsy or not.

Suggested presentation to the examiner:

My positive physical signs include facial angiofibromas, shagreen patches, and periungual fibromas. In this patient with a first-onset seizure, history of renal angiomyolipoma, and poor academic achievement, the diagnosis is tuberous sclerosis. A differential is alcohol withdrawal seizures, given her recent abstention from heavy alcohol use.

Don't forget: State the positive physical signs

> State your positive physical signs directly as specific marks are awarded for doing so. Do not gamble that as long as you arrive at the correct overall diagnosis of tuberous sclerosis, the examiner will assume that you have picked up the correct signs.

I will admit Ms Oh. Initial investigations include:
- MRI brain to demonstrate cortical tubers/harmatomas.
- Electroencephalogram (EEG).
- Blood tests to search for metabolic and electrolyte derangements (renal panel, calcium, magnesium, phosphate) and infective aetiologies (full blood count).
- Liver enzymes (important in view of alcohol use and if initiation of anti-epileptic drugs is being considered).

Management:
- Immediate management:
  - Close observation for further seizures.
  - Management of alcohol withdrawal including CIWA (Clinical Institute Withdrawal Assessment) charting, benzodiazepines, and thiamine supplementation.
- Anti-epileptic drugs (AEDs): there are grounds for and against starting AEDs at this point. It is reasonable to start AEDs given the strong association between epilepsy and tuberous sclerosis. On the other hand, it is also reasonable not to start AEDs while awaiting investigation results as this is the first episode of unprovoked seizure, and there are concerns of potential liver impairment.
- Counsel on alcohol use and refer for alcohol cessation programmes.
- Subsequent management of tuberous sclerosis may include:
  - Genetic testing and counselling.
  - Work-up for further manifestations of tuberous sclerosis: imaging of renal tumour, X-ray or CT thorax for lymphangioleiomyomas, slit lamp examination for retinal hamartomas, and formal cognitive testing.

Consultation Case 30

Mr H. Dumpty (Falls)

Use this case as practice! The pull-out booklet contains the candidate's information.

Information for the Candidate

Patient Details: Mr H. Dumpty, 70 years old

Your Role: Geriatric Clinic SHO

Referral Letter:
> Dear Colleague,
>
> Mr Dumpty was admitted for a right Colles' fracture which we have fixed. It seems that he has been having rather frequent falls. Could you please see him?
>
> Thank you.
>
> Dr Bone, Orthopaedic Surgeon

Vital Signs: BP 132/71 mmHg, HR 70/min, RR 12/min, SpO2 97% RA, T 35.9°C

Patient's Brief

Synopsis: *An elderly gentleman presents with falls, a magnetic gait, urinary dysfunction, and cognitive decline. The diagnosis is normal pressure hydrocephalus.*

Open the consult with: I don't know why I keep falling. I need to be more careful. *Do not volunteer any other information unless asked.*

History of current problem:

- One month ago, you fell on your outstretched right arm and sustained a wrist fracture, for which you required surgery.
- This fall occurred at home, in your living room. You were rushing to the toilet because you felt the urge to pass urine.
- You have been falling 2–3 times a month for the past few months. Apart from this wrist fracture, you have never injured yourself. You have not had other fractures.
- You find that you are not able to walk as fast as you used to. However, you have no weakness, numbness, leg stiffness, imbalance, or tremor. There is no change in the size of your handwriting.
- You have also been experiencing urinary urgency in the past 2–3 months. Occasionally, you wet yourself because you cannot reach the bathroom in time.

There is no pain on passing urine, slow stream, hesitation, or dribbling at the end of the stream.
- You will deny having any memory problems.
- You do not feel giddy or lightheaded, not even when standing up from a seated position.
- You have no neck pain or problems with your vision.

Past medical and surgical history:
- The 'urine problem' described above. A GP has given you some 'prostate' medication, but this does not seem to have helped.
- You have never had any head injury, brain bleed, or brain infections (meningitis).

Medication list:
- Tamsulosin 4 mg ON
- No drug allergies

Family history:
- Your late uncle had Parkinson's disease and was bedbound.

Relevant personal, social, occupational, and travel history:
- You are a retired lawyer. You used to spend your time doing charity work and investing in the stock market. In the last 3 months, you have terminated all volunteering commitments and stopped monitoring your investments. Instead, you spend your time at home doing very little. You are not able to give a reason why this is so.
- You are married and stay with your wife. Your children have moved out of your home.
- You have travelled to many exotic destinations in the past year. However, you have stopped travelling in the last 2 months.
- You neither smoke nor drink.

Relevant physical examination findings:
- Magnetic gait, turning in numbers. No reduced arm-swing or festination.
- No rest tremor, bradykinesia of upper limbs, or mask-like facies.
- Normal tone, reflexes, power, sensation, and cerebellar function.
- Postural blood pressure – no drop.
- Right wrist surgical scar.

You have some specific questions for the doctor at this consultation:
- Do I have Parkinson's disease? I don't want to be bedbound like my uncle.

Approach and Clinical Reasoning

Mr Dumpty presents with frequent falls. In clinical practice, falls in the elderly are usually multifactorial and can rarely be pinned down on a specific diagnosis. In PACES, however, a stem of 'falls' tends to lead to a specific neurological disorder or cause of postural hypotension (Table B4.27).

Table B4.27. Differentials to frequent falls in PACES.

These differentials are overrepresented in PACES. In real life, falls are usually multifactorial.

Category	Cause	Important clinical features
Neurological	Upper motor neuron (UMN): – Intracranial lesion – Spinal cord (e.g., cervical myelopathy)	UMN signs, stiffness Hemiparesis Hoffman's +ve, neck pain
	Lower motor neuron	Foot drop, peripheral neuropathy, etc.
	Extrapyramidal: – Advanced Parkinson's disease – Parkinson's-plus	Tremor, bradykinesia, rigidity Additional features (e.g., vertical gaze palsy)
	Ataxia: – Cerebellar ataxia – Sensory ataxia – Normal pressure hydrocephalus	Unsteadiness rather than weakness Cerebellar signs, underlying cause Loss of proprioception, vibration sense Triad of magnetic gait, cognitive impairment, urinary urgency or incontinence
Postural hypotension	Autonomic dysfunction	Postural giddiness, falls when getting up Longstanding diabetes, other autonomic failure syndromes
	Adrenal insufficiency	Postural giddiness Cessation of chronic steroid use, previous pituitary surgery or tumour History of other autoimmune disease
	Medications	Drug history (e.g., diuretics, beta blockers)
Metabolic	Hypoglycaemia	Giddiness, palpitations, diaphoresis, hunger; relief of symptoms when glucose is raised
	Hyponatraemia	Unlikely in PACES unless specific information about sodium levels are given
	Anaemia	Unlikely for stem to be 'frequent falls'

Acute presentation or new-onset falls: also consider cerebrovascular disease, intercurrent medical illness, drugs, etc.

As the differential is relatively broad, it is important to begin with open-ended questions and explore the circumstances around the falls, associated symptoms, and comorbids. This will clue you in to Mr Dumpty's urinary symptoms. It is necessary to explore the exact nature of his urinary symptoms and look for other neurologic symptoms and signs, so as to elicit the relationship between falls and urinary symptoms:

1. Conditions that cause both frequent falls and urinary symptoms:
   - Normal pressure hydrocephalus.
   - Upper motor neuron lesions, especially spinal cord lesions or bilateral cortical/subcortical lesion.
   - Causes of autonomic dysfunction, such as diabetes or multiple systems atrophy.
   - Note that falls and urologic dysfunction occur late in Parkinson's disease. A patient with early falls and Parkinsonism likely has atypical Parkinsonism (e.g., Parkinson-plus syndromes such as MSA-P) or other causes.

2. Falls as a complication of treatment of urinary or systemic disease:
   - Benign prostate hypertrophy (BPH), treated with alpha blockers and complicated by postural hypotension and falls. It becomes clear in this scenario that his urinary symptoms are atypical for BPH.
   - Diuretic use causing urinary urgency and postural hypotension.

Mr Dumpty does not have obvious cognitive impairment in the form of memory loss, apathy, or overt psychomotor slowing. He is cognitively high-functioning at baseline, so you will need to probe for a decline in executive function — Mr Dumpty inexplicably stopping charity work and investing — that provides subtle evidence of cognitive involvement. This makes the likely diagnosis normal pressure hydrocephalus, although postural hypotension from tamsulosin may also contribute to his falls.

Physical examination in this station will be challenging if you have not suspected the correct diagnosis and go in 'blind' or merely suspecting Parkinson's disease. Begin with the gait examination as that is where the money is. NPH classically causes a frontal gait disorder, which may include:

- Disequilibrium or truncal ataxia: patient's centre of gravity goes opposite to the direction the patient intends to move (e.g., patient keeps leaning backward when trying to get out of a chair).
- Gait apraxia and ignition failure whereby the patient has difficulty initiating steps. The classic gait of normal pressure hydrocephalus is described as 'magnetic' (look up some videos if you have not seen it in person). This can resemble a Parkinsonian gait especially in its slow movements, postural instability, and difficulty turning, but key differences are that (i) steps are not small and shuffling, (ii) arm swing is normal, and (iii) there is no asymmetry (with the patient still standing).

Other examination steps that should be done include:

- With the patient still standing, checking tandem gait and Romberg's to rule out cerebellar and sensory ataxia.
- Examining upper limb tone to confirm the absence of cogwheel and lead-pipe rigidity.

- Examining the lower limbs to confirm the absence of upper motor neuron signs and normal proprioception/vibration.
- Requesting for a postural blood pressure to rule out postural hypotension.
- Requesting for abdominal examination to exclude urinary retention, and offering a digital rectal examination.

Question and Answer

Suggested answer to the patient's concerns:

Thank you for sharing this concern with me. The prospect of being bedbound must be very scary. I don't think you have Parkinson's disease; instead I think you have something else called normal pressure hydrocephalus, which is a fancy term describing water ('hydro') accumulating in your brain ('cephalus'). The good news is that this condition is treatable and there is a good chance that you will be able to remain mobile. I will need to do some further tests to confirm what I think and see how we can get you better.

Suggested presentation to the examiner:

Mr Dumpty presents with the triad of gait dysfunction, urinary dysfunction, and cognitive decline. Examination is significant for a magnetic gait with no evidence of weakness, Parkinsonism, or cerebellar signs. The most likely diagnosis is normal pressure hydrocephalus. Differentials include other intracranial lesions causing obstructive hydrocephalus, previous subarachnoid haemorrhage or meningitis, and autonomic dysfunction such as that due to diabetes or multiple systems atrophy. Postural hypotension from tamsulosin may contribute to his falls.

I will like to confirm my diagnosis with:

- MRI brain looking for ventriculomegaly, and to exclude differentials of obstructive hydrocephalus and previous intracranial haemorrhage.
- Lumbar puncture with measurement of opening pressure.
- Assessment for any gait improvement after removal of 30–40 ml of cerebrospinal fluid (tap test).

If there is evidence of gait improvement, Mr Dumpty may benefit from a ventriculoperitoneal shunt. I will also involve the neurologist, neurosurgeon, physiotherapist, and occupational therapist in his management.

Consultation Case 31

Ms Alice (Muscle Cramps)

Use this case as practice! The pull-out booklet contains the candidate's information.

Information for the Candidate

Patient Details: Ms Alice, 50 years old

Your Role: Emergency Department SHO

Referral Letter:

> Dear Colleague,
>
> Thank you for seeing Ms Alice, who complains of persistent muscle cramps that did not resolve with rest and a muscle relaxant. She is on my follow-up for delusional disorder and is stable on risperidone 2 mg daily. There have been no dose changes in the past 5 years.
>
> Thank you.
>
> Dr Aaron Tang, Psychiatrist

Vital Signs: BP 137/84 mmHg, HR 70/min, RR 14/min, SpO2 98% RA, T 37.0°C

Patient's Brief

Synopsis: *Ms Alice has symptomatic hypocalcaemia after a total thyroidectomy.*

Open the consult with: I have been having these muscle cramps. I can't write because when I try to hold a pen, my hand just cramps up (demonstrate flexion of wrist and fingers). *Do not volunteer any other information unless asked.*

History of current problem:
- Your muscle cramps started a few days ago. Both hands and feet are affected. You have also had difficulty putting on your shoes this morning because your foot cramped up. They are not particularly associated with exercise or specific activities.
- You are also feeling some numbness around the mouth.
- You have been feeling somewhat anxious.
- No tremor, uncontrollable lip smacking, or abnormal movements.
- No abdominal pain or diarrhoea.
- No change in urine output, blood in urine, or frothy urine.
- No weight loss, night sweats, or neck/groin lumps.
- No seizure, chest pain, palpitation, or breathlessness.

Past medical and surgical history:

- Hypertension. Your baseline blood pressure is 140/90 mmHg, although you have been taking steps to control this.
- Hyperlipidaemia.
- Diabetes. Your most recent HbA1c is 7.0%.
- Kidney disease from diabetes, which you understand to be mild.
- Thyroid cancer, for which you underwent removal of the entire thyroid gland a week ago. The operation went smoothly, you did not require any blood transfusions and were discharged on the 3rd post-op day.
- You have also been seeing a psychiatrist for many years. You had some delusions when you were younger, but no longer have any psychiatric symptoms.

Medication list:

- Amlodipine 10 mg OM
- Atorvastatin 20 mg ON
- Dapagliflozin 5 mg OM
- Metformin 500 mg TDS
- Levothyroxine 100 mcg OM, newly started after your thyroid surgery
- Lisinopril 20 mg OM
- Risperidone 2 mg OM, no recent dose changes
- Supplements and herbal remedies: you take a daily multivitamin
- Drug allergy: nil
- No history of proton pump inhibitor use

Family history:

- Thyroid cancer.

Relevant personal, social, occupational, and travel history:

- You work as an accountant.
- You are single and unmarried.
- You do not smoke or drink.

Relevant physical examination findings:

This encounter will use a real, treated patient.

- Thyroidectomy scar.
- Hands – no tremor, tone normal.
- No Chvostek sign or Trousseau sign (inflate blood pressure cuff).
- No muscle weakness or percussion or grip myotonia.

You have some specific questions for the doctor at this consultation:
- Can you get rid of these cramps for me? I need to get on with my work as I have an important deadline to meet in a week.

Approach and Clinical Reasoning

Ms Alice presents with carpopedal spasm, which should be quite recognisable. This is pathognomonic of hypocalcaemia, and additionally she has circumoral numbness. Differentials to consider (Table B4.28) include extrapyramidal side effects from risperidone.

Table B4.28. Important causes of muscle cramps.

Cause	Examples
Electrolyte abnormalities	Carpopedal spasm – hypocalcaemia
Extrapyramidal disease	Parkinson's disease, Parkinson's-plus syndromes Drug-induced extrapyramidal side effects Wilson's disease
Focal dystonias	Affects only a specific body part (e.g., writer's cramp)
Myotonia	Myotonic dystrophy
Exercise-related	Exercise-associated cramps, heat cramps

Search for a cause of hypocalcaemia (Figure B4.3). Ms Alice's history points towards inadvertent parathyroid damage during thyroidectomy. While Ms Alice has chronic kidney disease, her kidney disease is mild and hypocalcaemia typically does not occur until late in the course of kidney disease. Screen and exclude the possibility of transfusion-related hypocalcaemia, malignancy-related hypocalcaemia, pancreatitis, and urinary or gastrointestinal losses leading to hypomagnesemia and hypocalcaemia. Vitamin D deficiency is less likely given the relatively acute onset.

Finally, exclude emergent complications of hypocalcaemia (i.e., arrhythmias and seizures).

Examination (there are unlikely to be many signs):
- Make a note of the thyroidectomy scar.
- Check thyroid status.
- Examine for features of extrapyramidal disease (tremor, lead-pipe and cog-wheel rigidity).
- You can offer to demonstrate the Chvostek sign (tap the facial nerve) and the Trousseau sign (inflate blood pressure cuff around the arm), but the patient in your exam is unlikely to have *untreated* hypocalcaemia.

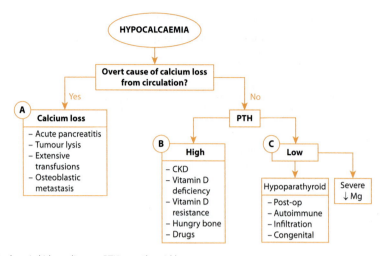

CKD: chronic kidney disease; PTH: parathyroid hormone

Figure B4.3. Approach to hypocalcaemia.

Question and Answer

Suggested answer to the patient's concerns:

Ms Alice, we should be able to help you with these cramps. I suspect that your calcium levels are low, perhaps as a complication of your recent thyroid surgery. I will admit you to do some blood tests and ECG. If your calcium is indeed low, I will give you calcium in a drip. The cramps should go away once your calcium levels are better. I will also ask your surgeon and the endocrine doctor to have a look at you. I hear that you have an important deadline and I will do my best to get you home as soon as possible. In the long term, it may be necessary for you to take calcium and vitamin D tablets.

Suggested presentation to the examiner:

Ms Alice presents with carpopedal spasm and perioral numbness, likely from hypocalcaemia post total thyroidectomy. My differentials for the muscle cramps include extrapyramidal side effects from risperidone. There is no evidence of Parkinsonism or other causes of hypocalcaemia such as calcium losses, transfusion or malignancy-related hypocalcaemia, or pancreatitis.

I will admit Ms Alice to a bed with continuous electrocardiographic monitoring.

Don't forget: Clear disposition

> State any need for admission and urgent treatment clearly. This is likely to be a marking point.

Investigations:

- I will confirm my diagnosis by checking calcium, albumin, phosphate, and parathyroid hormone levels.
- I will also check other electrolytes, as well as renal and thyroid function.
- I will look for complications by doing an ECG looking for QT prolongation and arrhythmias.

Management requires a multidisciplinary team involving the endocrinologist, thyroid surgeon, and allied health professionals. She will require intravenous calcium replacement acutely and long-term calcium and vitamin D replacement.

Consultation Case 32

Mr White (Anaemia)

Use this case as practice! The pull-out booklet contains the candidate's information.

Information for the Candidate

Patient Details: Mr White, 47 years old

Your Role: Medicine Clinic SHO

Referral Letter:
> Dear Colleague,
>
> Mr White came for routine health screening and was found to be anaemic. Would you please see him for further management?
>
> Thank you
>
> Dr Joyce Huang, GP

Vital Signs: BP 131/80 mmHg, HR 70/min, RR 11/min, SpO2 98% RA, T 37.0°C

Investigations:

Haemoglobin	9.8	g/dL	(13.0 - 17.0)
WBC	2.7	$\times 10^9$/L	(3.4 - 9.6)
Platelets	108	$\times 10^9$/L	(150 - 400)
Mean corpuscular volume	112	fL	(80 - 95)

Patient's Brief

Synopsis: *A middle-aged gentleman has pancytopenia and dorsal column dysfunction from B12 deficiency, as a consequence of a prior distal gastrectomy.*

Open the consult with: The doctor said that my blood counts are low, but I feel quite fine! *Also volunteer the history of sensory loss.*

History of current problem:

- You feel completely well. You do not have any light-headedness, chest pain, giddiness. You have been able to keep up with your weekly gym routine.
- You do not have any easy bruising or frequent infections.
- You have noticed that your fingertips are slightly numb. This does not bother you much. You have no memory problems, imbalance when walking, or falls.
- You eat a balanced diet with no restrictions. If asked, you do take a fair amount of meat (you particularly enjoy a good steak) as well as green leafy vegetables.

- You do not have any chronic abdominal pain or bloating, diarrhoea, rectal bleeding, change in stool frequency or calibre.
- You do not have any history of liver problems, jaundice, or change in urine colour. However, you have been warned to cut down your alcohol intake.
- There is no cold intolerance, constipation, or weight gain.
- You have no weight loss or night sweats.
- You do not have any kidney problems, decline in urine output, leg swelling, blood or bubbles in your urine.
- You do not have any chronic joint pains or rashes.

Past medical and surgical history:
- You have had part of your stomach removed. This was done 2 years ago for a bleeding stomach ulcer. You have made an uneventful recovery. You were supposed to return for follow up and blood tests but defaulted because you were busy with work and felt fine.

Medication list:
- PO Omeprazole 20 mg OM (longstanding > 5 years for 'gastric discomfort')

Family history:
- Your mother and sister both have had Hashimoto thyroiditis.
- There is no family history of blood cancers.

Relevant personal, social, occupational, and travel history:
- You work as a private banker.
- You drink heavily, often while entertaining clients. You consume approximately 1 bottle of wine or 5–6 shots of whisky per day. If asked, you have never felt guilty about drinking, annoyed when others criticise your drinking, or felt that you needed a drink first thing in the morning.
- You are single and not sexually active.
- You do not smoke.
- You travel extensively for business trips.

Relevant physical examination findings:

This encounter will use a real patient, although anaemia will be treated and conjunctivae are unlikely to be pale.
- No/mild conjunctival pallor.
- Presence/absence of glossitis *(quite rare)*.
- No weakness or wasting.
- Pinprick sensation grossly preserved.
- Loss of proprioception and vibration sense in limbs, Romberg's test is abnormal.
- Rest of lower limb neurological examination is normal, including tone and reflexes.

- Abdomen soft, non-tender; old midline laparotomy scar; no organomegaly.
- No lymphadenopathy.
- Rectal examination, if offered – empty rectum.

You have some specific questions for the doctor at this consultation:
- Is it my alcohol? Do I really need to cut down?
- What do I need to do now?

Approach and Clinical Reasoning

Mr White presents with macrocytic anaemia with borderline pancytopenia (mild leukopenia and thrombocytopenia). Your tasks in this station are to:

1. Identify the cause of macrocytic anaemia (Table B4.29). Explore diet and alcohol, gastrointestinal symptoms and disorders, thyroid symptoms, and drugs. Do not forget to exclude blood loss or haemolysis, which can lead to reticulocytosis and therefore increased mean corpuscular volume (as reticulocytes are larger than mature red cells).
2. Identify any symptoms or complications as a result of anaemia.
3. Look for any other manifestations, apart from anaemia, of the underlying disease.

Table B4.29. Major causes of macrocytic anaemia.

Differential	Important features
B12 or folate deficiency from:	May be pancytopenic in severe cases
Dietary insufficiency (eggs, meat, dairy, seafood)	B12 deficiency may also manifest with neurologic manifestations (peripheral neuropathy, dorsal column dysfunction, dementia)
Pernicious anaemia	
Malabsorption	Underlying malabsorption disorder e.g., proximal gastrectomy, terminal ileum resection, inflammatory bowel disease, chronic pancreatitis
	Reduced absorption of B12 due to anchlorohydria
	Other autoimmune disorders
Alcohol intake	Chronic, heavy alcohol intake
Hypothyroidism	Cold intolerance, weight gain, constipation
Drugs	Reduced absorption of B12 due to anchlorohydria with proton-pump inhibitors
	Impaired folate metabolism: metformin, methotrexate, hydroxyurea, anti-retroviral therapy
Reticulocytosis (pseudo-macrocytosis)	History of blood loss or features of haemolysis (jaundice, splenomegaly)
Myelodysplastic syndrome	Elderly, other cytopenias, family history; B symptoms rare.

History will reveal sensory loss in addition to pancytopenia, on a background of a previous gastrectomy and long term proton pump inhibitor (PPI) use. This is suggestive of vitamin B12 deficiency. There is also a significant history of alcohol consumption (which may also cause macrocytic anaemia and peripheral neuropathy), but otherwise no concern about blood loss, haemolysis, or hypothyroidism.

Patients with previous gastrectomy may also suffer from iron deficiency. Reduced gastric acidity post gastrectomy, exacerbated by PPI use, impairs iron absorption. In itself iron deficiency is more likely to present as microcytic rather than macrocytic anaemia, but it may coexist with B12 deficiency in this patient.

Key points on physical examination include:
- Examining conjunctivae for pallor (only present what you find, patient may have been treated and pallor may not be very obvious at a haemoglobin of 9.8).
- Neurological examination to check for features of B12 deficiency which may include: proprioception/vibration loss, spastic paraparesis with upper motor neuron signs in the lower limbs, peripheral neuropathy, or any combination of these. The combination of lesions can lead to interesting neurological phenomenon such as upgoing plantars with absent ankle jerks (see page 32).
- Looking in the mouth for glossitis (another feature of B12 deficiency).
- Examine abdomen; confirm the laparotomy scar and look for organomegaly.

Question and Answer

Suggested answer to patient's concerns:

Mr White, I suspect that your low blood count is due to vitamin B12 deficiency. This may be related to your previous stomach surgery, and continued use of omeprazole. It is also possible that your alcohol intake contributes to the low blood count and I will have to advise you to cut down – this much alcohol can lead to liver problems, nerve problems, and heart disease.

I will do some blood tests for you now to confirm what I suspect, and send you to the neurologists for a nerve study. I will see you again in a few days and if you indeed have vitamin B12 deficiency, we will give you B12 replacement. You will need a few shots of B12 injections and thereafter just tablets. We should also stop the omeprazole since you no longer have issues with gastric pains.

Suggested presentation to the examiner:

Mr White presents with macrocytic anaemia and in fact pancytopenia, on a history of previous gastrectomy, long term proton pump inhibitor use, and significant alcohol consumption. Physical examination is significant for loss of proprioception and vibration sense with preserved pinprick sensation, an old midline laparotomy scar, and the absence of conjunctival pallor or glossitis.

My principal diagnosis is vitamin B12 deficiency due to partial gastrectomy as well as omeprazole, associated with possible early subacute combined degeneration. His alcohol use could also have contributed to the macrocytic anaemia.

I will like to investigate by

- Confirming my diagnosis by repeating a blood count, checking B12 levels
- Checking ferritin and transferrin saturations to look for a concomitant iron deficiency
- Looking for pernicious anaemia by sending anti-intrinsic factor antibody[19] *(note: anti-parietal cell antibody is non-specific and not routinely sent)*
- For sensory findings: considering a nerve conduction study, and evaluating for other causes of neuropathy e.g., checking fasting glucose, thyroid function.
- Checking a liver function in view of alcohol intake.

Management: Mr White can be managed as an outpatient.

- For B12 deficiency, he will require intramuscular B12 replacement followed by long-term oral B12 and folate replacement.
- If there is pernicious anaemia, he will require either long-term intramuscular B12 or high-dose oral B12, and follow-up endoscopy due to the long-term risk of gastric cancer.
- He should be counselled on alcohol cessation.

---

[19] Anti-intrinsic factor antibody supports a diagnosis of pernicious anaemia, but its absence does not rule it out. A diagnosis of anti-intrinsic factor antibody negative pernicious anaemia may be made on clinical judgment (e.g., severity of B12 deficiency).

Consultation Case 33

Mdm Na (Hyponatraemia)

Use this case as practice! The pull-out booklet contains the candidate's information.

Information for the Candidate

Patient Details: Mdm Na, 70 years old

Your Role: Emergency Department SHO

Referral Letter:

> Dear Colleague,
>
> Mdm Na came to me last week complaining of lethargy. I decided to check her bloods and it turns out that she has rather significant hyponatraemia. Will you please see and manage her?
>
> Thank you.
>
> Dr Saw Tee, GP

Vital Signs: BP 130/70 mmHg, HR 72/min, RR 11/min, SpO2 98% RA, T 37.0°C

Investigations:

Na^+	119	mmol/L	(135 - 145)
K^+	4.0	mmol/L	(3.5 - 5.0)
Cl^-	88	mmol/L	(95 - 105)
HCO_3^-	23	mmol/L	(22 - 26)
Creatinine	72	umol/L	(normal)
Urea	10	umol/L	(normal)
Glucose	7.0	mmol/L	

Patient's Brief

Synopsis: *This lady has euvolemic hyponatraemia associated with weight loss, chronic cough, and haemoptysis. The concern is lung malignancy or tuberculosis, presenting with the syndrome of inappropriate antidiuretic hormone (SIADH).*

Open the consult with: I have been feeling unusually tired in the last 3 months. The GP says it is because my salt levels are low. *Do not volunteer any other information unless asked.*

History of current problem:

- You are alert; not confused or drowsy. You have not had any seizures.
- You have not had vomiting or diarrhoea.

- You are not feeling unusually thirsty, drinking excessive amounts of water, or passing inordinate amounts of urine.
- You have no leg swelling, breathlessness, abdominal swelling, jaundice, frothy urine, or blood in the urine.
- You have only one proper meal a day as you live alone and have difficulty accessing proper food. You snack on potato chips when you feel hungry.
- You do not have any giddiness when you stand up from a seated position.
- You do not have any cold intolerance or constipation.
- You have had some unintentional weight loss of 5–6 kg in the last 3 months.
- You have been having an irritating cough for the past 3 months. This started as a 'flu' but refused to go away. You have noticed that you cough out streaks of blood, but there is no breathlessness. You have not tried any antibiotics or medications for this cough.
- You have no fever, night sweats, or lumps in your neck or groin.
- You have not had any head trauma, chronic headache, weakness, or numbness.
- No rectal bleeding, muscle aches, joint pain, loud snoring, or low mood.
- You are menopausal.

Past medical and surgical history:
- Depression, diagnosed 2 years ago after your husband passed away from lung cancer.
- Nil. In particular, no history of tuberculosis, cancer, or psychiatric disease.

Medication list:
- Fluoxetine 20 mg ON, started 1 year ago
- Supplements and herbal remedies: nil
- Drug allergy: ibuprofen

Family history:
- Nil. No family history of lung cancer, tuberculosis, or kidney problems.

Relevant personal, social, occupational, and travel history:
- You are a retired teacher.
- You have been living alone in social housing (council flat/one-room rental flat) ever since your husband passed away from lung cancer 2 years ago.
- You have two children but they rarely visit. You have difficulty accessing hot food and sometimes make do with potato chips and instant meals when you are hungry.
- Your neighbour was recently diagnosed with tuberculosis.
- You smoke 1 pack a day since your teenage years. You do not drink.
- No travel history — you can't afford to travel.

Relevant physical examination findings:

This station is likely to be run with a patient surrogate.

- Generally comfortable; mild cachexia, no respiratory distress.
- No clubbing, nicotine stains ++.
- Hydration status normal.
- Respiratory examination – unremarkable.
- Neurological examination – unremarkable.
- No goitre.

You have some specific questions for the doctor at this consultation:

- Do I have cancer?
- Do I need to be admitted?

Approach and Clinical Reasoning

Pitfall: Do not 'force-fit' a generic approach when the stem is more specific.

> A common error is to apply a generic 'approach to fatigue' on this scenario. This is misguided as it ignores the additional information the stem provides — that Mdm Na has hyponatraemia. It is right to bear a healthy dose of scepticism that Mdm Na's fatigue may be due to a cause other than hyponatraemia, but this must not distract you.
>
> Certain PACES exam centres are known to set questions based on abnormal laboratory results; therefore, you should prepare these approaches unless you are sure that your exam centre eschews such questions.

Mdm Na presents with fatigue and hyponatraemia. Zoom in on the approach to hyponatraemia (Figure B4.4). Important history to identify possible causes include:

- Causes of non-hypotonic hyponatraemia — look for predisposition to hyperglycaemic crisis or any history of paraproteinemia.
- Fluid and salt intake (polydipsia, 'tea and toast diet', or beer potomania).
- Any suggestion of fluid overload (leg swelling), and medical history of conditions that could lead fluid overload (heart failure, nephrotic syndrome, renal failure, cirrhosis).
- Any suggestion of dehydration (postural giddiness), gastrointestinal and renal fluid losses (diarrhoea, vomiting, polyuria), or diuretic use.
- Symptoms of adrenal insufficiency and hypothyroidism.
- Causes of SIADH: tumours (especially lung, lymphoma), lung disease (pneumonia, tuberculosis), intracranial disease (meningitis, haemorrhage, trauma), and drugs (antidepressants, antipsychotics, etc.).

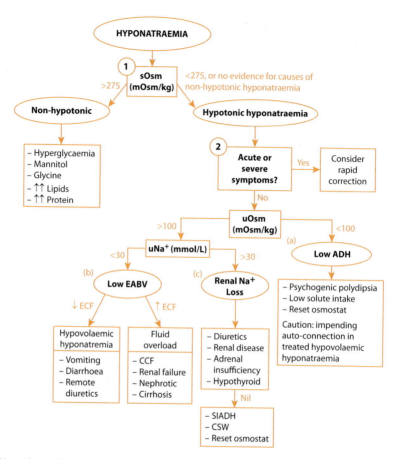

Figure B4.4. **Approach to hyponatraemia.**

Important differentials in Mdm Na include:

- SIADH from lung malignancy or tuberculosis, in view of significant weight loss and chronic cough with haemoptysis.
- SIADH from fluoxetine, a known cause of SIADH.
- Poor solute intake ('tea and toast diet') due to social isolation and difficulty accessing food is slightly less likely in view of her penchant for salty snacks.

Always exclude an emergency. Ensure that Mdm Na does not have any severe symptoms from hyponatraemia (e.g., drowsiness, seizures) that would require rapid correction of sodium.

Physical examination: hyponatraemia itself does not present with physical signs. Examination should search for the cause of hyponatraemia by checking the patient's fluid status and examining the respiratory system. A neurological and thyroid screen may also be helpful as these are differentials to hyponatraemia. Ensure that the patient is orientated and therefore not having severe symptoms from hyponatraemia.

Question and Answer

Suggested answer to the patient's concerns:

Mdm Na, thank you for sharing this concern with me. It must be really hard to lose your husband to lung cancer and now worry about it happening to yourself. I don't know for sure whether you have cancer. The salt level in your blood is low and what you have shared with me — that you have been coughing out blood and losing weight — is worrying. There are a number of reasons why this may be happening to you. Lung cancer is one possibility, but other possible causes include a lung infection or the drugs that you are taking. I will need to do further tests to figure out what is going on. Whatever the tests show, I want to tell you that we are here for you.

I think it's best that we admit you. Your salt levels are very low and this can be quite dangerous. We need to run the tests urgently and we need to monitor your salt levels closely as we treat you.

Don't forget: Present a disposition

> State the appropriate disposition clearly; that is, whether you will admit the patient or manage outpatient. If the latter, explain the follow-up plan and any advice (e.g., 'red flags' to come back to the Emergency Department). Recognising the need for admission is often a marking point.

Suggested presentation to the examiner:

Mdm Na presents with hyponatraemia, weight loss, and chronic cough with haemoptysis. On examination, she is euvolemic, her chest is clear, and there are no neurological deficits. My differentials include SIADH due to a lung malignancy, tuberculosis (given positive contact), fluoxetine, and poor solute intake due to social isolation and difficulty accessing food.

I will like to admit Mdm Na. Initial investigations include paired serum and urine sodium and osmolality, electrolytes, renal and liver biochemistries, thyroid function, and a ACTH stimulation (short synacthen) test. I will do a chest X-ray followed by CT thorax, and send sputum for gram stain and culture, acid-fast bacilli stain and culture and PCR.

Subsequent management depends on the result of these tests:

- If investigations confirm SIADH: Fluid restriction and/or sodium tablets, aiming for a rise in sodium of 8 mmol/L in 24 hours. I will also insert a urinary catheter for close monitoring of intake and output.

- If imaging finds a lung malignancy, I will obtain tissue diagnosis via transthoracic needle aspirate or bronchoscopic biopsy, and complete staging. I will also involve a multidisciplinary team including the oncologist, respiratory physician, and thoracic surgeon, and further treatment should be discussed at tumour board.

Consultation Case 34

Mr Choke (Dysphagia)

Use this case as practice! The pull-out booklet contains the candidate's information.

Information for the Candidate

Patient Details: Mr E. Choke, 40 years old

Your Role: Gastroenterology SHO

Referral Letter:
> Dear Colleague,
>
> Thank you for seeing Mr Choke for consideration of esophago-gastroduodenoscopy. He has been complaining of difficulty swallowing and has lost weight.
>
> Thank you.
>
> Dr Cai Jiashen, GP

Vital Signs: BP 100/60 mmHg, HR 60/min, RR 13/min, SpO2 100% RA, T 36.2°C

Patient's Brief

Synopsis: *This patient has myasthenia gravis with dysphagia, flaccid dysarthria, and fatigability.*

Open the consult with: I have been having difficulty swallowing in the last 2 months and it seems to be getting worse. *Do not volunteer any other information unless asked.*

History of current problem:

- It is not so much a sensation of food getting stuck in the throat, but rather a problem of the food remaining in the mouth and you can't get it down.
- You typically have toast for breakfast and sandwiches for lunch, which seem to be okay. However, you seem to have more trouble at dinnertime, when you have either a cut of meat or rice. There is no difference between solids and liquids.
- There is no pain when you swallow.
- You also occasionally cough when trying to eat and sometimes notice food coming up towards your nose when trying to swallow (nasal regurgitation).
- You are a teacher and you have been having difficulty projecting your voice for a full hour at a go. Towards the end of each lesson, students complain that they are unable to hear you.

- You have lost 3–4 kg in 2 months and often feel more tired than usual.
- You don't have weakness per se but have been finding it harder and harder to jog to school because you get tired and have to make repeated stops along the way. You do not get breathless; just a sense that your body is so heavy and wouldn't move any further.
- You have no numbness, tremors, double vision, droopy eyelids, facial droop, or blurred vision.
- You have no blood in your stools or sensation of feeling full with a small amount of food.
- You have no tightening of the skin in the fingers, fingers changing colour in a cold room, or rashes.
- You have no heat or cold intolerance, diarrhoea or constipation, tremor, leg swelling, anxiety or low mood.

Past medical and surgical history:
- Cancerous thyroid nodule, for which you had half your thyroid removed 3 years ago.

Medication list:
- Nil
- No supplements or alternative medicine
- No drug allergy

Family history:
- No neurologic disease, cancer, or thyroid problems.

Relevant personal, social, occupational, and travel history:
- You work as a teacher (as above).
- You are married with one child.
- You do not smoke or drink.
- No relevant travel history.

Relevant physical examination findings:
This encounter will use a real patient which may have been treated.
- Bilateral slight ptosis which is fatigable.
- Slurred and flaccid speech; bilaterally reduced palatal elevation.
- Tongue central, protrudes normally, no fasciculations.
- Rest of cranial nerves unremarkable.
- Proximal muscle power 4+/5, fatigable, neck flexion power 5/5.
- Tone, reflexes, sensation, and cerebellar normal.
- Neck scar, no goitre or cervical lymph nodes.

- Lungs clear bilaterally on auscultation.
- No sclerodactyly.
- No pallor.
- Gait normal.

You have some specific questions for the doctor at this consultation:

- Do I have cancer?

Approach and Clinical Reasoning

Begin the approach to chronic dysphagia by distinguishing between oesophageal (food getting stuck in the throat) and oropharyngeal dysphagia (difficulty initiating the swallow) (Figure B4.5).

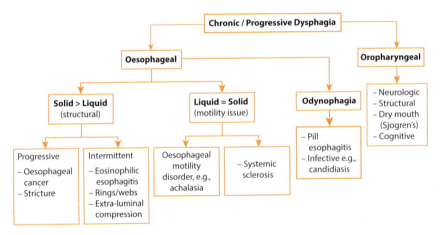

Figure B4.5. Approach to chronic dysphagia.

Mr Choke has oropharyngeal dysphagia, dysarthria, decreased effort tolerance, and weight loss. Recognise the syndrome of neurologic disease. Important differentials along the neuroaxis are:

(a) Lower motor neuron:
- Anterior horn cell (amyotrophic lateral sclerosis/progressive bulbar palsy): look for fasciculations and mixed upper and lower motor neuron signs.
- Neuromuscular junction (myasthenia gravis): look for fatigability.
- Nerve (post radiation or base of skull process): look for multiple lower cranial neuropathies.
- Muscle (certain myopathies).

(b) Upper motor neuron: ischaemic, demyelinating, neoplastic, etc.

(c) Extrapyramidal disease – Parkinson's disease

Mr Choke gives a history of fatigability, which must prompt suspicion of myasthenia gravis. Physical examination is critical as history alone cannot tell these causes apart. It will be reasonable to begin examining the cranial nerves, and quickly screen tone and reflexes in the limbs (for upper motor neuron and extrapyramidal disease). A jaw jerk is helpful but rarely performed correctly.

Apart from neurologic disease, important differentials are:

- Esophageal malignancy given his recent unintentional weight loss (although that can be explained by reduced oral intake alone).
- A compressive or infiltrative thyroid lesion given the previous history of thyroid cancer; and you should examine the neck for any masses.

Finish up by looking for complications of dysphagia, particularly

- Respiratory muscle weakness – you must rule out an emergency (i.e., impending respiratory muscle failure).
- Poor nutrition.
- Aspiration risk.

Question and Answer

Suggested answer to the patient's concerns:

Mr Choke, I don't think a cancer is the most likely diagnosis, although I will certainly need to do some tests to rule that out. I am concerned that you may have a nerve problem called myasthenia gravis, which has caused the muscles responsible for speaking and swallowing to become tired easily.

I need to do some tests urgently for you. This will include nerve and blood tests, and we will definitely need to make sure it is not a cancer. If the tests confirm what I think, I will start you on some medicine to make your speaking muscles stronger. If at any point you feel breathless or are so weak that you find it hard to talk or move, it is important that you come back to the A&E immediately.

Suggested presentation to the examiner:

Mr Choke presents with dysphagia, dysarthria, weight loss, and fatigability. My examination is significant for flaccid dysarthria with bilaterally reduced palatal elevation and bilateral fatigable ptosis. I do not note any tongue fasciculations. The jaw jerk is not brisk. He is coughing which makes me worry about aspiration. Neck flexion is strong which suggests that respiratory muscle weakness is less likely. I will like to complete my examination by checking gag and corneal reflexes, and performing a detailed examination of the upper and lower limbs.

My principal diagnosis is myasthenia gravis. Differentials include other neurological causes such as myopathy or progressive bulbar palsy and an esophageal neoplasm. There is no apparent compressive goitre.

My investigations will include:

- Checking negative inspiratory force/forced vital capacity if there is any question of respiratory compromise.
- Confirming the diagnosis of myasthenia: repetitive nerve stimulation test, anti-acetylcholinesterase receptor and anti-muscle specific kinase antibody, and CT thorax for thymoma.
- Esophagogastroduodenoscopy to exclude an esophageal neoplasm, and ultrasound thyroid to ensure that there is no recurrence of the thyroid nodule.
- Supportive investigations (e.g., haemoglobin, electrolytes, creatinine) in view of poor oral intake; further work-up for weight loss if necessary.

Management will involve:

- Treatment of myasthenia gravis – pyridostigmine, immunosuppression, consideration of thymectomy.
- If there is an acute flare – intravenous immunoglobulin, plasma exchange.
- Speech therapy referral to suggest diet consistency modifications.
- Dietician consult for nutrition advice in view of weight loss.

Consultation Case 35

Mr Philippe (Painful Hands)

Use this case as practice! The pull-out booklet contains the candidate's information.

Information for the Candidate

Patient Details: Mr P. Philippe, 40 years old

Your Role: Medicine Clinic SHO

Referral Letter:
> Dear Colleague,
>
> Mr Philippe has been complaining of joint pains affecting both hands. I would appreciate if you could see him.
>
> Thank you.
>
> Dr Joshua Yeo, GP

Vital Signs: BP 135/80 mmHg, HR 70/min, RR 11/min, SpO2 98% RA, T 37.0°C

Patient's Brief

Synopsis: *Mr Philippe had episodic inflammatory monoarthritis, which subsequently developed into chronic symmetrical small joint polyarthritis. The differential is gout versus rheumatoid arthritis.*

Open the consult with: My fingers have been painful, especially in the morning. *Do not volunteer any other information unless asked.*

History of current problem:

- You have been experiencing pain in the small joints of your fingers and in both wrists. This pain is worst in the morning, and gets better with activity during the day.
- You also experience bothersome hand stiffness in the mornings, which lasts for more than 2 hours. You have learnt that soaking your hands in a warm water bath helps greatly.
- These joint pains have been going on for the past year. Initially, it came as attacks lasting 2–3 days, and you were completely pain-free between attacks. In the last two months, however, your hands seem to be painful and stiff most days.
- You did not have any joint swelling in the past year. However, you recall an episode two years ago during which your right wrist became hot and swollen for two days.

- You did have recurrent right wrist sprains in the past, mostly while playing tennis, however the recent episodes of joint pains are not related to any injury or trauma.
- There is no relationship of joint pain with any food or drink intake.
- There has been no trauma or injury to your hands.
- You have otherwise been well with no fevers or weight loss.
- You have no pain in your back, knees, ankles, or feet.
- You have no rashes or nail deformities.
- You have no diarrhoea, blood in your stools, or abdominal pain.
- You have no penile discharge.
- You have no red eye, blurring of vision, breathlessness, chronic cough, mouth ulcers, hair loss, lumps in the neck or groin, abnormal bleeding, or blood or froth in urine (except for a previous episode of kidney stones).

Past medical and surgical history:
- Hypertension.
- High cholesterol.
- Diabetes, HbA1c 7.2%.
- Chronic gout with flares over 1st metatarsal joints or ankles about 2–3 times a year (never involved hands before), responds to colchicine PRN.
- Two episodes of kidney stones in the past 2 years; each episode resolved with painkillers.

Medication list:
- Atenolol, 50 mg OM
- Hydrochlorothiazide, 25 mg OM
- Metformin 500 mg BD
- Atorvastatin 10 mg ON
- No recent changes
- Supplements and herbal remedies: nil
- Drug allergy: nil

Family history:
- Your late mother had rheumatoid arthritis. You remember that she was quite disabled by it and had deformed 'piano key' hands.

Relevant personal, social, occupational, and travel history:
- You are a craftsman handling delicate and expensive luxury watches.
- You are married with two children. You do not have any sexual partners apart from your spouse.
- You smoke half a pack of cigarettes each day and have done so for the last 20 years.
- You drink at least 2 × 750 ml bottles of beer each day, occasionally with a stout or whisky.

Relevant physical examination findings:

This station can be run with a surrogate, or with a real patient with subtle signs. A patient with florid signs is unlikely at this encounter.

- Overweight.
- No obvious joint deformities, ulnar deviation, swan-neck or boutonniere deformity, nail pitting, or onycholysis.
- No overt/minimal swelling of the wrists or metacarpal-phalangeal and proximal interphalangeal joints.
- Normal range of motion of all small joints of the hands.
- No gouty tophi over hands or elbows, no rheumatoid nodules.
- Small gouty tophi over the earlobes.
- No psoriatic plaques over the hands, abdomen, back, or gluteal cleft.

You have some specific questions for the doctor at this consultation:

- I need to use my hands. Will I end up with the deformities that my mother had?

Approach and Clinical Reasoning

It is official advice[20] that scenarios in which patients present with classical histories and florid clinical signs are considered 'too easy'. Scenarios using patients with obvious signs may instead explore complications and nuances of disease. This scenario highlights the nuances in the clinical history of gout.

Mr Philippe has symmetrical, inflammatory chronic polyarthritis affecting the small joints of the hands. You will be familiar with the causes of a polyarthritis (Table B4.30) and their differentiators; that is, (i) the nature of pain — inflammatory vs. mechanical, (ii) distribution — axial vs. appendicular, symmetric vs. asymmetric, small- vs. large-joint, (iii) time course, and (iv) extra-articular features.

The closest differentials for Mr Philippe's joint pains are gout and rheumatoid arthritis (RA). The key here is to pay careful attention to the chronology of symptoms — notice that the nature of joint pain has changed over time. It is not always easy to tell gout from RA:

- Distribution: Mr Philippe's symmetrical small joint polyarthritis appears classical for RA. However, polyarticular gout can present in this manner particularly later in the course of disease.
- Time course:
  - The historical episode of acute monoarthritis, occurring in a joint with prior degenerative change, is classical for gout.

---

[20] MRCP(UK) Guidelines for Station 5 scenarios, last updated 2014. Available at https://www.mrcpuk.org/document/station-5-writing-guide. This document is likely to be updated as the new PACES format matures.

- Mr Philippe initially experienced intense inflammatory flares interspersed with asymptomatic intercritical periods. This favours gout over RA; while inflammation in RA may wax and wane, it tends not to become completely asymptomatic.
- Mr Philippe's current state of chronic arthropathy may be seen in both RA and late in the natural history of gout.
* Extra-articular manifestations: The history of 'kidney stones' may suggest urate nephrolithiasis. There are no extra-articular manifestations characteristic of RA.

Apart from considering gout vs. RA, screen through the other causes of inflammatory joint pain — rule out psoriasis, inflammatory bowel disease, axial symptoms, and other extra-articular manifestations of systemic rheumatologic illness.

Look for risk factors for gout. Recognise that Mr Philippe is using a thiazide diuretic, has significant alcohol intake, and is likely to have metabolic syndrome.

Table B4.30. Causes of polyarthritis.

Cause	Articular features	Extra-articular features
Mechanical joint pain		
Osteoarthritis	Tends to affect the hip, knee, and distal interphalangeal joints	Nil
Inflammatory Joint Pain		
Rheumatoid arthritis	Chronic symmetrical small joint arthropathy, characteristic deformities, atlantoaxial instability	Rheumatoid nodules, pulmonary fibrosis, scleritis, pyoderma gangrenosum
Spondyloarthritis (SpA)	Axial SpA: back pain, decreased spinal range of motion. Appendicular SpA: asymmetrical large > small joint oligo- or polyarthritis	Enthesitis, dactylitis, uveitis. Underlying psoriasis, inflammatory bowel disease, preceding diarrhoeal illness or urethritis (reactive arthritis)
Gout	Asymmetric mono- or oligoarthritis, episodic flares with asymptomatic intercritical periods	Gouty tophi. Urolithiasis
Systemic lupus erythematosus	Any pattern of inflammatory joint pain	Skin (oral ulcers, alopecia, rash), nephritis, serositis, cytopenias
Polyarticular septic arthritis	Acute-onset, may be severe (More commonly monoarticular; polyarticular involvement indicates haematogenous dissemination)	Fever, systemically unwell. May have endocarditis. Risk factors (e.g., IV drug use, immunosuppression)
Disseminated gonococcal infection	Acute presentation, migratory polyarthritis, risk factors	Tenosynovitis, rash (painless vesiculopustular or pustular). Genitourinary symptoms may be absent

Physical examination clinches the diagnosis of gout over rheumatoid arthritis. The observant candidate who inspects the patient early will notice the tophi upfront.

- Examination of the hands according to the look-feel-move schema; look particularly for tophi and deformities characteristic of rheumatoid arthritis, feel the joint lines for active synovitis, and move to assess range of motion.
- Functional assessment of the hands (e.g., using a pen, buttoning a shirt).
- Look for signs to suggest differentials (e.g., rashes, mouth ulcers, dactylitis).

Question and Answer

Suggested answer to the patient's concerns:

Thank you for sharing this with me. I am sorry to hear that your mother had such disabling deformities and I cannot imagine how worried you must be. I think you are much less likely to end up with the deformities that your mother had for two reasons. Firstly, I think you probably have gout, rather than rheumatoid arthritis. Gout can be serious, but it does not cause the piano-key deformities seen in rheumatoid arthritis. Secondly, even if you have rheumatoid arthritis, treatment has advanced greatly in the last 20 years — we now treat more aggressively and have many effective drugs, so it is uncommon with modern treatment to develop such severe deformities.

I will do some tests to confirm my diagnosis and we will start you on treatment. We should be able to bring down the joint pains and stop you from getting as many flares as you did. I want you to be able to use your hands without pain. On your part, it will be incredibly helpful to cut down on beer as this is well-known to make gout worse.

Suggested presentation to the examiner:

Mr Philippe first presented with an acute monoarthritis, then developed episodic inflammatory flares interspersed with asymptomatic intercritical periods, and now has chronic symmetrical small joint polyarthritis. This is on a background of significant beer intake, thiazide use, and a suggestion of possible nephrolithiasis. On examination, there are small gouty tophi over the earlobes. There are no joint deformities characteristic of deforming rheumatoid arthritis, rheumatoid nodules, or psoriatic rash. There is no evidence of active joint swelling, and his range of motion is full. Function appears intact. My principal diagnosis is gout. The differential diagnosis is rheumatoid arthritis.

I will investigate to confirm my diagnosis, look for differentials, and assist management.

- To confirm my diagnosis:
  - The ideal diagnostic test for gout is synovial fluid microscopy for negatively birefringent needle-shape crystals. This may not be possible as there is no joint effusion to tap.
  - Imaging such as plain hand X-rays looking for joint erosions.

- To look for differentials:
  - I will do blood tests such as inflammatory markers, rheumatoid factor and anti-citrullinated peptide antibodies.
  - I may consider an MRI which is more sensitive for synovitis.
- To assist in management:
  - I will check urate levels to guide uric acid lowering therapy[21].
  - I will check a blood count and renal biochemistry.

Management will involve a multidisciplinary team including the rheumatologist, urologist, GP, dietitian, and allied healthcare professionals. This includes:

- Uric acid lowering therapy (allopurinol) with counselling about side effects, particularly the risk of Stevens-Johnson-syndrome (note: a uricosuric agent is contraindicated given the history of urate nephrolithiasis).
- Analgesia, favouring colchicine or non-steroidal anti-inflammatories over prednisolone, in view of diabetes.
- Thiazides increase urate resorption and may be switched to an alternative antihypertensive. Given this patient's diabetes, an angiotensin-converting enzyme inhibitor or angiotensin receptor blocker (ARB) would be first line. Losartan, in particular, has a uricosuric effect and may be the ARB of choice in this patient.
- Dietician counselling, particularly on alcohol intake, avoidance of trigger foods, and weight loss.
- Optimisation of management for his comorbids.

---

[21] Elevated uric acid increases the risk of gout but does not diagnose gout, and normal uric acid does not rule it out (levels may be falsely low during attacks). The main role of checking uric acid is to establish a baseline to guide uric acid lowering therapy, which will subsequently be titrated against a uric acid target.

Consultation Case 36

Ms S. L. Ee (Mouth Ulcers)

Use this case as practice! The pull-out booklet contains the candidate's information.

Information for the Candidate

Patient Details: Ms S. L. Ee, 33 years old

Your Role: Rheumatology Clinic SHO

Scenario: Ms Ee is on follow up for systemic lupus erythematosus. She has brought forward her appointment, complaining of mouth ulcers. She is worried of a lupus flare.

Vital Signs: BP 115/66 mmHg, HR 67/min, RR 10/min, SpO2 97% RA, T 37.0°C

Patient's Brief

Synopsis: *A young lady with known lupus presents with mouth ulcers due to methotrexate toxicity. She has been incorrectly taking methotrexate daily instead of weekly.*

Open the consult with: My mouth is full of ulcers! My lupus has never been so bad. *Apart from the opening lines above, do not volunteer any other information unless asked.*

History of current problem:

- Oral ulcers first appeared 3–4 weeks ago but have gotten bigger and more in number. They are painful and troublesome when you eat. You have tried various mouth gels, which numb the ulcers for a short while but do not yield any lasting benefit.
- You do not have a history of recurrent oral ulceration.
- You have no genital ulcers.
- In the past month, you have also been having up to 5 loose stools a day. You notice small streaks of blood in your stools, but you think that this is because of haemorrhoids. This is associated with mild, crampy abdominal colic, relieved by defecation.
- You have also been feeling tired; in particular, you feel lightheaded and breathless when going out of the house even on a short errand.
- You are having your menstrual period now and it seems unusually heavy (8–9 pads a day, from 4–5 usually).

Consultation Case 36   421

- You have lost 4–5 kg in the past month.
- You do not have any joint pain, fever, rashes, painful hands, colour changes in your hands when exposed to the cold, blood in urine, eye pain, blurring of vision, or mood symptoms.
- No jaundice, abdominal pain, or change in urine colour.

Past medical and surgical history:
- Systemic lupus erythematosus. You first presented five years ago with fatigue, malar rash, pain and colour changes in your hands especially when exposed to the cold, and blood in your urine. You have been maintained on low-dose prednisolone, hydroxychloroquine, and azathioprine. Your last flare was 3–4 months back, mainly with joint pain.
- Three months ago, the rheumatologist switched azathioprine to methotrexate for better control of joint pains, given that you have completed your family.
- Haemorrhoids.

Medication list:
- Methotrexate 20 mg, which you have been taking daily. If asked, your next follow-up visit is in 4 months, but you appear to be running out of medicine.
- Hydroxychloroquine, 200 mg daily
- Prednisolone, 5 mg daily
- Off-the-shelf multivitamin tablet, daily
- You recall that the rheumatologist also prescribed a 'vitamin tablet'. You have not been taking this, as you prefer to use your own multivitamin.
- Drug allergy: nil

Family history:
- Nil

Relevant personal, social, occupational, and travel history:
- Married with two daughters, 2 years old and 7 months old.
- You used to work as a retail sales assistant, but are currently a full-time mother.
- No smoking or alcohol intake.
- You are sexually active only with your husband.

Relevant physical examination findings:
- Multiple 1–1.5 cm ulcers all over oral mucosa, no vesicles/blisters/lip mucosal ulcerations *(note: a patient listed for the PACES exam may no longer have ulcers)*.
- Conjunctival pallor +, no scleral icterus.
- No malar rash or psoriatic plaques.
- Lungs clear.
- Abdomen soft, non-tender, no masses.

- Digital rectal examination (if offered) – empty rectum.
- Calves supple, no pedal oedema.

You have some specific questions for the doctor at this consultation:

- Will these ulcers go away? I can't stand them any longer!

Approach and Clinical Reasoning

Ms Ee presents with persistent mouth ulcers on a background of systemic lupus erythematosus. The differential list for mouth ulcers (Table B4.31) is long, but for the purposes of MRCP PACES you should focus on systemic causes. It is helpful to begin with open-ended questions and associated symptoms, which can quickly narrow the differentials.

Table B4.31. Differentials to severe/recurrent mouth ulcers.

Category	Cause	Important clinical features
Idiopathic	Recurrent aphthous stomatitis	Exclusion of secondary causes
Systemic causes	Behcet syndrome	Recurrent oral and genital ulcers May have systemic involvement
	Systemic lupus erythematosus	Skin: malar rash, cutaneous lupus Systemic involvement: fever, cytopenias, joint involvement, nephritis
	Inflammatory bowel disease	Colitis – abdominal pain, bloody diarrhoea
	Neutropenia Antimetabolite drugs (e.g., methotrexate, chemotherapy)	Antecedent drug/chemo exposure May have gastrointestinal mucositis (e.g., diarrhoea), cytopenias, or sepsis
	Acute HIV infection	Painful mucocutaneous ulceration and sore throat
Dermatologic causes	Oral lichen planus	May have reticular white papules and plaques alongside erosions
	Mucosa ulcerations: Stevens-Johnson syndrome, pemphigus vulgaris	Extensive cutaneous rashes/erosions/bullae on trunk/limbs Lips often involved Painful haemorrhagic oral erosions in the Stevens-Johnson syndrome
	Infections (e.g., herpes simplex (HSV), syphilis)	HSV – painful small ulcers and vesicles Syphillis – painless chancre Exposure history

Apart from mouth ulcers, Ms Ee also has bloody diarrhoea, menorrhagia, lethargy, and decreased effort tolerance. The drug history must ring alarm bells — methotrexate is newly started, she is taking it *daily*, and she has omitted the co-prescribed 'vitamin' (folic acid supplementation). Methotrexate overdose causes mucositis (bloody diarrhoea, ulcers) and cytopenias (thrombocytopenia presenting as menorrhagia, symptomatic anaemia).

Don't forget: Methotrexate toxicity

> Methotrexate for non-malignant conditions is usually prescribed as a 10–25 mg weekly dose (not daily) with folic acid supplementation. It is prone to inadvertent overdose.

A possible differential is Crohn's disease, which can explain bloody diarrhoea and mouth ulcers but not menorrhagia. Lupus flare is less likely given the use of high-dose methotrexate and symptoms that differ from previous flares. In every rheumatology patient, it is important to enquire what the first presentation and usual flares are like — patients often flare with similar disease manifestations.

Physical examination should focus on:

- Looking at the oral ulcers – excluding vesicles, haemorrhagic erosions (Stevens-Johnsons syndrome), or other lesions.
- Searching for other manifestations of lupus (e.g., malar rash, cutaneous lupus, arthropathy, fluid overload from nephritis).
- Ensuring that the abdomen is soft (in view of the history of bloody diarrhoea).
- Offering a rectal examination for rectal bleeding.

Question and Answer

Suggested answer to the patient's concerns:

Ms Ee, these ulcers must be bothering you so much. The ulcers are likely to go away, but we need to get a few things done. I suspect that you may have inadvertently taken too much methotrexate. I will like to admit you and we will give you an antidote for methotrexate overdose. This will help the ulcers get better, although it may take a few days.

Suggested presentation to the examiner:

Ms Ee presents with a 2-week history of oral ulcers, bloody diarrhoea, menorrhagia, weight loss, and constitutional symptoms after taking 20 mg daily methotrexate without folic acid supplementation. Examination is remarkable for multiple oral aphthous ulcers without other cutaneous stigmata of lupus. My primary diagnosis is methotrexate toxicity presenting with mucositis and cytopenias. There is no evidence of hepatitis. Differentials include Crohn's disease and less likely a lupus flare.

I will like to admit her. Investigations include:

- Confirming my diagnosis by checking methotrexate levels.
- Looking for organ involvement by checking liver function for transaminitis, full blood count for cytopenias, iron studies if there is anaemia, coagulation studies in view of menorrhagia, and renal function.
- If symptoms do not improve with cessation of methotrexate, I will also need to investigate for differentials including performing fecal calprotectin and referring for colonoscopy, as well as pelvic ultrasound and gynaecological referral for work-up of menorrhagia.

Management will include:

- Stopping methotrexate.
- High-dose folinic acid (leucovorin) rescue.
- IV hydration and management of symptoms.
- Generally not to restart methotrexate (as toxicity can be idiosyncratic instead of dose-dependant), but this decision should be made by the rheumatology specialist.

Consultation Case 37

Mdm Yang (Itch)

Use this case as practice! The pull-out booklet contains the candidate's information.

Information for the Candidate

Patient Details: Mdm Yang, 49 years old

Your Role: Dermatology Clinic SHO

Referral Letter:
> Dear Dermatologist,
>
> I have been seeing Mdm Yang for a persistent generalised itch which does not respond to moisturiser creams or topical steroids. A trial of scabies treatment was also unsuccessful.
>
> Would you please see her? Thank you.
>
> Dr Shawn Lin, GP

Vital Signs: BP 120/72 mmHg, HR 60/min, RR 12/min, SpO2 95% RA, T 37.0°C

Patient's Brief

Synopsis: *This lady with aquagenic pruritus and splenomegaly likely has polycythaemia vera.*

Open the consult with: I have been feeling really itchy for the past 2 months. The GP gave me some creams but they don't work one bit. *Do not volunteer any other information unless asked.*

History of current problem:
- Itch is severe and noticeable over your entire body.
- You have never noticed any rash, even transiently.
- You have tried various creams including moisturisers, steroids, and even scabies treatment (which the GP proposed because of your occupational exposure), but none of them resulted in any relief.
- Interestingly, you have noticed that a hot shower makes the itch worse.
- As a scrub nurse, you use rather strong disinfectant soaps to wash your hands many times a day. There is no rash over your hands, and the itch is not worse over the hands.

- You have been feeling slightly lethargic.
- No jaundice, change in urine colour, or abdominal pain.
- No blood in urine, frothy urine, leg swelling, decreased urine output, or breathlessness.
- No weight loss, night sweats, or lumps in your neck or groin.
- No diarrhoea, heat intolerance, or weight loss.
- Last menstrual period was 2 weeks ago; menses are not unusually heavy or light, and there is no changes in your menses.
- You have been vaccinated against hepatitis B and your last hepatitis B/C/HIV check a year ago (an occupational requirement) was negative.
- No episodes (even transient) of headache, giddiness, weakness, numbness, or blurring of vision.
- No burning pains in the feet or hands.
- No pain or swelling in the legs.

Past medical and surgical history:
- Nil

Medication list:
- Nil
- Supplements and herbal remedies: nil
- Drug allergy: nil

Family history:
- Nil

Relevant personal, social, occupational, and travel history:
- Works as a scrub nurse in the hospital.
- Married with two teenage children.
- Non-smoker.
- No alcohol intake.

Relevant physical examination findings:
- No jaundice, pallor, cyanosis, or xanthelasma.
- No peripheral stigmata of chronic liver disease.
- Abdomen soft non-tender. 2 cm splenomegaly, and no hepatomegaly or ascites.
- No lymphadenopathy.
- No goitre, proptosis, or tremor.
- No pedal oedema.

You have some specific questions for the doctor at this consultation:

- Why am I feeling so itchy? Is it because of the soap that I use to scrub up in the operating theatre? It is affecting my work because I feel so itchy but I can't scratch when I am scrubbed up.

Approach and Clinical Reasoning

The approach to pruritus begins by determining whether there is or is no rash. While Mdm Yang has no rash, her concern about contact dermatitis is fair given her occupational exposure. Verify that there was *never* a rash — transient rashes like urticaria may not be visible at the point of consult. Major causes of generalised pruritus without a rash include dysfunction of the renal, hepatic, haematological, and thyroid systems (Table B4.32).

Table B4.32. Causes of generalised pruritus without rash[22].

Cause	Important clinical features
Uraemia	Fluid overload (dyspnoea, leg swelling), decrease in urine output, underlying cause of renal disease (e.g., longstanding diabetes, haematuria in glomerulonephritis)
Cholestasis, particularly primary biliary cholangitis	Jaundice, tea-coloured urine, ± right hypochondrial pain Xanthelasma in primary biliary cholangitis
Polycythaemia rubra vera[23]	Aquagenic pruritus (itch worst after a hot bath) ± splenomegaly ± vasomotor symptoms (hand or feet pain) ± symptoms of hyperviscosity (e.g., headaches)
Other hematologic malignancy (e.g., Hodgkin lymphoma)	Weight loss, night sweats, anaemia, lymphadenopathy
Thyrotoxicosis	Heat intolerance, diarrhoea, goitre, proptosis
Drugs	Drug history – especially opiates

Mdm Yang has a classical history of aquagenic pruritus which is suggestive of polycythaemia vera. Secondary causes of polycythaemia typically are asymptomatic incidental findings and tend not to cause aquagenic pruritus.

---

[22] Other causes which are less relevant for PACES include: skin xerosis, psychogenic (delusion of parasitosis).

[23] While aquagenic pruritus is most classical in polycyemia vera, it may less commonly be present in other myeloproliferative neoplasms (e.g., essential thrombocytosis).

Look for other manifestations and complications of polycythaemia vera:

- Thrombotic complications:
  - Erythromelalgia: burning hand/feet pain with erythema due to microvascular thrombosis.
  - Arterial thrombosis (e.g., stroke, myocardial infarction).
  - Venous thrombosis (e.g., deep venous thrombosis, pulmonary embolism).
- Haemorrhagic complications, seen in polycythemia rubra vera patients with very high platelet counts due to acquired Von Willebrand disease.
- Hyperviscosity symptoms, particularly frequent headaches and transient visual disturbances.
- Constitutional symptoms – loss of appetite and weight.

Examination should focus on:

- Looking for ruddy complexion, cyanosis.
- Identifying splenomegaly (common) ± hepatomegaly (uncommon).
- Evidence of thrombotic complications (e.g., unilateral leg swelling).
- Searching for differentials – ensuring that there is no lymphadenopathy, jaundice, stigmata of chronic liver disease, xanthelasma (primary biliary cholangitis), or goitre.

Question and Answer

Suggested answer to the patient's concerns:

Mdm Yang, I'm sorry to hear that this has been affecting you so badly. It must be bothersome. I don't think the itch is because of the soap; instead, I suspect that this is due to an overproduction of red blood cells in your body. I will need to do some tests to confirm the diagnosis. I don't have to admit you, but we should get the tests done today and I will see you in a week to review the results. In the meantime, let me give you some medications to help with the itch.

Suggested presentation to the examiner:

Mdm Yang presents with aquagenic pruritus and splenomegaly. My principal diagnosis is polycythaemia vera. There are no thrombotic, haemorrhagic, or hyperviscosity symptoms at the moment. There is no evidence to support differential diagnoses such as uraemia, liver disease, lymphoma, or hyperthyroidism.

Investigations:

- I will confirm my diagnosis by doing a full blood count and, if the haemoglobin is elevated (>16.5 g/dL in men, >16 g/dL in women), check erythropoietin levels (suppressed) and JAK2 mutation.
- Bone marrow aspiration and trephine (sometimes omitted in patients with a classic presentation, suppressed erythropoietin levels, and positive JAK2 mutation).

- Screen for other cardiovascular and thrombotic risk factors.
- Screen for differentials by checking renal, liver, and thyroid function.

Management of polycythaemia vera may be beyond the level expected of a PACES candidate. Knowing that aspirin and phlebotomy are potential management options is likely adequate.

(Additional information) The treatment of polycythaemia vera takes a risk-stratified approach. Mdm Yang, being 49 years old without a history of thrombosis, falls into the low risk category and will benefit from:

- Phlebotomy to maintain haematocrit < 45%.
- Low-dose aspirin.
- Treatment of cardiovascular risk factors.
- Adjuncts (e.g., vaccination, patient education).

Cytoreductive therapy (hydroxyurea, busulfan) will only be indicated if her symptoms are refractory to phlebotomy and aspirin, if she has elevated platelet counts, or if she develops a thrombosis event (and thereby enters the high risk category).

Consultation Case 38

Ms Poo (Diarrhoea)

Use this case as practice! The pull-out booklet contains the candidate's information.

Information for the Candidate

Patient Details: Ms Poo, 47 years old

Your Role: Gastroenterology Clinic SHO

Referral Letter:
> Dear Colleague,
>
> Thank you for seeing Ms Poo. She has had a 1-month history of diarrhoea which does not resolve on symptomatic treatment.
>
> Thank you.
>
> Dr Loo, GP

Vital Signs: BP 107/60 mmHg, HR 111/min, RR 12/min, SpO2 98% RA, T 37.0°C

Patient's Brief

Synopsis: *This lady presents with signs and symptoms of hyperthyroidism which may be amiodarone-induced thyrotoxicosis.*

Open the consult with: Nothing seems to be helping my diarrhoea. It just doesn't stop! *Do not volunteer any other information unless asked.*

History of current problem:
- This diarrhoea started gradually and has gotten worse over the past month. The GP has given you a course of oral antibiotics, charcoal tablets, and anti-diarrhoea medicine, but this has not worked.
- You have 4–5 watery stools a day. There is no blood in the stools. The stools are not foul-smelling, large in volume, and do not float on water.
- There is no association with any particular foods.
- You have occasional cramping abdominal pain which comes with the urge to pass motion, but this is mild.
- You have lost 5 kg over the past month despite eating well.
- You have noticed that you often feel very hot, even in a cold room.
- You have also been somewhat more anxious and hot-tempered than usual. Your hands shake a little sometimes.

- Your period the past 2 months have been unusually light. Your last period was 3 weeks ago.
- No joint pains, rashes, tightening of the skin over your fingers, or change in colour of the fingers on entering a cold environment.
- No leg swelling, decrease in urine output, blood or bubbles in the urine.
- No fever or no lumps in your neck or groin.

Past medical and surgical history:
- You had a heart attack 6 months ago and had your heart vessel ballooned. You were also told that you had an irregular heartbeat and were given amiodarone to control your heart rhythm.
- Hypertension.
- You have not had prior abdominal surgery.

Medication list:
- Aspirin 100 mg OM
- Amiodarone 200 mg OM, started 5 months ago
- Atorvastatin 20 mg ON
- Bisoprolol 5 mg OM
- Clopidogrel 75 mg OM
- Rivaroxaban 20 mg OM
- Valsartan 40 mg ON
- No traditional medicine, supplements, or herbal remedies
- No drug allergy

Family history:
- Nil

Relevant personal, social, occupational, and travel history:
- You have no relevant travel history.
- You are married with 2 teenage children. Your spouse is your only sexual partner.
- You do not smoke or drink.
- You are a housewife.

Relevant physical examination findings:
This encounter may use either a real or a surrogate patient. The history and physical signs will be simulated to mimic an acute presentation.
- Irregularly irregular pulse.
- Tremor on outstretched arms.
- No proximal muscle weakness.

- No goitre.
- Lid lag present, no exophthalmos or ophthalmoplegia.
- Abdomen soft, non-tender.
- Calves supple, no oedema.

You have some specific questions for the doctor at this consultation:
- What is wrong with me?

Approach and Clinical Reasoning

Ms Poo presents with a history of chronic diarrhoea. A number of important causes have to be considered (Table B4.33), but often the best strategy is to ask the patient open-ended questions about his/her associated symptoms.

Table B4.33. Important differentials in chronic diarrhoea.

Cause	Stool	Important considerations
Infective	Usually watery	Particularly parasites and viruses (e.g., CMV)
		Look for immunocompromised state (especially HIV*)
Inflammatory	Blood-stained, with significant abdominal pain	Inflammatory bowel disease* – look for skin tags, ulcers, arthritis, uveitis, pyoderma, etc.
		Ischaemic colitis – abdominal angina, atrial fibrillation
		Radiation colitis
		Particular invasive infections
Malabsorptive	Steatorrhoea or watery, with weight loss	Chronic pancreatitis, cystic fibrosis
		Celiac disease
		Bacterial overgrowth – may have underlying scleroderma* or abnormal gastrointestinal motility
		Post-surgical (e.g., short gut, post-cholecystectomy)
Drug-related	–	Antimetabolites (e.g., chemotherapy, methotrexate*)
		Alteration of gut flora (e.g., antibiotics)
		Osmotic effects (e.g., electrolyte salts)
Metabolic	–	Hyperthyroidism* – look for systemic features
		Carcinoid syndrome – episodic diarrhoea, flushing, bronchospasm
Malignancy and infiltrative	–	Colonic neoplasia
		Amyloidosis* – underlying chronic inflammatory disease, plasma cell dyscrasia, multi-organ involvement (e.g., hepatomegaly, nephrotic syndrome, cardiomyopathy, neuropathy)
		Gastrointestinal lupus

*PACES favourites.

Pitfall: Time management

> For presenting complaints with a large number of differentials, a balance has to be struck between comprehensively considering all possibilities and going into adequate depth for key differentials (e.g., in cases of inflammatory bowel disease — exploring the patient's extra-intestinal manifestations).

It becomes apparent that Ms Poo has watery diarrhoea and weight loss associated with heat intolerance, oligomenorrhoea, tremors, and worsening tachycardia (despite being on amiodarone). This is suggestive of hyperthyroidism. Proceed to examine thyroid status and for a goitre.

Practice makes perfect: The thyroid examination

> You should have a well-rehearsed routine for thyroid examination. A possible routine that can be completed in 2–3 minutes includes:
> (1) Examining thyroid structure[24]:
> - Inspect for a goitre. Have the patient sip water and observe the goitre ascending on swallowing.
> - Palpate from behind – determine if the goitre is smooth and diffuse, or nodular.
> - Percuss for retrosternal extension.
> - Auscultate for a thyroid bruit.
>
> (2) Determining thyroid status:
> - Examine outstretched hands for tremors.
> - Feel the pulse for tachycardia and atrial fibrillation.
> - Check proximal muscle strength.
> - Demonstrate lid lag.
>
> (3) Examining for manifestations of underlying disease and complications:
> - Examine for exophthalmos ± ophthalmoplegia (Graves' disease).
> - Palpate lower limbs for oedema (heart failure).
> - Look for thyroid acropachy (Graves' disease).

The next step is to identify a cause of hyperthyroidism. Important causes include:

- Graves' disease – exophthalmos and thyroid bruit are specific to Graves' (but are not necessarily present in all cases).
- Early thyroiditis, such as hashi-toxicosis.
- Toxic multinodular goitre.
- Drugs: iodine (as in amiodarone, radiocontrast medium), lithium, immune checkpoint inhibitors.
- Secondary hyperthyroidism due to a thyroid-stimulating hormone (TSH)-secreting adenoma (rare).

---

[24] Note: As this is not a surgical examination, it would typically be unnecessary to check whether the goitre ascends on tongue protrusion or to examine cervical lymph nodes.

Unusually, Ms Poo does not have a goitre. The drug history — that she has been started on amiodarone five months ago — should ring alarm bells. Note that the temporal sequence is important — it could be that (a) the hyperthyroidism precipitated atrial fibrillation, necessitating amiodarone use, or (b) the amiodarone caused hyperthyroidism.

Amiodarone can cause a variety of thyroid disorders:

- Hypothyroidism.
- Hyperthyroidism – Amiodarone-induced thyrotoxicosis (AIT).
  - Type 1 AIT: arises from increased synthesis of thyroid hormone in patients with pre-existing thyroid disease. Typical onset within months of starting amiodarone therapy. Patients may have features of underlying thyroid disease, such as thyroid eye disease or thyroid nodules.
  - Type 2 AIT: a drug-induced destructive thyroiditis. This is typically late-onset (years after starting amiodarone).
  - You should not be expected to distinguish between type 1 and 2 AIT in PACES.

Finally, ensure that Ms Poo is well and not in frank *thyroid storm*.

Question and Answer

Suggested answer to the patient's concerns:

Ms Poo, it seems like you may have high thyroid hormone levels, which is driving your diarrhoea, weight loss, tremors, constant feeling of heat, and anxiety. At the moment it is not clear what the high thyroid hormone levels are due to, but this could be related to the drug amiodarone you are taking for your heart rhythm, or it could be an autoimmune process in which your body mistakenly recognises your thyroid gland as something foreign and triggers it to make more thyroid hormone. I will like to do some blood tests to confirm what I suspect, after which I will be able to have more information for you.

Suggested presentation to the examiner:

Ms Poo presents with clinical hyperthyroidism with diarrhoea, weight loss, heat intolerance, and anxiety. Physical examination is significant for tremors, atrial fibrillation, and lid lag, but the absence of a goitre or signs of Graves' ophthalmopathy. Differentials for her hyperthyroid state include amiodarone-induced hyperthyroidism, Graves' disease, and thyroiditis.

Investigations will include:

- Checking serum TSH, free T4 to confirm the hyperthyroid state.
- Sending thyroid receptor antibodies (TRAb).
- Ultrasound thyroid to look for hypervascularity (suggests underlying Graves' disease – type 1 AIT), nodules (type 1 AIT), or hypovascularity (type 2 AIT).

- Radioiodine uptake scan useful in differentiating type 1 AIT (normal or high uptake) and type 2 AIT (little or no uptake).
- Checking a blood count, renal function, and electrolytes as these may be deranged due to diarrhoea.

Management is best handled by a multidisciplinary team involving the endocrinologist and cardiologist.

- Type 1 AIT is treated with antithyroid drugs, while type 2 AIT is treated with steroids. The distinction between type 1 and type 2 AIT is challenging.
- Amiodarone is ideally discontinued, but this will have to be done in consultation with the cardiologist. An alternative rate or rhythm control strategy for her atrial fibrillation will be necessary.

Consultation Case 39

Ms L. Sai (Abdominal Pain)

Use this case as practice! The pull-out booklet contains the candidate's information.

Information for the Candidate

Patient Details: Ms L. Sai, 30 years old

Your Role: Emergency Department SHO

Scenario: Ms Sai, who is on follow up for Crohn's disease, complains of abdominal pain.

Vital Signs: BP 100/60 mmHg, HR 111/min, RR 10/min, SpO2 99% RA, T 39.0°C

Patient's Brief

Synopsis: *A young lady with Crohn's disease is unwell with fever, abdominal pain, and fecaluria. The main concern is urosepsis from an enterovesical fistula.*

Open the consult with: I haven't been able to go to work for the past two days. I'm just lying in bed with fever and chills. My tummy hurts. I can't eat much. *Do not volunteer any other information unless asked.*

History of current problem:
- Your fever started two days ago. The temperature has been in the 38.5°C to 39.5°C range, despite paracetamol. You have not had any antibiotics.
- You have also been having severe lower abdominal pain, localised in the right lower abdomen, which does not radiate anywhere. It is constant, does not come and go, and is better when you lie still in bed. This is the most severe pain you remember ever having in your history of Crohn's disease.
- You have not had significant diarrhoea or rectal bleeding. You have passed two slightly loose stools today, which is your baseline.
- You feel that your tummy is 'bloated' but have not noticed it to be distended.
- You feel nauseous but have not vomited.
- In the past 24 hours, you have been having frequent urges to pass urine, and you experience a 'burning sensation' when you pass urine. Unusually, your urine seems to contain bubbles of gas and brown solid matter — you are quite puzzled by this.
- You have no vaginal bleeding or discharge. Your last menstrual period just ended a week ago, and you are sure that you are not pregnant.

- You feel generally unwell.
- You have no jaundice, vaginal bleeding or discharge, cough, difficulty breathing, headache, leg swelling, lumps in your neck or groin, rashes, joint pain, or mouth ulcers.

Past medical and surgical history:
- Crohn's disease. You first presented with bloody diarrhoea 2 years ago, and a colonoscope confirmed that you had Crohn's disease affecting the small and large intestines. In the past six months, you have been admitted thrice for a Crohn's flare, each of which presented with fever, bloody diarrhoea, and abdominal pain which comes and goes. You have never had surgery for this condition; each admission was treated with intravenous medicines. At baseline, you pass 2–3 loose stools a day.
- Urinary tract infection. You have had two urinary tract infections in the past 3 months. Each resolved with a course of oral antibiotics.

Medication list:
- Azathioprine 100 mg OM
- Infliximab 5 mg/kg IV infusion every 8 weeks. The last dose was given 6 weeks ago.
- Hyoscine (scopolamine) butylbromide 10 mg TDS PRN for stomach cramps.
- Supplements and herbal remedies: nil
- Drug allergy: nil

Family history:
- Nil

Relevant personal, social, occupational, and travel history:
- You work in a sedentary office job.
- You are not married and are not sexually active.
- You do not smoke or drink.
- No relevant travel history.

Relevant physical examination findings:

This encounter may use either a real or a surrogate patient. The history and physical signs will be simulated to mimic an acute presentation.

- General condition well, non-toxic.
- Abdomen soft with lower abdominal tenderness, no guarding or rebound.
- No abdominal scars, stomas, or masses.
- Bowel sounds present.
- Renal punch negative.
- No pallor or jaundice.
- Rectal examination, if offered: empty rectum.

- No mouth ulcers, perianal skin tags, joint swelling/pain, red eye, rashes.
- Rest of examination normal.

You have some specific questions for the doctor at this consultation:
- Doctor, is this another flare of my Crohn's disease? I am sick and tired of it!
- Do I need to be admitted?

Approach and Clinical Reasoning

Ms Sai presents with abdominal pain on a background of Crohn's disease with frequent flares. Consider the complications of Crohn's disease (Table B4.34), as well as the causes of acute abdominal pain in general. You must demonstrate a safe clinical approach by considering all emergent causes of abdominal pain, including gynaecological (particularly ectopic pregnancy) and urologic causes in addition to gastrointestinal and hepatobiliary causes of pain. You may only pick up her urinary symptoms if you consider urological causes of abdominal pain.

Table B4.34. Complications of Crohn's disease and ulcerative colitis (UC) presenting with abdominal pain.

Crohn's/UC	Cause	Important features
Both	Disease flare	Colicky pain with bloody diarrhoea ± systemic toxicity (fever, tachycardia) in severe flares; typically gradual onset over days to weeks
UC	Toxic megacolon	Severe toxic symptoms and >10 stools a day in UC
UC > Crohn's	Intestinal perforation	Acute, constant, severe pain, exacerbated by movement; guarded, rigid abdomen; unwell patient
		May be preceded by disease flare/toxic megacolon
Crohn's	Enterovesical fistula	Cystitis (dysuria, frequency) or pyelonephritis (fever, flank pain), may be recurrent; pneumaturia, fecaluria
Crohn's	Intestinal obstruction	Abdominal pain, distension, nausea/vomiting, and inability to pass stool or flatus. The full quartet of symptoms may not be present in partial or early obstruction. Vomiting is early and constipation late in a proximal obstruction, while constipation is early and vomiting late in a distal obstruction.
Crohn's	Abscess	Localised, constant pain, fever, may have palpable mass; can be difficult to discern clinically without imaging
Both	Infective colitis, (e.g., C. difficile)	Diarrhoea
		Systemic malaise in severe disease
Both	*Always consider the general causes of abdominal pain including urological and gynaecological causes (e.g., ectopic pregnancy).*	

This case illustrates these complications of inflammatory bowel disease. Ms Sai's presentation differs from a typical Crohn's flare in several aspects. She does not have diarrhoea. Her pain is not colicky, but instead constant and worse on movement — suggesting peritonitis, which may be localised (from an abscess) or generalised (from perforation); you need to check for guarding and rebound on examination. She also gives a history of frequent episodes of cystitis, pneumaturia, and fecaluria (recognise that this is the 'brown solid material' she describes), which is worrisome for an enterovesical fistula. This has probably caused not just cystitis but frank urosepsis and she is unwell.

As you examine Ms Sai, take particular care to uphold patient welfare given that she has abdominal pain.

- Focus on the abdomen, looking for scars, tenderness, signs of peritonitis (guarding, rigidity), and masses.
- Examine for systemic features of toxicity and offer a rectal examination.
- If time permits, look briefly for extra-intestinal manifestations of Crohn's disease – arthritis, uveitis, cutaneous (erythema nodosum, pyoderma gangrenosum), jaundice (sclerosing cholangitis).

There will obviously not be a patient with frank peritonitis in the PACES exam (and therefore these signs will be absent or simulated). However, there is sufficient clinical suspicion in this encounter to raise concern of peritonitis for which you must admit her.

Question and Answer

Suggested answer to patient's concerns:

Ms Sai, I am sorry to hear how frustrating this Crohn's disease has been. I can't imagine what you have been through. You are right that this is probably related to your Crohn's disease, but I am also concerned that it may be more than a typical flare. It does not sound right that you have such severe pain and are passing gas and brown matter in your urine. There may be a collection of pus in your abdomen, or an abnormal connection between your intestines and your bladder.

I will need to admit you. We will have to do some blood tests, X-ray, and scans of your tummy, after which I will start you on intravenous antibiotics. I will call in the surgeon and your gastroenterologist, and depending on what the scans find, you might also need surgery. We will do our best to get you better.

Suggested presentation to the examiner:

This is a young lady with Crohn's disease who presents with fever, tachycardia, severe abdominal pain, fecaluria, and recurrent cystitis. I am concerned about urosepsis from an enterovesical fistula, intra-abdominal abscesses, or the possibility of frank perforation, although I do note that the abdomen is soft and not guarded.

I will admit her. Investigations include:

- Bloods: blood cultures, a full blood count for anaemia and leucocytosis, inflammatory markers, and renal and liver biochemistries to guide treatment.
- Urine microscopy and cultures.
- Urine pregnancy test.
- Imaging: immediately an erect chest X-ray looking for air under the diaphragm, and subsequently a CT scan of the abdomen looking for enterovesical fistula and focal abscesses.

Management must involve the surgeons, gastroenterologist, and allied healthcare professionals.

- I will keep her nil by mouth and begin broad-spectrum intravenous antibiotics and IV fluids.
- In view of acute sepsis, I will temporarily withhold her immunosuppression until further discussion with her gastroenterologist (note: if she were on steroids, this should not be withheld; instead, stress doses should be given).
- I will arrange for surgical consult. She may require surgical drainage of an abscess or repair of an enterovesical fistula.
- She will need to continue long-term immunosuppression after this acute episode.

Consultation Case 40

Ms Jackson (Abnormal Movement)

Use this case as practice! The pull-out booklet contains the candidate's information.

Information for the Candidate

Patient Details: Ms Jackson, 23 years old

Your Role: Emergency Department SHO

Referral Letter:
> Dear Colleague,
>
> Thank you for seeing this young lady with abnormal movements who is understandably very anxious.
>
> Thank you.
>
> Dr Wei Ting, GP

Vital Signs: BP 103/60 mmHg, HR 71/min, RR 11/min, SpO2 98% RA, T 37.0°C

Patient's Brief

Synopsis: *A young lady presents with an acute onset of unilateral choreoathetosis, which may be precipitated by a hyperglycaemic crisis or estrogen exposure from oral contraceptives.*

Open the consult with: I can't control my hands, they just keep moving and I don't know why. *Do not volunteer any other information unless asked.*

History of current problem:

- Your left arm has been making odd involuntary 'dancing' movements. You are bothered but is unable to voluntarily stop them
- This started approximately 3 days ago and seems to have been getting worse.
- You have never had similar encounters.
- You also noticed that you have been feeling very thirsty and passing large amounts of urine over the last 3 days.
- No neck lump, tremor, weight loss, heat intolerance, or change in appearance.
- No weakness, numbness, slurred speech, blurred vision, or facial droop.
- No joint pain, rash, hair loss, mouth ulcers, or blood or bubbles in your urine.

- No headache.
- No nausea, vomiting, jaundice, change in urine colour, or abdominal pain.

Past medical and surgical history:
- Nil

Medication list:
- Oral contraceptive pill, started 1 week ago

Family history:
- Your grandmother had Parkinson's disease, and you recall that she was disabled for a number of years before she passed on. There is no family history of Huntington's disease or stroke.
- Type 1 diabetes runs in your family and a number of your cousins have it.

Relevant personal, social, occupational, and travel history:
- You are working as an accounts assistant.
- You are unmarried but have a steady boyfriend.
- Your last menstrual period is 5 days ago.
- You neither drink nor smoke.

Relevant physical examination findings:

This encounter will use a real patient.
- Spontaneous quasi-purposeful, writhing movements predominantly affecting the left upper limb.
- Milkmaid's grip (when asked to grip the examiner's fingers in her hand, patient squeezes and releases).
- Darting tongue (when asked to stick out tongue and hold it there, the tongue alternately protrudes and withdraws).
- Dish-spooning of hands (motor impersistence — when asked to hold both forearms extended, the forearm pronates).
- No joint deformities, synovitis, or rash.
- No jaundice.
- No focal weakness or numbness.
- No rigidity or bradykinesia.
- No goitre.

Note: If acting out this scenario for a colleague, consider looking up videos of hemichorea (e.g., https://www.youtube.com/watch?v=GzRV5HCyVl4. Video by N Engl J Med).

You have some specific questions for the doctor at this consultation:
- Is this Parkinson's disease? My grandmother had Parkinson's disease and it was especially awful towards the end.

Approach and Clinical Reasoning

Begin by characterising the 'abnormal movement'. The movement disorders in the PACES examination are often easy to spot and discern (spot diagnosis).

- Tremor – rhythmic oscillations caused by alternating contractions of agonist and antagonist muscles:
  - Rest tremor – for example in patients with Parkinsonism.
  - Postural tremor, occurring with hands outstretched – essential tremor, hyperthyroidism.
  - Intention tremor – cerebellar dysfunction.
- Myoclonus: sudden, brief, intermittent jerks.
- Chorea: unpredictable, irregular, and dance-like movement of the limb or limbs.
- Athetosis: continuous, slow, flowing, writhing, involuntary movement, often affecting the hands and feet.
- Hemiballismus: violent, involuntary flinging of one limb.
- Tics: paroxysmal, stereotypic movements and vocal expressions, may be suppressible (sensory tricks).
- Dystonia: abnormal, involuntarily sustained muscular contraction resulting in abnormal posturing affecting various body parts (e.g., torticollis, limb dystonia, facial dystonia); may be suppressible using sensory tricks (geste antagoniste).
- Myotonia: inability to relax after sustained and strong voluntary muscular contraction.

The classic description of chorea is given in the case vignette above. You must consider the causes of chorea (Table B4.35) — helpful distinguishing features include: (a) time-course of onset, (b) unilateral vs. generalised chorea, (c) family history, (d) drug exposures, and (e) associated symptoms (e.g., of thyroid disease, autoimmune disease, osmotic symptoms in diabetes).

Ms Jackson has unilateral chorea of acute onset, which makes hereditary causes less likely as their onset is usually insidious and progressive. Additionally, she complains of polydipsia and polyuria with a significant family history of type 1 diabetes, suggestive of a possible hyperglycaemic state. She also has a significant medication history of new oral contraceptive pill use, which could have precipitated chorea (although that would classically be generalised rather than unilateral).

Question and Answer

Suggested answer to the patient's concerns:

Ms Jackson, I'm sorry to hear about your grandmother. What she went through sounds awful. However, I do not think that you have Parkinson's disease. Your involuntary movement is different from those seen in patients with Parkinson's disease. These movements you have now, which in medical terms we call chorea, may be due to high blood sugar, especially when you have frequent thirst and urination. They may also be due to the oral contraceptive pills you've been taking recently. Let me first check your blood sugar and hold off your oral contraceptive pills, and we can discuss our next course of action.

Table B4.35. Common causes of chorea.

Distribution	Differential	Key examples
Unilateral	Focal basal ganglia structural abnormality or lesion	Infarct
		Haemorrhage
		Space occupying lesion/tumour
	Hyperglycaemia	Diabetic ketoacidosis/hyperglycaemic hyperosmolar state^
Generalised*	Hereditary#	Huntington's disease
		Wilson's disease
	Endocrine	Hyperglycaemia
		Hyperthyroidism
	Oestrogen-related	Pregnancy, contraceptive pill
	Autoimmune	Autoimmune/paraneoplastic encephalitis (e.g., anti-NMDA, anti-Hu, anti-Yo)
		Systemic lupus erythematosus
		Coeliac disease
	Infectious and post-infectious	Post-streptoccal (Sydenham chorea, usually in childhood)
		Prion disease (Creutzfeldt-Jakob disease)
		HIV infection
	Drugs	Dopaminergic drugs (e.g., antipsychotics and metoclopramide); may be tardive dyskinesia (oro-bucco-lingual movements) which may not resolve on cessation of drug
		Anti-epileptic medications
		Stimulants (e.g., amphetamines)
		Thyroxine

^Diabetic crises such as diabetic ketoacidosis and hyperosmolar hyperglycaemic state more commonly causes hemichorea than generalised chorea. This laterality is not completely understood but thought to be due to selective perturbations over the basal ganglia contralateral to the side of hemichorea.

*A helpful mnemonic for the generalised causes of chorea is C for CHOREA – Copper (Wilson's), Chemicals (Drugs), Huntington's, Oestrogen, Rheumatic fever, Endocrine, and Autoimmune.

#There are many more hereditary causes of chorea which will not be discussed here.

Tip: Gathering more information to address the patient's concerns

> If you did not examine for extrapyramidal signs during the physical examination, when asked specifically "is this Parkinson's disease", it may be wise to spend a few seconds to examine specifically for cogwheel rigidity and bradykinesia, which (a) demonstrates your attention to the patient's concern and (b) may have been a marking point. It is perfectly acceptable to go back and forth between history, examination, and addressing the patient's concerns.

Suggested presentation to the examiner:

Ms Jackson presents acutely with unilateral choreoathetosis as evidenced by spontaneous quasi-purposeful, writhing movements of both upper limbs, as well as motor impersistence as demonstrated by the dish-spooning of hands and a milkmaid's grip. This may be precipitated by hyperglycaemia given the concomitant history of polyuria and polydipsia, or by her recent initiation of oral contraceptives.

I will first like to check her capillary glucose. I am concerned about the possibility of diabetic ketoacidosis given significant osmotic symptoms. If so, I will admit her for management of diabetic ketoacidosis. Additionally, I will stop her oral contraceptive pills and advise on non-hormonal contraceptives such as barrier contraception.

I will concomitantly investigate for other causes of chorea, including:

- MRI brain for focal basal ganglia lesions[25].
- Thyroid function tests.
- Work-up for autoimmune and paraneoplastic causes.

---

[25] Additional information not expected in PACES: In chorea due to hyperglycaemia, MRI typically demonstrates T1 hyperintense and T2 hypointense signal changes affecting the putamen and/or caudate. CT brain findings are usually subtle.

Consultation Case 41

Ms Mabok (Giddiness)

Use this case as practice! The pull-out booklet contains the candidate's information.

Information for the Candidate

Patient Details: Ms. Mabok, 34 years old

Your Role: Emergency Department SHO

Referral Letter:
> Dear Colleague,
>
> Thank you for seeing Ms Mabok. She complains of a one-day history of giddiness.
>
> Warm regards,
>
> Dr Hallpike, GP

Vital Signs: BP 127/80 mmHg, HR 80/min, RR 14/min, SpO2 98% RA, T 37.0°C

Patient's Brief

Synopsis: *This young lady with a history of recurrent miscarriages presents with central vertigo, slurred speech, and neck pain. This is concerning for transient ischaemic attack with underlying antiphospholipid syndrome, as well as vertebral artery dissection.*

Open the consult with:

- I felt giddy all of a sudden today. The GP insisted that I come to the emergency department, but I feel okay now and I want to go home.
- *Apart from the opening lines above, volunteer the history of neck pain, which you are bothered by.*

History of current problem:

- This occurred today at approximately 8am (more than 4.5 hours ago). You were standing at the bus stop waiting for the bus when this dizziness started suddenly. It seemed as though everything was spinning around you and you felt nauseated. It lasted for approximately 30 minutes before resolving.
- The giddiness was not worsened with changes to your posture and head position.
- During the episode, you found it difficult to speak clearly or walk straight. You can speak and walk normally now.

Consultation Case 41

- Additionally, when the dizziness started, you felt a sharp, tearing pain at the right side of your neck. This was quite painful (pain score 7/10) when it started but improved slightly afterwards. It is still bothering you now (pain score 4/10).
- During this episode, you did not experience weakness or numbness, visual disturbances, headaches, hearing difficulties, tinnitus, chest discomfort, breathlessness, palpitations, or diaphoresis.
- This is your first time experiencing giddiness of this character.
- You have no other significant complaints.

Past medical and surgical history:

- Nil

Medication list:

- Nil
- Supplements and herbal remedies: nil
- Drug allergy: nil

Family history:

- Your mum had recurrent episodes of giddiness. She was told that this was due to 'stones in her ears'.
- Your dad is on long-term warfarin for repeated 'blood clots in the leg'.
- No other family history of note.

Relevant personal, social, occupational, and travel history:

This station may be run with a patient surrogate or with a real (but treated) patient.

- You are working as an office clerk.
- You are married but without children. You have had 4 miscarriages in the past 2 years.
- You have not travelled out of the country before.
- You do not smoke or drink.
- You do not use intravenous drugs.

Relevant physical examination findings:

- Cranial nerve examination yielded no abnormal findings:
    - Pupils equal and reactive to light.
    - Ocular movements normal (both pursuits and saccades).
    - Nystagmus absent.
- No sensorimotor and cerebellar deficits over the bilateral upper and lower limbs.
- Gait normal.
- Pulse regular in rate, rhythm, and volume.
- No carotid bruit.
- Praecordial auscultation: first and second heart sounds; no murmur.

- No palpable lymphadenopathy.
- No pedal oedema.
- No other remarkable examination findings.

You have some specific questions for the doctor at this consultation:
- Is this similar to the ear problem my mum had?

Approach and Clinical Reasoning

Ms Mabok presents with a transient episode of giddiness. Characterise this episode further — in particular, explore whether it is vertiginous or non-vertiginous, its time course, provoking factors, and associated symptoms (Table B4.36).

Table B4.36. Important causes of episodic giddiness in PACES.

Mechanism	Key features	Important aetiologies
Central vertigo	Brainstem signs and symptoms: facial droop, dysarthria, dysphagia, diplopia, cerebellar dysfunction, Horner's syndrome Lasts minutes-hours (not seconds) Does not fully resolve when immobile	Brainstem stroke/TIA Vestibular migraine Steal syndrome (giddiness provoked by upper limb use, see Consultation Case 44)
Peripheral vertigo	Worsened by changes in head position May have hearing loss or tinnitus; no other neurologic deficits Nausea and vomiting may be severe Variable duration of vertigo	BPPV (classically lasts seconds) Vestibular neuritis (likely to still be present, albeit less severe when the head is kept still) Ototoxic drugs Meniere's disease
Postural giddiness	Lightheadedness provoked by postural change Diaphoresis Darkening of vision Low/borderline low blood pressure Lethargy, features of underlying disease	Adrenal insufficiency Autonomic failure (e.g., diabetes, multiple system atrophy) Drugs (e.g., diuretics, anti-cholinergics, levodopa) Reduced cerebral blood flow (e.g., severe basilar artery or bilateral carotid artery stenosis)
Cardiovascular disease (Case 28)	Sudden-onset especially during exertion or at rest Palpations, cardiac murmur May have positive family history	Outflow obstruction (e.g., critical aortic stenosis, HOCM) Arrhythmias Channelopathy (e.g., long QT)
Anaemia	Exertional dyspnoea, lethargy Features of cause of anaemia	Blood loss Haemolysis Decreased production

BPPV: benign paroxysmal positional vertigo; HOCM: hypertrophic cardiomyopathy

Ms Mabok has transient vertigo which has associated cerebellar features. This is worrisome for central vertigo — a posterior circulation transient ischaemic attack (TIA).

Pitfall: Keep asking 'why'

> Don't stop at the diagnosis of a TIA — explore why this patient had a TIA. PACES favourites that can present with a TIA stem include Graves' disease (atrial fibrillation), atrial septal defect (paradoxical embolism), and more. Be curious!

TIA is a PACES favourite (often as a backup station involving a surrogate patient) and you must look for secondary causes (Table B4.37). The patient's neck pain is an important red flag.

Table B4.37. Secondary causes of young stroke/TIA.

Mechanism	Differential	Important features
Cardio-embolic	Atrial fibrillation (isolated or secondary; e.g., hyperthyroidism)	Irregular pulse
	Paradoxical embolism through an atrial septal defect or patent foramen ovale	Abnormal cardiac exam (e.g., murmur, split second sound, displaced apex)
	Endocarditis: infective and non-infective	Fever, intravenous drug use in infective endocarditis
	Left ventricular thrombus	Features of thyrotoxicosis
	Valvular disease (e.g., rheumatic heart disease, prosthetic heart valves)	
Hyper-coagulable state	Hereditary prothrombotic disorder	Family history
	Hyperviscosity (e.g., polycythaemia, sickle cell anaemia)	Venous thromboembolism, recurrent miscarriages
	Antiphospholipid syndrome, primary or secondary to rheumatologic disease	Features of systemic illness (e.g., aquagenic puritus, joint pain, rashes)
Small vessel disease	Young hypertension – look for underlying cause	Blood pressure
	Hyperlipidaemia (isolated, familial, or secondary; e.g., nephrotic syndrome)	Family history
	Diabetes mellitus	Features of underlying illness (e.g., glomerulonephritis, acromegaly, Cushing's syndrome)
	Cerebral vasculitis or arteriopathy	
	Substance use (e.g., cocaine)	
Large vessel disease	Large vessel atherosclerosis	Neck pain (dissection)
	Carotid/vertebral artery dissection	Carotid bruit, poorly felt peripheral pulses
	Vasculitis (e.g., Takayasu arteritis)	
Haemorrhagic*	Bleeding diathesis	Systemic bleeding
		Drug history

*Will not present with TIA.

Important underlying causes of young TIA that Ms Mabok's history raises include:
- Vertebral artery dissection, given history of neck pain.
- Antiphospholipid syndrome, in view of the history of recurrent pregnancy loss and family history of recurrent deep venous thrombosis.

Examination may include:
- Features of endocrinopathies – in particular, inspect for a spot diagnosis (e.g., Graves' disease).
- Neurological examination to assess for persistent neurologic deficits (obviously, untreated acute stroke will not feature in PACES).
- Palpate the pulse for atrial fibrillation.
- Cardiac examination.
- Auscultation for a carotid bruit.

Question and Answer

Suggested answer to the patient's concerns:

Ms Mabok, your giddiness appears to be quite different from what your mum had. You had not only giddiness, but also difficulty speaking and balancing. Although these are resolved at present, I am worried that you may have had a 'warning stroke', also known as a transient ischaemic attack. I am concerned about a tear in the blood vessel supplying blood to your brain, or whether you have unusually thick blood that clots easily. This is potentially dangerous as you are at risk of having a stroke. You will need to be admitted for further tests, such as scans of your brain and heart, and blood tests to investigate the cause of your giddiness and fever. We will also need to start you on urgent treatment to reduce the risk of you having another stroke.

Suggested presentation to the examiner:

Ms Mabok presents with an episode of central vertigo, slurred speech, and incoordination. This is associated with neck pain, recurrent miscarriages, and a family history of recurrent deep vein thrombosis. I am worried about a transient ischaemic attack secondary to either vertebral artery dissection or the prothrombotic complications of antiphospholipid syndrome. Examination is otherwise unremarkable.

I will admit Ms Mabok to the acute stroke unit. Investigations will include:
- An urgent CT brain and CT angiogram looking for features of vertebral artery dissection, cerebral infarction, or haemorrhage.
- This should be followed by MRI brain with MR angiography.
- I will investigate for antiphospholipid syndrome with a full blood count, clotting times, and lupus anticoagulant titres. I will also look for underlying rheumatologic illness by sending autoantibodies such as antinuclear and anti-double-stranded DNA antibodies.

- Bloods for fasting glucose, lipids, and thyroid panel.
- Young stroke work-up.
  - Thyroid panel.
  - Antinuclear antibody, anti-double-stranded DNA antibody, lupus anticoagulant titres (as above).
  - Anti-cardiolipin IgM and IgG titres.
  - Antithrombin III, protein C and S levels, homocysteine.
  - Factor V Leiden (omit if the patient is ethnically Chinese).
  - Holter study.
  - Transthoracic echocardiogram, with agitated saline (bubble study).
  - *Note that an ultrasound doppler of the carotid artery is less relevant in a posterior fossa stroke/TIA, as in this scenario.*

Treatment will depend on the above investigations and will require guidance of a specialist neurology service. Options include:

- For treatment of vertebral artery dissection, anticoagulation or antiplatelet therapy.
- For antiphospholipid syndrome (fulfilling Sapporo criteria), warfarin anticoagulation.
- General measures: statin, control of diabetes, blood pressure.

Consultation Case 42

Ms Campbell (Giddiness)

Use this case as practice! The pull-out booklet contains the candidate's information.

Information for the Candidate

Patient Details: Ms Campbell, 41 years old

Your Role: Rheumatology Outpatients SHO

Scenario: Ms Campbell, who is on follow up for systemic sclerosis, brought forward her scheduled appointment because of giddiness and diarrhoea.

Vital Signs: BP 180/108 mmHg, HR 90/min, RR 16/min, SpO2 95% RA, T 36.0°C

Investigations: Haemoglobin 9.8 mg/dL, WBC 4.2×10^9/L, Platelets 90×10^9/L
Creatinine 180 umol/L (baseline 70 umol/L)
Urine dipstick – blood 1+, protein, and nitrites negative

Patient's Brief

Synopsis: *This patient with known systemic sclerosis presents in scleroderma renal crisis following a diarrhoeal illness.*

Open the consult with: I had diarrhoea after eating some cheap sashimi and now feel awfully giddy. *Volunteer the past medical history of systemic sclerosis.*

History of current problem:

- You started having watery diarrhoea, vomiting, and lethargy a week ago after having cut-price sashimi from a less-than-reputable food outlet. The diarrhoea and vomiting has since resolved, although you still feel lethargic and have not been eating well. You have had no diarrhoea.

- What's really bothering you now is the giddiness, which started 3 days ago and has gotten worse since. It is more a sensation of lightheadedness than one of the room spinning. You feel giddy throughout the day; it does not occur in discrete episodes. This is worst when you stand up suddenly from a seated position or when you get out of bed in the morning.

- You are still able to walk and you do not fall to one side. You have no weakness or numbness, blurring of vision, double vision, slurring of speech, facial droop, difficulty hearing, or ringing in your ears.

- You have never lost consciousness, fallen, or injured yourself.

Consultation Case 42

- You have no headache, chest pain, breathlessness, palpitations, leg swelling, or blood or bubbles in your urine.
- You notice that the amount of urine you are passing has decreased in the past week.
- You have not noticed any abnormal bleeding or easy bruising.

Past medical and surgical history:
- Systemic sclerosis. You first presented 3 years ago with pain and colour changes in your hands when exposed to the cold. You have also had ulcers of your fingers, tightening of the skin, difficulty swallowing, and some lung involvement. Your disease is stable and under control. You are compliant to medication and follow up.
- Your blood pressure has always been normal and you have never had kidney problems from systemic sclerosis.

Medication list:
- Calcium with vitamin D
- Omeprazole 20 mg BD
- Mycophenolate mofetil 1 g BD
- Nifedipine 30 mg OM
- Supplements and herbal remedies: for the past 6 months, you had been taking a health supplement purchased online. The GP said that this "probably contained steroids" and advised you to stop, which you did 2–3 weeks ago.
- You have also been having mefenamic acid (Ponstan), purchased over the counter, for period cramps. You last took this a week ago (a day before the diarrhoea occurred).
- Drug allergy: nil

Family history:
- Nil

Relevant personal, social, occupational, and travel history:
- You work as a receptionist in a law firm.
- You are not married and do not have children.
- You do not smoke or drink.
- No significant travel history.

Relevant physical examination findings:
- Postural BP (if requested): 180/108 > 140/79.
- Cranial nerves normal, pupils equal and reactive, no pronator drift, no cerebellar signs.
- Sclerodactyly (Photos 29 and 30), extending to above the elbows.
- Amputation of right index finger at the metacarpophalangeal joint.

- Digital pulp atrophy and pseudoclubbing (Photo 29).
- Telangiectasia on hands (Photo 30), neck, and chest.
- Microstomia.
- Fine end-inspiratory crepitations in both lung bases.
- Hydration status fair.
- No stigmata of Cushing's syndrome.
- Rectal examination, if offered: normal.
- Fundoscopy: not to proceed.

Photos to be shown to candidate upon request (use colour plates for full-colour photos).

Photo 29

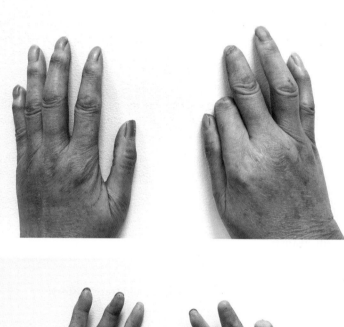

Photo 30

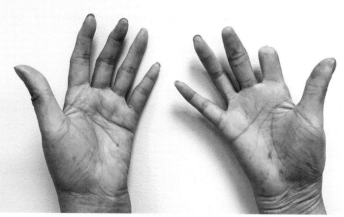

Clinical photos generously provided by Dr Jon Yoong Kah Choun, Singapore General Hospital

Consultation Case 42

You have some specific questions for the doctor at this consultation:

- I regret eating the sashimi. Please give me some strong medicine and I will go home to rest.

Approach and Clinical Reasoning

This is a challenging case, but the battle is won outside the room if one reads the candidate's information carefully — it gives away the diagnosis of scleroderma renal crisis. Recognise the presentation of new-onset renal impairment and thrombocytopenia (urine sediment may be bland or show new haematuria or proteinuria). There may also be microangiopathic haemolytic anaemia (anaemia, thrombocytopenia), as in this case, heart failure and pulmonary oedema, as well as seizures from hypertensive encephalopathy. Further history will reveal that Ms Campbell has two risk factors for scleroderma renal crisis: steroid use and diffuse skin involvement.

Note that some exam centres may NOT provide the history of scleroderma in the candidate's information. You will need to spot the diagnosis as you enter the room and confirm it by asking the patient. Rarely, some exam centres will coach the patient *not* to reveal the history of scleroderma even when asked, requiring that you come to the diagnosis by recognising its physical features (although there may be otherwise unexplained immunosuppressants in the medication list).

Even if you recognise the likely diagnosis, you must have a reasonable approach to Ms Campbell's presentation and consider differentials. Characterise her giddiness further but do not simply use the standard approach to giddiness — you must take into account Ms Campbell's presenting features *in toto*. She has new-onset renal impairment, hypertensive urgency, postural giddiness, anaemia, and thrombocytopenia on a background of systemic sclerosis. There is a preceding episode of gastroenteritis with an identifiable trigger — eliciting the time course of events and that diarrhoea has since resolved is helpful.

This is not a straightforward case. Some candidates will find enumerating a problem list helpful to reduce cognitive load and connect the various abnormalities. Whichever way this is done, important differentials include:

- Scleroderma renal crisis, which is the best unifying diagnosis.
- Haemolytic uraemic syndrome from diarrhoeal illness, presenting with acute kidney injury and microangiopathic haemolytic anaemia.
- Adrenal insufficiency from sudden cessation of long-term steroids.
- Other differentials to acute kidney injury (e.g., hypovolemia from diarrhoea, NSAID use).
- Other differentials to anaemia (e.g., gastrointestinal bleeding from NSAID use).

Physical examination should focus on:

- Demonstrating the classical features of systemic sclerosis (e.g., sclerodactyly, acro-osteolysis, digital ulcers and pitting, calcinosis, salt and pepper rash, microstomia and telangiectasia). While this does not contribute towards evaluating the

cause of the patient's current complaint, most examiners expect these signs to be presented.
- Screening for focal neurology given the complaint of giddiness (at the very least, checking pupils, pronator drift, coordination, facial droop, and speech).
- Looking for other features of renal impairment (e.g., signs of fluid overload).
- Looking for differentials (e.g., checking for pallor, offering to do rectal examination for PR bleed, checking for palpable bladder (post-renal obstruction)).

Recognise that scleroderma renal crisis is an emergency; Ms Campbell requires admission and urgent intervention with angiotensin-converting enzyme inhibitors to prevent further deterioration.

Question and Answer

Suggested answer to the patient's concerns:

Ms Campbell, I am very sorry but you seem quite unwell and I can't let you go home now. I must admit you for treatment. Your blood pressure is very high, your kidney function has taken a hit, and your cell counts are low. I don't think this is just because of diarrhoea from the sashimi. I am concerned about a complication of systemic sclerosis which is affecting your kidneys. If left untreated, this can lead to long-term kidney failure and even death. I will get the rheumatology team and the renal team on board. We will need to do some tests and start treatment urgently.

Suggested presentation to the examiner:

Ms Campbell presents with hypertensive urgency, acute kidney injury, anaemia, and thrombocytopenia on a background of systemic sclerosis. Physical examination is significant for features of systemic sclerosis such as sclerodactyly extending above the elbows, right index finger amputation, digital pulp atrophy and pseudo-clubbing, telangiectasia, and fine inspiratory lung crepitations. There is also pallor. There is no focal neurology and no pedal oedema. I will complete my examination by doing a rectal exam for PR bleed and fundoscopy for retinal changes of hypertensive encephalopathy.

My principal diagnosis is scleroderma renal crisis, especially given the risk factors of diffuse skin disease and steroid use. Other considerations include haemolytic uraemic syndrome, gastroenteritis causing acute kidney injury, and postural giddiness from dehydration, as well as adrenal insufficiency from cessation of steroid use.

She is unwell and requires admission. Further work-up includes:
- The diagnosis of scleroderma renal crisis is clinical, but I will look for supportive features such evidence of microangiopathic haemolytic anaemia (schistocytes, fragments).
- Looking for complications including checking electrolytes for hyperkalaemia, acidosis, and chest X-ray for pulmonary oedema.

- 8am serum cortisol followed by a short synacthen test looking for adrenal insufficiency.
- Looking for differentials – checking inflammatory markers and blood culture, doing ultrasound kidneys to exclude post-renal obstruction, etc.

Management must involve a multidisciplinary team including the rheumatologist, nephrologist, and allied healthcare professionals. Principles are:

- Reversal of scleroderma renal crisis with angiotensin-converting enzyme inhibitors, classically captopril. Addition of other antihypertensive agents may be required.
- Avoiding nephrotoxins, hypovolemia, and dehydration.
- Replacement doses of steroids if there is a component of adrenal insufficiency[26].
- Treating complications such as hyperkalaemia, fluid overload.

---

[26] Prescribing corticosteroids in this scenario is not straightforward. On the one hand, corticosteroid use is associated with an increased risk of scleroderma renal crisis. On the other hand, this is an acutely unwell patient in whom adrenal insufficiency has not been excluded (although hypertension makes it less likely). It is reasonable to give steroids until adrenal insufficiency is excluded.

Consultation Case 43

Mrs Drowsy (Confusion)

Use this case as practice! The pull-out booklet contains the candidate's information.

Information for the Candidate

Patient Details: Mrs Drowsy, 64 years old

Your Role: Oncology Unit Walk-In Clinic SHO

Referral Letter:
> Dear Colleague,
>
> Mrs Drowsy is on home hospice support for metastatic ovarian cancer. We have found her to be intermittently confused over the past week. She is struggling to manage at home. Please kindly see her.
>
> Warm regards,
>
> Dr G. Reaper, Eternal Life Home Hospice

Vital Signs: BP 125/82 mmHg, HR 77/min, RR 8/min, SpO2 96% RA, T 36.0°C

Patient's Brief

In this scenario, the history is taken from a surrogate (the patient's daughter) and not the actual patient.

Synopsis: *A patient with metastatic ovarian cancer presents with constipation, myoclonus, and decreased urine output. Key differentials include morphine toxicity, hypercalcaemia of malignancy, and acute kidney injury.*

Open the consult with: *Mum has been drowsy and vomiting and I don't know what to do.* Introduce yourself as Mrs Drowsy's daughter and volunteer the history of metastatic ovarian cancer.

History of current problem:
- Mum was relatively well and able to care for herself and move around the house until a week ago.
- In the past week, however, she has been lethargic and intermittently 'sleepy'.
- She has also been feeling nauseous and has vomited several times. The contents of the vomitus are undigested food; there is no blood, dark-coloured solids, or green liquid.

Consultation Case 43

- She has been feeling constipated. She usually passes one stool a day, but the last time she passed stool was 4 days ago. She is still able to pass gas.
- Her tummy has been distended for several months. The doctors told you that this was because of cancer. There is no noticeable increase in distension.
- She does have abdominal pain but this is longstanding, baseline cancer pain.
- She seems to have been passing less urine in the past week. There is no blood or bubbles in the urine.
- She has also complained of giddiness when getting up from the bed or a chair.
- Mum has had odd jerking movements of the right hand in the past 2–3 days.
- She has no fever, cough, diarrhoea, change in urine colour, pain on passing urine, or increase in urinary frequency.
- She has no jaundice, breathlessness, weakness or numbness, headache, slurred speech, blurring of vision, seizures, vaginal bleeding, or abnormal bruising.

Past medical and surgical history:

- Metastatic ovarian cancer. Mum first presented with abdominal bloating and significant weight loss 3 years ago. She underwent surgery to remove the uterus and ovaries, as well as many rounds of chemotherapy.
- Unfortunately, the cancer recurred six months ago, presenting with abdominal distension. The cancer had also spread to liver and bones. You are unsure about whether there is any spread to the brain.
- It is understood that mum's cancer cannot be cured. She last received chemotherapy 3 months ago and there was no response. She chose to stop all treatment and has been on palliative care.
- She has made an advanced care plan – her preferred place of death is at home. She is amenable to hospital admission if needed, but will not want cardiopulmonary resuscitation or admission to the intensive care unit.

Medication list:

- PO morphine sustained release 80 mg twice a day. This was recently increased a week ago from 40 mg twice a day due to inadequate pain control. She does not use any breakthrough doses.
- Naproxen 550 mg twice a day, started 3 weeks ago.
- Supplements and herbal remedies: nil
- Drug allergy: nil

Family history:

- Mum's sister had breast cancer in her 50s, her mother (your grandmother) had ovarian cancer at age 40, and an aunt had breast cancer in her 30s.

Relevant personal, social, occupational, and travel history:

- You stay with mum and dad. You have another sister.

- No relevant travel history.
- No smoking or drinking.

Relevant physical examination findings:

The actual patient — not the surrogate — is examined.

- General condition non-toxic.
- Hydration status – mucous membranes dry, skin turgor reduced; no oedema.
- Abdomen soft, distended, with positive shifting dullness; non-tender without guarding or rebound.
- Neurology normal.

You have some specific questions for the doctor at this consultation:

- Is this the end? Is mum going to die?

Approach and Clinical Reasoning

Tip: Surrogate patients in PACES

> This scenario introduces the use of a surrogate patient for history taking, although physical examination is performed on the actual patient. MRCP permits such an arrangement should the actual patient not speak English or is otherwise unable to give a history. The surrogate may be a relative/caregiver or a professional actor appointed by the examination centre. It may be a surprise and disorientating to some candidates, so do be mentally prepared!

Mrs Drowsy presents with a 1-week history of altered mental state on a background of metastatic ovarian cancer. There are many causes of altered mental state, but particular attention must be paid to the causes that an oncology patient would be predisposed to (Table B4.38). There may be more than one contributory cause. A detailed history of her underlying cancer, including sites of disease (local and metastases), previous complications, and treatment history (chemotherapy, radiation therapy, and surgery) is important. You should also go into some detail about her analgesia use, including any recent dose adjustments and breakthrough doses.

In addition to altered mental state, Mrs Drowsy has constipation, nausea/vomiting, borderline low respiratory rate (provided in the stem), myoclonus, and decreased urine output. This is on a background of metastatic ovarian cancer with peritoneal and bone metastases, and recent NSAID use. Important differentials for her presentation include:

- Morphine toxicity which explains her gastrointestinal symptoms, myoclonus, and decreased respiratory rate. This may have been precipitated by a dose increase, as well as decreased clearance from acute kidney injury.

- Hypercalcaemia of malignancy given known bone metastases. This can explain the constipation, vomiting, and confusion.
- Uraemia from acute kidney injury, which may be a result of pre-renal (dehydration from vomiting), renal (NSAID use), and post-renal (obstructive uropathy from peritoneal disease) causes.
- Other differentials include hepatic encephalopathy (given liver metastases), hyponatraemia, and sepsis.

Table B4.38. Causes of altered mental state in an oncology patient.

Category	Cause	Important clinical features
Complications of treatment	Sepsis, including neutropenic sepsis	Fever, localising symptoms Suspect neutropenia if there has been recent chemotherapy (especially 10–14 days after), marrow infiltration, other cytopenias
	Drug toxicity, especially opioids and chemotherapy	Increase in opioid dose or decrease in renal clearance Pin-point pupils, myoclonic jerks, decrease in respiratory rate
Complications of disease	Electrolyte abnormality, especially $\downarrow Na^+$, $\uparrow Ca^{2+}$	Gastrointestinal or renal losses Hypercalcaemia: constipation, vomiting, renal stones, bone metastases
	Dehydration Renal insufficiency/uraemia	Poor oral intake, decreased urine output, nephrotoxic drugs, peritoneal metastases (post-renal obstruction)
	Hepatic encephalopathy	Jaundice, tea-coloured urine, liver metastases
	Hypoxia, hypercapnia	Dyspnoea, lung cancer/metastases, respiratory depressants (e.g., opioids)
Underlying disease	Brain metastases, seizures	Headache, vomiting, known brain cancer/metastases
	Intracranial haemorrhage	Headache, focal neurological deficits, brain metastases, coagulopathy
Others	Depression	Low mood, loss of interest
	General medical causes of altered mental state remain relevant.	

Physical examination should cover:
- Examining for pinpoint pupils (morphine toxicity).
- Checking hydration status (given suspicion of acute kidney injury).
- Examining the abdomen – look for tenderness, masses, or ascites.
- Looking for other differentials, such as checking for jaundice and screening neurology to rule out focal deficits (brain metastasis).

Question and Answer

Suggested answer to the patient's concerns:

You must be very worried about how mum is doing as she has not been well. I don't know at the moment which way this is going to go — whether mum will or will not pull through. It is very possible that these may be her last days, or that there may be something treatable that we can address to get her better. It may be best if we admit her. I will like to do some tests to find out what is happening. If there is something that we can treat without too much difficulty and get her better, we will do so. If this is just the cancer getting worse and we can't undo that process, we will do our very best to keep her comfortable and ensure that she does not suffer.

While this is not explored in this encounter, note the strong family history of breast and ovarian cancers. She is likely to have BRCA mutation or other genetic cancer syndrome.

Suggested presentation to the examiner:

Mrs Drowsy presents with a 1-week history of altered mental state, nausea, vomiting, constipation, myoclonus, and decreased urine output on a background of metastatic ovarian cancer. My key considerations are:

- Morphine toxicity precipitated by a dose increase.
- Hypercalcaemia of malignancy.
- Acute kidney injury due to dehydration, NSAID use, and possibly obstructive uropathy due to peritoneal metastases.
- Other differentials include hepatic encephalopathy, sepsis, and hyponatraemia.

I will admit Mrs Drowsy. My immediate management will include:

- Confirming the diagnosis by checking electrolytes, calcium, and renal function, looking for a cause of kidney injury by doing urine microscopy, and abdominal imaging.
- Ruling out differentials by checking full blood count and infective markers for signs of infection, assessing liver biochemistry. I will also like a CT brain to rule out brain metastases, but this will require contrast and is preferably deferred until her renal function recovers. Ascitic tap to rule out spontaneous bacterial peritonitis can be considered but may not be within the goals of care.
- IV hydration, temporarily holding off of morphine, and stopping NSAIDs.
- If there is hypercalcaemia, she will also need anti-resorptives (bisphosphonate or denosumab) and intranasal calcitonin.

Moving forward:

- Re-staging (including abdominal and brain imaging) is likely of limited benefit in this patient who is on best supportive care.

- Her analgesia should be optimised, for instance by switching morphine to fentanyl to reduce the risk of accumulation in renal impairment, and co-prescribing laxatives with morphine.
- I will also pay attention to whether the patient has adequate psychosocial support, and ensure early involvement of the palliative care team.

Ultimately, management should be guided by consideration of goals of care. If it becomes clear that her prognosis is guarded, focus should shift towards comfort care (symptom relief, minimise investigations) and honoring the patient's advance care plan (terminal discharge to her preferred place of death: home).

Consultation Case 44

Ms Claudia (Leg Pain)

Use this case as practice! The pull-out booklet contains the candidate's information.

Information for the Candidate

Patient Details: Ms Claudia, 35 years old

Your Role: Emergency Department SHO

Referral Letter:
> Dear Colleague,
>
> Ms Claudia migrated from East Asia 2 years ago. She has been on my follow up since then for difficult-to-control hypertension. Today she came to see me with a new complaint of right leg pain. Would you please see her to exclude deep vein thrombosis?
>
> Thank you.
>
> Dr Dorothy Huang, GP

Vital Signs: BP 155/82 mmHg, HR 48/min, RR 10/min, SpO2 99% RA, T 37.0°C

Patient's Brief

Synopsis: *This young lady likely has Takayasu arteritis, presenting with lower limb claudication, resistant hypertension, and steal syndrome.*

Open the consult with: I don't know what's wrong with my right leg. I can't walk for more than a minute without this terrible ache. To get to the bus stop I have to stop to rest multiple times. *Readily volunteer the history of lightheadedness (below) even if not asked.*

History of current problem:
- You feel a cramping pain, worst over the right thigh but felt in the entire leg; you have no back pain or shooting pain radiating down to the foot.
- Leg pain is exacerbated by walking. 2–3 months ago, you could walk 300–400 meters before the pain started, but in the past 2 weeks you have consistently only been able to walk 100 meters before having to rest.
- Leg pain is worst walking uphill and better walking downhill, and relieved by rest.
- There is no rest pain and you are able to stand for prolonged periods of time without any issue.

- Leg pain is not triggered by specific movements of the hip or knee.
- There is no leg swelling, redness, ulcers, numbness, or weakness. You have no fever.
- In the last 6 months, you have been feeling more tired than usual and have lost 6 kg.
- You have also noted mild lightheadedness whenever you do house chores (e.g., sweeping the floor) using your right upper limb. Interestingly, you are able to use your left upper limb for similar tasks without any difficulty. This lightheadedness is not worse when standing up from a seated position or with head movements.
- No difficulty seeing, slurred speech, or facial droop.
- No chest pain, dyspnoea, or post-meal stomach pain.
- No decrease in urine output, bubbles, or blood in the urine.
- No history of immobilisation, long-haul flights, or recent surgery.

Past medical and surgical history:
- Hypertension diagnosed 3 years ago on routine health screening. Your blood pressure has been difficult to control even though you have been 100% compliant to medication and religiously follow a low-salt diet.
- No diabetes or hyperlipidaemia, last screened 1 year ago.
- You are not obese.

Medication list:
- Nifedipine extended-release 60 mg BD that was recently increased from 30 mg BD 1 month ago.
- Hydrochlorothiazide 50 mg OM
- Telmisartan 80 mg OM
- Supplements and herbal remedies: nil
- Drug allergy: nil

Family history:
- Your father had a left below-knee amputation for an infected diabetic foot ulcer.

Relevant personal, social, occupational, and travel history:
- You are a housewife.
- You are married with 2 teenage children.
- You do not smoke or drink.

Relevant physical examination findings:
- Weak right femoral, dorsalis pedis, and posterior tibial pulse with radial-femoral delay.
- Bilateral carotid bruit.
- 4-limb blood pressure: right upper limb 155/82 mmHg; left upper limb 102/64 mmHg, right lower limb 90/50 mmHg, left lower limb 124/52 mmHg.

- Right lower limb – calves supple with no ulcers, pedal oedema, weakness, or numbness.
- Straight leg raise negative.
- No heart murmur.
- No cushingoid features.

You have some specific questions for the doctor at this consultation:

- The GP said that I have a clot in my leg veins that can travel to my lungs and kill me. Is this serious?

Approach and Clinical Reasoning

This is a difficult case which has repeatedly appeared in MRCP PACES (with a variety of presenting complaints including hypertension and giddiness). Always begin with open-ended questions because a complicated patient like Ms Claudia is often primed to quickly volunteer key information. Ms Claudia has a triad of limb claudication, an odd complaint of lightheadedness exacerbated by use of the right upper limb, and resistant hypertension. Your task is to demonstrate a reasonable approach to each complaint and propose a unifying diagnosis.

Begin with the complaint of leg pain. First rule out musculoskeletal joint pain — pain felt in the joints and occurs from the first step. Then differentiate between vascular and neurogenic claudication:

- Claudication distance is fixed and reproducible in vascular claudication, but variable in neurogenic claudication.
- The pain in neurogenic claudication may be described as 'shooting' from the back into the feet, while that in vascular claudication predominantly occurs in the affected limb.
- Vascular claudication is worst walking uphill and relieved by rest; neurogenic claudication is worse walking downhill and relieved by spine flexion.

Ms Claudia has vascular claudication with a decreasing claudication distance. This should start you thinking — peripheral arterial disease typically occurs in older patients with multiple vascular risk factors and is quite unusual in a 35-year-old woman.

Pitfall: 'Surgical' complaints

> Do not forget the approach to 'surgical' complaints — being able to approach a 'surgical' complaint is very much expected. On the other hand, a condition predominantly managed by surgeons is unlikely to be the final diagnosis in MRCP PACES — you must search for the underlying 'medical' condition.

The complaint of lightheadedness exacerbated by the use of the right upper limb is a classic description of the subclavian steal syndrome. This phenomenon is seen in patients with subclavian artery stenosis proximal to the vertebral artery origin, such that blood flows in a retrograde fashion from the brain through the vertebral artery into the limb. Exercise of that upper limb therefore compromises posterior fossa cerebral blood flow, causing brainstem symptoms such as giddiness.

These symptoms should prompt you to examine the vasculature of all 4 limbs, including requesting for a 4-limb blood pressure (demonstrating discordant blood pressure in 4 limbs), palpating all peripheral pulses, looking for radial-radial and radio-femoral delay, and auscultating for carotid bruit. If time permits, examining the back and checking a straight leg raise to exclude neurogenic claudication will also be ideal. You can also consider auscultating the heart for aortic regurgitation in aortitis.

Putting together Ms Claudia's vascular occlusions in two locations, resistant hypertension, constitutional symptoms (tiredness, weight loss), and absent peripheral pulses, the unifying diagnosis is Takayasu arteritis. Her East Asian ancestry is an additional hint. Takayasu arteritis is a large vessel vasculitis that causes inflammatory occlusion of large vessels (e.g., the branches of the aorta and the renal arteries, causing renovascular hypertension). Differentials include atherosclerotic disease, infectious aortitis, and other vasculitic disorders (e.g., giant cell arteritis).

Question and Answer

Suggested answer to the patient's concerns:

Ms Claudia, the past 3 months must have been really scary for you. I do not think that you have a clot in your leg veins. However, I suspect that you have a problem with the arteries in your body — some of these are becoming inflamed and blocked. This is likely to be an autoimmune condition called Takayasu arteritis in which the immune cells in your body cause inflammation of the vessels. I need to do some tests to confirm this diagnosis. I will admit you and expedite the necessary tests so that we can get you treated as soon as possible.

Suggested presentation to the examiner:

Ms Claudia presents with lower limb vascular claudication, right upper limb steal syndrome, resistant hypertension, and constitutional symptoms. Examination is significant for discordant 4-limb blood pressure, weak right femoral pulse with radial-femoral delay, and a carotid bruit. The unifying diagnosis is Takayasu arteritis, although differentials include atherosclerotic disease, infectious aortitis, and other vasculitides.

I will like to admit her for investigations and treatment. Investigations include:

- Confirming the diagnosis by imaging the vascular tree (MR or CT angiography, and Doppler ultrasound of the renal arteries).
- Evaluating differentials by performing MRI of the lumbar spine and checking for other causes of resistant hypertension (e.g., creatinine and electrolytes, urine microscopy for haematuria, further history and examination for Cushing's syndrome).
- Searching for other cardiovascular risk factors, in particular repeating the lipid and diabetes screens.

- It will be reasonable to perform an ultrasound scan of the deep veins on the painful leg to address the patient's concern of deep vein thrombosis.

She should be managed by a multidisciplinary team including a rheumatologist, vascular surgeon, and allied healthcare professionals. Principles of management include:

- Immunosuppression with systemic glucocorticoids and steroid-sparing agents (e.g., methotrexate, azathioprine).
- Vascular intervention if necessary.
- Treatment of hypertension.
- Supportive measures such as patient education, treatment of comorbids, healthy lifestyle habits, and physiotherapy.

Consultation Case 45

Mr Pee (Frequent Urination)

Use this case as practice! The pull-out booklet contains the candidate's information.

Information for the Candidate

Patient Details: Mr P. Pee, 30 years old

Your Role: Internal Medicine SHO

Referral Letter:
> Dear Colleague,
>
> Thank you for seeing Mr P. Pee who complains of frequent urination. He is too young to have a prostate problem.
>
> Thank you.
>
> Dr S. Shee, Urology

Vital Signs: BP 120/70 mmHg, HR 55/min, RR 13/min, SpO2 99% RA, T 37.0°C

Investigations: Urine microscopy – normal
Fasting glucose 5.0 mmol/L
Uroflowmetry – normal

Patient's Brief

Synopsis: *This young gentleman has symptomatic hypercalcaemia presenting as polyuria. With a background of pituitary adenoma and a family history of parathyroid adenoma, the underlying diagnosis is likely multiple endocrine neoplasia type 1.*

Open the consult with: I keep peeing every hour, but the urologist says that everything is OK with my prostate and bladder. *Do not volunteer any other information unless asked.*

History of current problem:

- Your bladder is full each time you go to the toilet and you actually feel an urge to pee.
- You do not have any discomfort when you pass urine, foul smelling urine, urgency, poor stream, hesitancy, double voiding, or incontinence.
- In the past 3 months, you have felt constantly thirsty and drink at least one 500 ml bottle of water each hour. Even if you do not drink water (e.g., if you are outside and don't have water on you), you find yourself passing urine just as frequently.

- You have no blood or bubbles in your urine at present. However, 3 months ago, you had an episode of blood in the urine and severe flank pain. You went to the emergency department and were told that you had a kidney stone. This resolved with intravenous fluids and painkillers. You did not need surgery.
- The GP checked your glucose recently and told you that you do not have diabetes.
- You occasionally feel 'bloated' and constipated for the past 2 months. You think this is because of irregular meal habits. There is no blood in your stool.
- You have no bony aches or previous fractures.
- You do not have any head injury, headache, giddiness, blurring of vision, nausea or vomiting, cold/heat intolerance, weight gain/loss, or decreased libido.

Past medical and surgical history:
- Brain tumour. You were diagnosed with a 'brain tumour' 5 years ago after you kept bumping into things on the sides. You did not need surgery. You understand that the tumour shrank with medicine and you no longer bump into things on the sides. An MRI scan and blood tests 2 months ago was normal, and you have been cleared to drive normally in the last 4 years.
- Kidney stone, as described above.

Medication list:
- Cabergoline 0.5 mg twice weekly. You are compliant to this.
- Supplements and herbal remedies: nil
- Drug allergy: nil

Family history:
- Your older brother had surgery for a nodule in the pancreas. You know that this was not cancer but do not know too much else about his medical condition.
- No family history of kidney problems, brain tumour, or hormone problems.

Relevant personal, social, occupational, and travel history:
- You are a construction site supervisor. This entails working outdoors under the sun for long hours. You ensure that you always have water with you.
- You are single and have no children.
- You do not smoke or drink.
- No relevant travel history.

Relevant physical examination findings:

This encounter may be run with a patient (who will have been treated) or a surrogate.
- Tongue moist, no leg swelling.
- Visual fields normal.
- No goitre.
- Abdomen soft, non-tender.

- No neck mass.

You have some specific questions for the doctor at this consultation:
- Is this because of my brain tumour?
- Is there anything I need to be careful of?

Approach and Clinical Reasoning

This is a complex case but a systemic approach will lead you to the answer. First, clarify what Mr Pee means by 'frequent urination' — distinguish between lower urinary tract symptoms and polyuria. The urologist has helpfully ruled out urological causes. Consider the causes of polyuria (Figure B4.6). Exclude primary polydipsia by taking a psychiatric history and asking if urine volume falls if he does not drink water. Enquire for a drug history (particularly lithium and diuretics) and ask about symptoms of hypercalcaemia (constipation, renal colic) and pituitary adenoma (headache, bitemporal hemianopia).

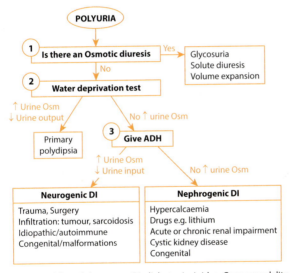

ADH: antidiuretic hormone; DI: diabetes insipidus; Osm: osmolality

Figure B4.6. Approach to polyuria.

Important differentials to consider in this case are:

- Nephrogenic diabetes insipidus from hypercalcaemia – he has vague abdominal symptoms and recent nephrolithiasis, which raises suspicion for hypercalcaemia. Consider the causes of hypercalcaemia.
- Neurogenic diabetes insipidus from pituitary adenoma (presumably a prolactinoma, for which surgery is almost never indicated) – think of tumour recurrence or non-compliance to medication. This is less likely as a recent MRI brain and blood tests (presumably a prolactin level) were normal.

Appreciate that Mr Pee has multiple endocrine derangements — a history of pituitary adenoma, hypercalcaemia (parathyroid adenoma), and a family history of 'pancreatic nodule'. This is suspicious of multiple endocrine neoplasia type 1.

Think this through: The MEN syndromes

> The MEN syndrome is a PACES favourite.
> MEN 1: <u>P</u>ituitary, <u>P</u>arathyroid, <u>P</u>ancreatic (endocrine)   (3P)
> MEN 2A: <u>P</u>haeochromocytoma, <u>P</u>arathyroid, <u>M</u>edullary thyroid   (2P + 1M)
> MEN 2B: <u>P</u>haeochromocytoma, <u>M</u>edullary thyroid, <u>M</u>arfanoid,
>   <u>M</u>ucosal neuroma   (1P + 3M)
> What are the possible ways by which the MEN syndrome can present?

Examination can include:

- Examining hydration status – look for dehydration from polyuria.
- Examining for recurrence of pituitary adenoma – check visual fields for bitemporal hemianopia.
- Feel the abdomen, in view of his non-specific abdominal complaints.
- Check for other features of MEN syndrome – feel the thyroid.

Remember to address the safety issues here:

- Rule out pituitary apoplexy (headache, visual disturbances, vomiting, hypoglycaemia).
- Mr Pee works outdoors under the sun for long hours. This puts him at risk of dehydration and hypernatraemia, especially if he neglects to drink sufficient water.

Question and Answer

Suggested answer to the patient's concerns:

Possibly, a brain tumour you had could be one reason why your body might be producing too much urine. However, when I examined you, there is no indication of it coming back, and reassuringly, your recent MRI brain and blood tests were normal. There are some other reasons why your body might be producing too much urine. I suspect that you may have an overgrowth of another of the hormone glands in your body, which causes high calcium levels and excessive urine production.

Let me do some blood tests for you now. If the salt levels in your body are abnormal, I will need to admit you. If possible, try to avoid working under the hot sun for too long. If you ever develop severe headache, vomiting, and visual problems, come in to emergency immediately.

Suggested presentation to the examiner:

Mr Pee presents with symptoms of hypercalcaemia including polyuria, constipation, and urolithiasis. Given the background of previous pituitary adenoma and family history of a possible pancreatic neuroendocrine tumour, multiple endocrine neoplasia type 1 is a consideration, in which case the hypercalcaemia may be due to primary hyperparathyroidism. A differential is neurogenic diabetes insipidus from recurrence of pituitary adenoma, but this appears less likely. Examination reveals clinical euvolaemia, a soft abdomen, and no bitemporal hemianopia.

Investigations:
- I will check his creatinine and electrolytes including calcium, sodium, serum and urine osmolality.
- Classically the next step is a water deprivation test to distinguish nephrogenic vs. neurogenic diabetes insipidus. However, I would not do this if there is hypercalcaemia.
- Then, I will administer vasopressin (ddAVP).
  - If there is no change in urine osmolality, he has nephrogenic diabetes insipidus.
  - If urine output falls and osmolality rises, he has neurogenic diabetes insipidus and my next step will be an MRI of the pituitary gland.
- As for the hypercalcaemia, I will check his parathyroid hormone levels, which I expect to be high[27], and subsequently look for a parathyroid adenoma by doing a parathyroid uptake (sestamibi) scan.
- I will also check his prolactin levels and the other pituitary hormonal axes.

Management requires a multidisciplinary team including the endocrinologist and neurosurgeon. Principles are:
- If he has significant hypercalcaemia or hypernatraemia, I will admit him for intravenous hydration ± bisphosphonates.
- Parathyroidectomy as primary treatment of parathyroid adenoma.
- Adjuncts include patient education focusing on adequate hydration, genetic testing, and counselling (autosomal dominant inheritance pattern).

---

[27] If parathyroid hormone is low, the next step is to search for a malignancy.

Consultation Case 46

Mr Kuning (Deranged Liver Enzymes)

Use this case as practice! The pull-out booklet contains the candidate's information.

Information for the Candidate

Patient Details: Mr Kuning, 32 years old

Your Role: Gastroenterology SHO

Referral Letter:

> Dear Colleague,
>
> Thank you for seeing Mr Kuning for abnormal liver function tests detected on health screening.
>
> Regards,
>
> Dr Kelly Chng, GP

Vital Signs: BP 120/70 mmHg, HR 60/min, RR 15/min, SpO2 95% RA, T 36.0°C

Investigations:

Bilirubin	30	umol/L	(3 - 17)
Alanine aminotransferase (ALT)	160	IU/L	(5 - 35)
Aspartate transaminase (AST)	334	IU/L	(5 - 35)
Alkaline phosphatase (ALP)	70	IU/L	(30 - 150)
Albumin	37	g/L	(35 - 50)

Full blood count, creatinine, electrolytes – normal

Patient's Brief

Synopsis: *This young man has deranged liver enzymes and neuropsychiatric symptoms. He has a history of alcohol use and a family history of liver and neurological problems. The differentials are alcohol use disorder and Wilson's disease.*

Open the consult with: The GP told me that my liver enzymes are not normal, but I feel fine. *Also volunteer the history of low mood and hands shaking.*

History of current problem:

- You have no jaundice, abdominal pain, or change in urine or stool colour.
- You have no rectal bleeding, vomiting of blood, abnormal bruising, or leg or abdominal swelling.
- You have lost 5 kg in the past 6 months and your appetite is poor. You think this is because your mood has been low.

Consultation Case 46

- You do not feel lethargic or lightheaded, and there is no decrease in exercise tolerance.
- You have not eaten raw shellfish or had any diarrhoeal illness.
- You have no sexual partners apart from your spouse. You do not have any history of intravenous drug abuse. You have not received any blood transfusions or tattoos.
- You drink 5–10 shots of hard liquor each night, usually while entertaining clients. You feel guilty about your drinking, but unfortunately this is part of the banking culture. You do not drink in the morning. You feel annoyed that your wife keeps bugging you about your alcohol intake.
- Your wife has often commented that your speech is slurred, and you have noted that your hands tend to shake.
- The relationship with your wife has been rocky in the past year. Because your mood has been low, you have preferred to spend time alone rather than with her, and you have felt uncontrollably irritable with her.
- You have not been doing well at work. Somehow you have difficulty focusing. You have been put on a performance improvement plan.

Past medical and surgical history:

- Nil

Medication list:

- Nil
- Supplements and herbal remedies: none
- Drug allergy: nil

Family history:

- Your uncle was told that he had Parkinson's disease in his late 30s. He died from liver failure quite suddenly in his early 40s. You do not know the cause of his liver failure.

Relevant personal, social, occupational, and travel history:

- You work as a junior banker.
- You are married without children.
- You do not smoke.
- There is no relevant travel history.
- You have not had vaccinations against hepatitis A and B.

Relevant physical examination findings:

There may be a real patient or a surrogate at this encounter.

- No jaundice.
- No stigmata of chronic liver disease.
- No Dupuytren's contracture or parotidomegaly.

- Abdomen soft, non-tender; no masses.
- No tremor, dystonias, chorea, or ataxia.
- Speech not slurred.
- Gait normal.

You have some specific questions for the doctor at this consultation:
- Is my liver problem because of alcohol?
- What should I do now?

Approach and Clinical Reasoning

Pitfall: Barking up the wrong tree

> Laboratory results are provided upfront in this encounter and this must guide your approach. Do not use a generic approach to jaundice or abnormal liver enzymes. Rather, identify the correct clinical syndrome and focus on the appropriate differentials. Spending too much time to pursue the causes of obstructive jaundice would be barking up the wrong tree.

Interpret the provided laboratory results before entering the station. Recognise the clinical syndrome of an asymptomatic patient who has a hepatocellular pattern of deranged liver enzymes. Initial causes to consider will include:

- Infective: chronic viral hepatitis, other viral infections.
- Toxic: alcohol or drug-induced liver injury.
- Metabolic: fatty liver disease.
- Vascular: congestive hepatitis.
- Autoimmune hepatitis.
- Hereditary: haemochromatosis, Wilson's disease.

Mr Kuning has a constellation of liver disease (abnormal liver enzymes), neurologic disease (dysarthria, tremor), and psychiatric disease (personality change, depression). Key differentials are:

- Alcohol use disorder which can explain the 2:1 ratio of AST:ALT, tremor, dysarthria, and personality change.
- Wilson's disease, particularly given the family history involving his uncle.

Screen for complications of liver disease including gastrointestinal bleeding (esophageal varices), coagulopathy (thrombocytopenia, inadequate clotting factor synthesis), abdominal distension (ascites), and confusion.

Physical examination should focus on:

- Looking for any signs of chronic liver disease, hepatomegaly, or splenomegaly.

- Examining neurology for tremor, Parkinsonism, dysarthria, and cerebellar signs.
- Looking for specific signs of Wilson's disease (Kayser-Fleischer rings) or alcohol use (Dupuytren's contracture, parotidomegaly).

Question and Answer

Suggested answer to the patient's concerns:

Mr Kuning, indeed alcohol use is a possible cause of your liver inflammation, slurred speech, and shaking hands. However, I will also have to consider other causes of these symptoms. Given what you told me about your uncle, I am also worried about a disorder in which your body accumulates copper, called Wilson's disease.

I need to do some further blood and urine tests to find out what exactly is happening. I don't have to admit you, but we should get these tests done today and see you again in a week. I will send you to the eye doctor to have a look at your eyes. We may or may not need to do a liver biopsy. On your end, it would be best to stop drinking alcohol to prevent further liver damage.

Suggested presentation to the examiner:

Mr Kuning presents with a hepatocellular pattern of deranged liver enzymes, tremor, dysarthria, personality change, and depression. There is a history of significant alcohol use and a family history of liver and neurological problems. Examination is unremarkable for any signs of chronic liver disease, hepatomegaly, or splenomegaly. There is no tremor, extrapyramidal signs, or cerebellar signs, and no Kayser-Fleischer rings. My principal diagnosis is Wilson's disease. My differential includes alcohol-use disorder.

He can be investigated outpatient with a close follow-up involving:

- Confirmation of my diagnosis by:
  - Repeating liver studies.
  - Checking serum copper (low), ceruloplasmin (low), and 24 h urinary copper (high).
  - Giving an ophthalmology referral to look for Kayser-Fleischer rings.
  - Considering liver biopsy.
- Searching for other causes of deranged liver enzymes such as doing hepatitis viral serology.
- Looking for complications by checking full blood count, clotting, glucose, elastography (fibroscan), and doing a liver ultrasound to look for evidence of cirrhosis.

Treatment will involve a muldisciplinary team including a gastroenterologist, psychiatrist, and neurologist. Principles are:

- Chelation therapy for Wilson's disease (penicillamine) if this is diagnosed.
- Avoidance of further liver insult through alcohol cessation, avoiding hepatotoxins, and vaccination against hepatitis.

- Screening for and treating complications (e.g., esophagogastroduodenoscopy for varices).
- Adjuncts include cognitive behavioural therapy for psychiatric disease.
- Patient education, family screening, and genetic counselling.

Consultation Case 47

Ms Fairchild (Raised aPTT)

Use this case as practice! The pull-out booklet contains the candidate's information.

Information for the Candidate

Patient Details: Ms Fairchild, 32 years old

Your Role: Medicine Outpatients SHO

Referral Letter:

> Dear Colleague,
>
> Thank you for seeing Ms Fairchild for raised aPTT.
>
> She saw me to do a face lift. Unexpectedly, the routine pre-op work-up found an elevated aPTT. I am hoping that you will be able to investigate and let me know whether I can proceed with the procedure.
>
> Thank you,
>
> Dr W. Wu, Plastic Surgery

Vital Signs: BP 110/62 mmHg, HR 65/min, RR 10/min, SpO2 99% RA, T 36.0°C

Investigations:
Prothrombin time (PT)	12.0 s (normal)
Activated partial thromboplastin time (aPTT)	80.2 s (30 - 50 s)
Full blood count	normal

Patient's Brief

Synopsis: *This young lady has isolated prolonged aPTT without clinical bleeding, associated with unprovoked deep vein thrombosis and recurrent early pregnancy loss. The diagnosis is antiphospholipid syndrome.*

Open the consult with: Dr Wu said that one of my 'bleeding tests' is abnormal and I will bleed if I do a face lift. *Volunteer the information of blood clots in the leg.*

History of current problem:
- You do not have any lip/gum bleeding, easy bruising, or joint swelling/pain. Your periods are not unusually heavy (4 pads/day at its peak).
- You have had two wisdom teeth extracted some time ago and you did not have any problems with prolonged bleeding thereafter.
- You have had 4 miscarriages in the past 5 years; all of them happened in the first trimester.

- You have no weakness, numbness, giddiness, slurred speech, or double vision.
- You do not have any rashes. Your hands do not change colour in a cold environment.
- You have no breathlessness, leg swelling, or blood or bubbles in the urine.
- You have a balanced, healthy diet and are of normal body mass index.
- You have no liver problems, jaundice, abdominal pain, or change in urine colour.
- You saw the plastic surgeon purely for cosmetic reasons because you were upset that your jaw line did not look pretty.

Past medical and surgical history:

- Two years ago, you had a blood clot in your right calf which was not provoked by any long flight or period of immobility. You took blood thinners for 3 months and were told that they were not necessary thereafter.
- No other medical problems.

Medication list:

- No long term medications
- No blood thinners (now)
- No traditional medicine, supplements, or contraceptive pill
- NKDA

Family history:

- Your mother had lupus and passed away from kidney failure.

Relevant personal, social, occupational, and travel history:

- You have been married for 5 years. You have no children, having miscarried 4 times during your marriage.
- You are a retail store assistant.
- You do not smoke or drink.

Relevant physical examination findings:

This encounter may use either a real or a surrogate patient.
- Comfortable.
- No leg swelling.
- No bruises or rashes.
- Normal neurological examination.
- No joint swelling or pain.
- No jaundice.

You have some specific questions for the doctor at this consultation:
- Do I have haemophilia? I've heard that people with haemophilia can't do surgery because they will bleed uncontrollably.

Approach and Clinical Reasoning

Ms Fairchild presents with isolated prolonged aPTT. The approach to prolonged aPTT begins with (a) ruling out prolonged aPTT due to sample contamination or anticoagulant use, and (b) taking a bleeding history to determine if the patient has a bleeding or non-bleeding phenotype (Figure B4.7). Although you will not be able to do this in the exam, the next step is a mixing study (50% patient's serum + 50% normal plasma) to distinguish between factor deficiency (correctable) vs. factor inhibitor (non-correctable).

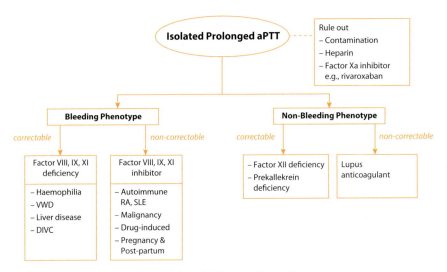

DIVC: disseminated intravascular coagulation; RA: rheumatoid arthritis; SLE: systemic lupus erythematosus; VWD: Von Willebrand disease

Factor XII deficiency does not cause bleeding.

Figure B4.7. Approach to isolated prolonged aPTT.

Ms Fairchild does not have any significant bleeding history and instead has a history of unprovoked distal deep vein thrombosis. This should raise suspicion of a lupus anticoagulant, which artificially prolongs aPTT and is associated with thrombosis rather than bleeding (the differentials of factor XII or prekallerein deficiency are not expected knowledge in PACES). The lupus anticoagulant is part of antiphospholipid syndrome (APS) and you should ask about pregnancy losses — Ms Fairchild does have recurrent pregnancy losses and clearly fulfils the diagnostic criteria of APS (see Box).

Sapporo criteria (Sydney revision) for antiphospholipid syndrome (APS).

Definite APS = ≥1 clinical + ≥1 laboratory criteria	
Clinical criteria	Laboratory criteria

• Arterial or venous thrombosis
• Pregnancy morbidity not explained by other causes:
  a) ≥1 fetal loss ≥10 weeks
  b) ≥1 premature birth ≤34 weeks due to pre-eclampsia or placental insufficiency
  c) ≥3* early pregnancy loss (<10 weeks)
  *≥3 required as early pregnancy loss is common
	Consecutive (>12 weeks apart) positive tests for:
	• Lupus anticoagulant
	• Anti-cardiolipin IgG/IgM
	• Anti β2-glycoprotein 1 IgG/IgM

APS can be primary or accompany systemic lupus erythematosus (SLE); if time permits, you should briefly ask for features of SLE such as Raynaud's syndrome, rash, or haematuria, which Ms Fairchild does not have.

Physical examination should cover:

- Looking for any cutaneous ecchymosis.
- Examining for livedo reticularis, which is common in APS.
- Screening for arterial and venous thrombosis such as calf swelling (deep vein thrombosis) or hemiparesis (cerebral infarct).
- Examining briefly for signs of SLE including malar rash, scarring alopecia, or synovitis.

Question and Answer

Suggested answer to the patient's concerns:

Ms Fairchild, I don't think you have haemophilia and I don't think you are more likely to bleed than anyone else. While you are right that the abnormal blood test, called a clotting time, can indicate haemophilia, in your case actually I suspect another disease called antiphospholipid syndrome. This can cause the same test to be abnormal but instead of bleeding, it causes blood clots and miscarriages. I will need to do additional tests to confirm this and if so, we do need to treat you with a blood thinner.

Suggested presentation to the examiner:

Ms Fairchild has the antiphospholipid syndrome with isolated prolonged aPTT, recurrent early pregnancy loss, and a previous episode of unprovoked deep vein thrombosis. There is no clinical suggestion of underlying SLE at present.

I will investigate by:

- Repeating the PT/aPTT to confirm that it is abnormal.

- Checking for lupus anticoagulant and other antiphospholipid antibodies: anticardiolipin and anti β2-glycoprotein 1 and then repeating the positive test >12 weeks later to document persistence of the antibodies.
- Checking for underlying SLE by sending autoantibodies such as an antinuclear antibody and double-stranded DNA, as well as evaluating for other organ manifestations (e.g., serum creatinine, urine microscopy and protein quantification to check for renal involvement).

Management will involve a haematologist, obstetrician specialising in high-risk pregnancy, and allied healthcare professionals. This patient is likely to require long-term anticoagulation ideally with warfarin.

484 A STRATEGY TO AND WORKED PRACTICE FOR THE MRCP PACES

Consultation Case 48

Ms Clot (Low Platelets)

Use this case as practice! The pull-out booklet contains the candidate's information.

Information for the Candidate

Patient Details: Ms Rachel Clot, 47 years old

Your Role: Haematology Clinic SHO

Referral Letter:

> Dear Colleague,
>
> Thank you for seeing Ms Clot early for thrombocytopenia.
>
> She has a history of systemic lupus erythematosus, diabetes, and hypertension. She was admitted last week for exertional chest pain and underwent a coronary angiogram. This showed minor coronary artery disease which we will treat medically.
>
> She made an unscheduled clinic visit today complaining of right thigh swelling. An ultrasound confirmed deep vein thrombosis of the right superficial femoral vein. Unfortunately, her platelets were low, so I was unable to start anticoagulation.
>
> Would you please see her for further management?
>
> Thank you.
>
> Dr B. Loon, Cardiology

Vital Signs: BP 106/64 mmHg, HR 80/min, RR 10/min, SpO2 97% RA, T 37.0°C

Investigations: Haemoglobin 12.2 g/L (12 - 16)
White cell count 4.0×10^9/L (2.5 - 10)
Platelets 40×10^9/L (150 - 400), previously normal

Patient's Brief

Synopsis: *This lady with known lupus likely has heparin-induced thrombocytopenia, presenting with thrombocytopenia and new deep vein thrombosis after heparin exposure. There is no other evidence of a lupus flare.*

Open the consult with: The cardiologist said that I have a clot in my leg but he can't treat me because my platelets are low. *Do not volunteer any other information unless asked.*

History of current problem:

- One week ago, you were admitted for central, crushing chest pain triggered by exertion, which you never had before. A coronary angiogram showed only minor blockages of your heart vessels. You were discharged with aspirin and cholesterol medication.
- However, in the last two days, you noticed that your right thigh was swollen and painful.
- You made an unscheduled visit to the cardiologist today and he sent you for an ultrasound. You understand that this ultrasound showed that you had a clot in your thigh.
- You are quite surprised as you remember receiving blood thinners and also an injection of 'strong blood thinner' during the angiogram.
- You have otherwise been well since the angiogram, moving about and doing your usual daily routines.
- You have no breathlessness, chest pain, palpitations, bleeding, lightheadedness, or decrease in effort tolerance.
- You have no fatigue, lethargy, joint pains, rashes, fever, decrease in urine output, blood or bubbles in your urine, jaundice, or change in urine colour.
- You have no recent air travel.
- You are currently having your period.

Past medical and surgical history:

- Lupus, diagnosed 3 years ago. You first presented with fatigue, rashes, joint pains, and blood in your urine. Your disease has been stable and your last flare was more than 12 months ago while tapering prednisolone. You usually flare with increased blood and protein in the urine. You have not had any low cell counts, bleeding, or anaemia with your previous flares.
- Diabetes, well controlled, HbA1c 7.0%.
- Hypertension on medications.
- No history of liver or kidney disease.

Medication list:

- Aspirin 100 mg OM
- Atorvastatin 40 mg ON
- Enalapril 10 mg BD
- Glipizide 5 mg OM
- Hydroxychloroquine 200 mg OM
- Metformin 850 mg BD
- Mycophenolate mofetil 500 mg BD
- Prednisolone 10 mg every other morning
- No supplements or traditional medicine
- No drug allergy

Family history:

- Rebecca, your older sister, is on blood thinners for deep vein thrombosis.

Relevant personal, social, occupational, and travel history:

- You are not married and have never been pregnant. You are not sexually active.
- You work as an insurance agent.
- You do not smoke or drink.

Relevant physical examination findings:

This encounter is likely to use a real patient whose deep vein thrombosis has been treated.

- Lupus malar rash or photosensitive rash ± oral ulcers, alopecia.
- May have livedo reticularis.
- Right thigh not swollen.
- No cutaneous ecchymoses.
- No pallor.
- No lymphadenopathy.
- No splenomegaly.

You have some specific questions for the doctor at this consultation:

- Is this my lupus giving trouble again?

Approach and Clinical Reasoning

Tailor the differentials to Ms Clot's thrombocytopenia to her known systemic lupus erythematosus (SLE) (Table B4.39).

Table B4.39. Causes of thrombocytopenia in SLE.

Cause	Important features
SLE flare with immune mediated platelet destruction	Other manifestations of SLE flare (rash, arthralgia, haematuria, fever, constitutional symptoms), raised ESR and dsDNA Thrombocytopenia being a feature of previous SLE flares ± other cytopenias or Evan's syndrome (autoimmune haemolytic anaemia + autoimmune thrombocytopenia)
Marrow suppression	± Other cytopenias Use of myelosuppressive immunosuppressants; watch for recent dose increases or overdose (e.g., inadvertent daily dosing of methotrexate)

(Cont'd)

Cause	Important features
Drug-induced thrombocytopenia	Many drugs can cause drug-induced immune thrombocytopenia Heparin-induced thrombocytopenia presents with thrombosis rather than bleeding
Platelet consumption	Microangiopathic haemolytic anaemia (e.g., thrombotic thrombocytopenic purpura, catastrophic antiphospholipid syndrome)
Hypersplenism	Splenomegaly, usually with mild anaemia and leukopenia
General causes of thrombocytopenia	Infection: HIV, hepatitis viruses, dengue Myelodysplasia, haematologic malignancy Liver disease with hypersplenism

SLE: systemic lupus erythematosus

It is important to find out the cumulative disease manifestations of Ms Clot's SLE and what her previous flares were like — SLE patients tend to have a 'signature' flare pattern with similar clinical manifestations. As Ms Clot has no features of an SLE flare, apart from low cell counts which were never a feature of her previous flares, one would be cautious in ascribing her current thrombocytopenia to an SLE flare.

The smoking gun in this scenario is that Ms Clot has developed new thrombosis and thrombocytopenia 5 to 10 days after a diagnostic coronary angiogram during which intravenous heparin was used. This is suspicious for heparin-induced thrombocytopenia (HIT).

The 4Ts score is a helpful guide (you are not expected to memorise this, but should understand what are the 'high risk' features). Ms Clot fulfils all 4 criteria of the '4Ts' score (low risk: score 1–3, moderate risk: score 4–5, high risk: score 6–8).

- Platelet fall > 50% and nadir ≥ 20×10^9/L (2 points).
- Time of onset day 5–10 since starting heparin (2 points).
- New thrombosis event (2 points).
- No other clear cause of thrombocytopenia (2 points) – there is no evidence of microangiopathic haemolytic anaemia and no recent increase in immunosuppression to suggest marrow suppression.

Physical examination should focus on:

- Eliciting features of deep vein thrombosis (these may be absent as the patient would have been treated).
- Looking out for bleeding manifestations (unlikely as HIT presents with thrombosis, not bleeding).
- Evaluating for other clinical features of lupus (e.g., rash, arthralgia).
- Palpation of the spleen.

Question and Answer

Suggested answer to the patient's concerns:

Ms Clot, this may not be due to lupus as it is quite different from your previous lupus flares. I'm wondering if it is a complication of the blood thinners you were given. Unusually some patients react to the blood thinner by developing low platelets and clots.

I will need to admit you. I will send off some blood tests including antibodies against the blood thinner. We will start you on other forms of blood thinner to deal with the clot you have. If you develop any bleeding, breathlessness, or chest pain, you must let me know immediately.

Suggested presentation to the examiner:

Ms Clot presents with thrombocytopenia and a new deep vein thrombosis after recent intravenous heparin exposure. This is suggestive of heparin-induced thrombocytopenia (HIT). Differentials include thrombocytopenia as a result of lupus flare, but there is no other evidence of a lupus flare. There is no other cause of platelet consumption such as microangiopathic haemolytic anaemia.

Investigations:

- I will perform a 4T score to assess the probability of HIT, and confirm my diagnosis by sending anti-platelet factor 4 (anti-PF4) antibody.
- I will assess for other evidence of lupus activity (blood count, renal function, liver function, urine protein/creatinine ratio, complement levels, dsDNA, etc.).
- I will send a blood film to look for evidence of microangiopathic haemolysis.
- In preparation for anticoagulation I will check her clotting profile.

Management:

- I will stop all heparins immediately (first thing to be done if she is at intermediate or high risk of HIT).
- Ms Clot should instead receive a non-heparin anticoagulant such as a direct oral anticoagulant (not warfarin as it takes time to effect therapeutic anticoagulation).
- I will admit her and refer urgently to a haematologist and also involve a rheumatologist in her management.

Consultations

5 | How Examiners Grade

This section illustrates the examiner's perspective of how PACES is marked. Understanding what examiners look for will help you to strategise and maximise your marks.

Examiners begin the day by calibrating each station. This entails rehearsing the history and verifying the physical signs present, then completing the calibration sheet (Table B5.1) which serves as a marking rubric. An example of a completed calibration sheet for Consultation Case 03 (Ms Sniffles) is given in Table B5.2. While examiners may vary in what they deem 'key points' for a satisfactory candidate, both examiners must agree on the points to include in the calibration sheet before the carousel starts.

Table B5.1. Blank calibration sheet (consultations).

Clinical communication	What key elements of history must a satisfactory candidate consider?
Physical examination	What key components of physical examination should a satisfactory candidate undertake?
Managing patient concerns	How should a satisfactory candidate respond to the patient's concerns?
Identifying physical signs	What physical signs should a satisfactory candidate detect?
Differential diagnosis	What diagnoses should a satisfactory candidate consider?
Clinical judgement	What key steps in management should a satisfactory candidate consider?
Maintaining patient welfare	Treats patient respectfully, sensitively, and ensures comfort, safety, and dignity.

Table B5.2. Sample calibration sheet for Consultation Case 03 (Ms Sniffles).

Synopsis: *A young lady with known myasthenia gravis presents with worsening shortness of breath, weakness, and diplopia. She has a myasthenia flare precipitated by an upper respiratory tract infection as well as levofloxacin.*

Clinical communication	What key elements of history must a satisfactory candidate consider? – History of upper respiratory tract infection – Proximal weakness/difficulty climbing up the stairs on background of myasthenia gravis – Diplopia worse in evenings – History of levofloxacin use
Physical examination	What key components of physical examination should a satisfactory candidate undertake? – Examination of extraocular eye movements – Examination of muscle power and testing for fatigability
Managing patient concerns	How should a satisfactory candidate respond to the patient's concerns? – To acknowledge the patient's concerns of having to be at the important presentation – However not to agree to discharge the patient but instead to admit for treatment (safety issue)
Identifying physical signs	What physical signs should a satisfactory candidate detect? – Ptosis – Ophthalmoplegia – Proximal myopathy – Fatigability
Differential diagnosis	What diagnoses should a satisfactory candidate consider? – Flare of myasthenia gravis – Reasonable differentials: pulmonary embolism, asthma
Clinical judgement	What key steps in management should a satisfactory candidate consider? – Rule out respiratory failure (e.g., blood gas, test negative inspiratory force, or equivalent) – Chest X-ray – Stop levofloxacin but treat infection – Consider intravenous immunoglobulin or plasma exchange
Maintaining patient welfare	Treats patient respectfully, sensitively, and ensures comfort, safety, and dignity.

Candidates are marked against this predetermined calibration sheet. Typically, only a few key points are listed for each skill — for instance, a reasonable history will certainly be far more comprehensive than the few points listed, but a candidate must hit all the required points to be awarded a 'satisfactory' grade (2 marks) for the skill. A candidate who misses one point is likely to be 'borderline' (1 mark), while missing more than one point will likely be deemed 'unsatisfactory' (0 marks). You will realise that it is quite easy to miss specific points and hence lose marks.

Two worked cases are provided in the subsequent pages, each with a sample calibration sheet. Our recommendation is that you should go through each case twice — first attempting it as a candidate (with a tutor or colleague who has previously attempted the case), and a second time acting as the examiner. When acting as the examiner, create your own calibration sheet before comparing against our sample, then practice grading a colleague attempting the case as the candidate.

Consultation Case 49

Mr Beer (Acute Kidney Injury)

The focus of this case is to illustrate the examiner's perspective of how PACES is marked. **Please read the introduction 'how examiners grade' (page 489) if you have yet to do so**.

Information for the Candidate

Patient Details: Mr Beer, 50 years old

Your Role: Medicine Clinic SHO

Scenario: Mr Beer was found to have a creatinine of 242 umol/L on routine laboratory investigations, up from 128 umol/L two months ago.

Vital Signs: BP 150/83 mmHg, HR 75/min, RR 10/min, SpO2 98% RA, T 37.0°C

Patient's Brief

Synopsis: *This patient with known gout develops acute kidney injury due to NSAID use and possible urate urolithiasis.*

Open the consult with: What's wrong with my kidneys, doc? I feel just fine! *Do not volunteer any other information unless asked.*

History of current problem:
- You feel quite yourself and have not been unwell.
- You have not had any fever, diarrhoea, vomiting, or lethargy; and have been eating and drinking normally.
- However you try to limit your water intake – as a taxi driver, you have limited access to toilets for a large part of the day and cannot afford to be running to the bathroom too frequently.
- You do not have any leg swelling, breathlessness, drowsiness, or confusion.
- You do not have any pain on passing urine, sense of urinary urgency, poor urine stream, hesitancy, or dribbling towards the end of urination.
- If specifically asked, you do recall an episode two weeks ago where you had right flank pain and blood-tinged urine. This went away after a day and you are no longer bothered by it.
- You do not have any frothy urine or decreased urine output.

- You have frequent gout flares which typically present as sudden episodes of knee and foot pain which resolve after a few days.
- You do not have any rashes or mouth ulcers.
- You do not have any back pain, constipation, or abdominal pain.
- You do not have any asthma, cough, coughing out blood, or blocked nose/ears.

Past medical and surgical history:
- Hypertension.
- Hyperlipidemia.
- Diabetes for 20 years. This was poorly controlled in the initial days but you have since made huge efforts to do better. Your latest HbA1c taken 2 months ago is 7.5%.
- Gout for >15 years. It tends to flare often – once a week – despite regular medication. You found panadol and colchicine ineffective and in the past 2–3 weeks needed to buy additional medication over the counter (Ponstan – mefenamic acid).

Medication list:
- Allopurinol 200 mg OM
- Amlodipine 5 mg OM
- Atorvastatin 20 mg ON
- Dapagliflozin 10 mg OM
- Colchicine 500 mcg TDS as needed
- Linagliptin 5 mg OM
- Metformin 1 g BD
- Valsartan 160 mg OM
- You are compliant to all medications, with no recent changes to dosages
- If specifically asked – in the past 2–3 weeks you have also been taking over-the-counter Ponstan (mefenamic acid) for joint pains
- Drug allergy: nil

Family history:
- Your mother had kidney failure due to diabetes and was on dialysis from 60 years old until she passed away in her 70s.
- No family history of autoimmune disorders.

Relevant personal, social, occupational, and travel history:
- You work as a taxi driver.
- You are single and unmarried.
- You drink heavily – mainly beer, approximately 4–5 330 ml cans a night, along with friends.
- You do not smoke.

Relevant physical examination findings:

This station will be run with a real patient.

- Gouty tophi over the right elbow and multiple gouty tophi over the hands (e.g., right thumb and ring finger, left index finger). No gouty tophi over the earlobes.
- No joint deformities, subluxation, ulnar deviation, or swan-neck or boutonniere deformity. No nail pitting or onycholysis.
- No active swelling of the wrists or metacarpal-phalangeal and proximal interphalangeal joints.
- Normal range of motion of all small joints of the hands.
- Abdomen soft, renal punch negative, no ballotable kidneys
- Lungs clear.
- Skin tugor fair, no oedema.

Photos to be shown to candidate upon request (use colour plates for full-colour photos).

Photo 31 **Photo 32**

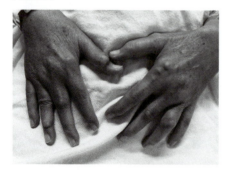
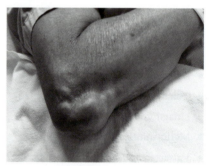

You have some specific questions for the doctor at this consultation:
- Will my kidney get better?

Approach and Clinical Reasoning

This is a reasonably straightforward case of acute kidney injury in a patient with tophaceous gout. The approach to acute kidney injury, which should be familiar ground, will not be rehashed here. Work through pre-renal, renal, and post-renal causes, paying particular attention to differentials with a PACES flavour such as:

- Glomerulonephritis – particularly those secondary to systemic diseases.
- Drugs – direct nephrotoxicity as well as allergic interstitial nephritis.
- Infiltrative – myeloma and amyloidosis.
- Renovascular disease – renal artery stenosis, Takayasu arteritis.
- Polycystic kidney disease.
- Microangiopathic haemolytic anaemia (e.g., thrombotic thrombocytopenic purpura).

The precipitants of acute kidney injury in this case include:

- NSAID use for poorly controlled tophaceous gout.
- Urolithiasis (flank pain and haematuria) – possibly urate stones on a background of gout. His attempts to limit water intake will exacerbate this problem.
- The differential of glomerulonephritis can be considered given the history of haematuria.

Physical examination should focus on (1) physical signs of gout, (2) physical findings of potential causes of kidney dysfunction, and (3) physical findings of complications of kidney dysfunction. Recall that the hands are to be examined according to the look-feel-move schema:

- Look for tophi and deformities. The observant candidate may get the diagnosis at first glance at the patient. Apart from the hands and elbows, check the ear lobe for tophi.
- Feel joint lines for active synovitis.
- Move to assess range of motion. If time permits, it will be good to do functional assessment of the hands (e.g., using a pen, buttoning a shirt).
- Look for signs to suggest differentials (e.g., rashes, mouth ulcers, dactylitis).

Question and Answer

Suggested answer to the patient's concerns:

This news that your kidney isn't working as it should must come as a shock. I think I have an idea of what is hurting the kidneys and once we address this, there is a good chance that your kidneys will get better. First, the painkillers you are taking are very effective but they may not be good for the kidneys, so we will need to stop them. Second, you may be having kidney stones that are related to gout; I will do some tests to see if this is the case and then we will decide on how to manage it.

Suggested presentation to the examiner:

Mr Beer has acute kidney injury. Likely precipitants include NSAID use and possible urate urolithiasis. Physical examination is significant for multiple gouty tophi over the hands and elbows without active joint swelling. He is euvolemic.

My investigations will include:

- Repeating renal function, electrolytes.
- Urine microscopy and protein/creatinine ratio; urine phase contrast.
- Non-contrast CT kidneys/ureter/bladder looking for hydronephrosis and stones, and assessing kidney size.
- Serum urate levels to guide uric acid lowering therapy.
- Considering autoimmune studies if phase contrast shows dysmorphic haematuria.

Management plan:
- Immediate management:
  - Ensure no urgent indication for dialysis.
  - Stop NSAIDs, metformin, valsartan.
  - Trial of hydration.
  - If CT shows hydronephrosis or urolithiasis, consideration of urological intervention to relieve obstruction/remove stones.
- Subsequent measures:
  - May eventually require to increase allopurinol aiming for a serum uric acid target of <300 mmol/L (note: uricosuric agents are contraindicated and may exacerbate stones). He is at higher risk of severe cutaneous adverse reactions given his renal impairment so titration of allopurinol should be done slowly (e.g., 50 mg increments).
  - Patient education to avoid NSAIDs; may offer alternate analgesia such as colchicine (prednisolone likely not ideal given diabetes history).
  - Diet modification – low purine.

Sample Marking Scheme

Attempt to craft your own marking scheme before referring to this sample!

Clinical communication	What key elements of history must a satisfactory candidate consider? – History of flank pain and haematuria – History of NSAID use – History of poorly controlled gout
Physical examination	What key components of physical examination should a satisfactory candidate undertake? – Examination of hands and tophi – Examination of fluid status
Managing patient concerns	How should a satisfactory candidate respond to the patient's concerns? – Explain that the kidney will likely improve when precipitants are stopped
Identifying physical signs	What physical signs should a satisfactory candidate detect? – Gouty tophi

(Cont'd)

Differential diagnosis	**What diagnoses should a satisfactory candidate consider?** – AKI due to NSAID use – Urolithiasis – Glomerulonephritis (history of haematuria)
Clinical judgement	**What key steps in management should a satisfactory candidate consider?** – Stop NSAIDs – Renal imaging – Relief of obstruction/stones – Increase allopurinol at a later date after recovering from AKI
Maintaining patient welfare	**Treats patient respectfully, sensitively, and ensures comfort, safety, and dignity.**

Consultation Case 50

Mr Ezekiel (Fractures)

The focus of this case is to illustrate the examiner's perspective of how PACES is marked. **Please read the introduction 'how examiners grade' (page 489) if you have yet to do so.**

Information for the Candidate

Patient Details: Mr Ezekiel, 58 years old

Your Role: Ward SHO

Referral Letter:
> Dear Medical Colleague,
>
> Mr Ezekiel has had two fractures this year (proximal humerus and distal radius). Is there anything you can do to reduce his risk of fracture recurrence?
>
> Thank you.
>
> Dr Saw, Orthopaedic Surgeon

Vital Signs: BP 165/80 mmHg, HR 73/min, RR 12/min, SpO2 98% RA, T 37.0°C

Patient's Brief

Synopsis: *This patient with end-stage kidney failure on haemodialysis has tertiary hyperparathyroidism presenting with pathologic fractures and vascular disease. He is non-compliant to phosphate binders and had declined parathyroidectomy.*

Open the consult with: I'm not sure how I fractured my arm. I didn't fall or injure myself! *Do not volunteer any other information unless asked.*

History of current problem:

- While reaching out to pick up a 6-pack of canned drinks at the supermarket yesterday, you heard a sudden crack and felt a sharp pain in your right arm. You were sent to the emergency department where the doctors told you that you had broken the arm bone.

- A similar episode happened three months ago when you fractured your left wrist while cooking.

- You did not require surgery for both episodes. You have just completed 6 weeks of wearing an arm sling.

- You have otherwise been well with no bone pain or back pain.
- You have not gained or lost weight.
- Your bowel movements are normal with no diarrhoea or constipation, and you have no weight loss.
- You do not have any tremors or heat intolerance.
- You no longer engage in sexual intercourse but still experience morning erections.
- You have never done a bone mineral density test.
- Your kidney doctors have told you that your 'bone health' is not good and that your phosphate control leaves much to be desired. You are on multiple medications for 'bone health' and phosphate control, and have seen the dietitian multiple times to talk about 'low phosphate diet'. However, you have not always been taking the required medications (especially the mid-day dose; see next page).
- The kidney doctors have also told you that you need surgery for a gland in your neck. You are reluctant to do any surgery and have been putting it off.

Past medical and surgical history:
- End stage kidney failure from diabetes. You have been on dialysis for twelve years – first peritoneal dialysis for 7 years, then converted to haemodialysis in the past 5 years. You attend in-centre haemodialysis three times a week, four hours each time.
- Diabetes; HbA1c is 8.7%.
- Hypertension.
- Ischaemic heart disease. You had a heart attack and required stenting of your heart vessels last year.
- Peripheral vascular disease. You had a non-healing foot ulcer requiring angioplasty of the leg vessels two years ago.
- Stroke. This happened four years ago, and you made a good recovery.

Medication list:
- IV Alfacalcidol, 1mcg 3× a week
- IV Epoetin-Beta (Recormon), 4000 units every 5 days
- IV Iron sucrose (Venofer), 100 mg every month
- PO Aspirin 100 mg OM
- PO Atorvastatin 40 mg ON
- PO Bisoprolol 5 mg OM
- PO Nifedipine 30 mg ON
- PO Renal vitamin, 1 tablet OM
- PO Sevelamer 1600 mg TDS with each meal
- PO Valsartan 80 mg OM on non-dialysis days
- SC Insulin Glargine 18 units ON

- SC Insulin Aspart 6 units TDS
- Drug allergy: Amoxicillin
- You find the number of medications quite burdensome, especially those which you must take three times a day. You admit to not carrying these medications with you out of the house, and usually skip mid-day doses (while you are at work) and at times also evening doses (especially if you eat out).
- You do not take any traditional medicines or supplements.

Family history:
- No family history of frequent fractures or kidney disease.

Relevant personal, social, occupational, and travel history:
- You manage your own business – a small company in the import-export trade.
- You do not drink or smoke.
- You stay with your spouse. You have one son who has recently moved out.

Relevant physical examination findings:
This station will be run with a real patient.
- Left wrist (radiocephalic) arteriovenous fistula (Photo 33).
- Terminal phalanx resorption of both upper limbs (Photo 34).
- Genu valgum (bowing of legs).
- Lungs clear.
- No pedal oedema.
- No conjunctival pallor.
- No blue sclera.

Photos to be shown to candidate upon request (use colour plates for full-colour photos).

Photo 33

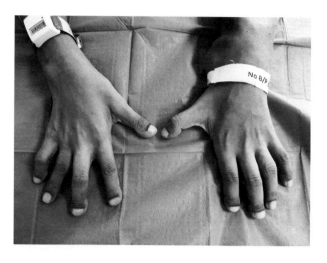

Consultation Case 50

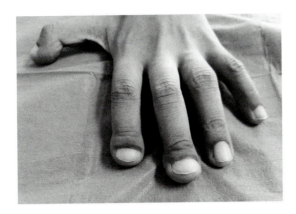

Photo 34
(close up)

You have some specific questions for the doctor at this consultation:
- Why do I keep getting fractures?

Approach and Clinical Reasoning

Mr Ezekiel, a patient with kidney failure on haemodialysis, presents with recurrent atraumatic fractures. While the diagnosis of renal bone disease is relatively apparent, do due diligence to work through the differentials for recurrent fractures/secondary osteoporosis (Table B5.3).

Table B5.3. Important causes of recurrent fractures/secondary osteoporosis.

Cause	Examples
Endocrine disease	Hyperparathyroidism, including primary (parathyroid adenoma) or secondary/tertiary (renal bone disease)
	Hypogonadism, primary or secondary
	Hypercortisolism
	Vitamin D deficiency
	Hyperthyroidism
Malignancy	Multiple myeloma
	Bony metastases
Connective tissue disease	Osteogenesis imperfecta (look for blue sclera)
	Marfan syndrome
	Ehler-Danlos syndrome
Drugs	Alcohol
	Glucocorticoids
	Antiepileptic drugs (e.g., carbamazepine, phenytoin)
	Cyclosporin
	Antidepressants (SSRI, tricyclics)

The pathophysiology of renal bone disease is complex; bone turnover may be high due to overactive parathyroid hormone (PTH) (secondary and tertiary hyperparathyroidism) or low (adynamic bone disease) due to oversuppression of PTH. Mr Ezekiel has numerous features in keeping with tertiary hyperparathyroidism including long dialysis vintage, non-compliance to phosphate binder sevelamer (uncontrolled hyperphosphatemia drives PTH secretion), as well as numerous vascular complications (stroke, ischaemic heart disease, and peripheral vascular disease) contributed by extraskeletal calcification. He has been offered — but declined — parathyroidectomy.

Tip: The giveaway medication list

> Mr Ezekiel's medication list is a giveaway — but only to those in the know! He is on cinacalcet — a calcimimetic that *mimics* the effect of *calcium* to inhibit the calcium-sensing receptor and inhibit PTH production. It is *only* given to patients with tertiary hyperparathyroidism. Pay attention to the medication list!

Eliciting the physical signs of tertiary hyperparathyroidism may be unfamiliar, but all that has to be done is to observe and describe! Physical findings may include:

- Bone abnormalities — most characteristically resorption of terminal digits (as in this case), genu valgum, fractures, and brown tumours on imaging.
- Calciphylaxis (not present in this case) — painful skin necrosis due to microvascular occlusion. This is a condition with high mortality.
- Extraskeletal calcification and sequelae — look for lower limb ulcers and neurologic deficits from previous strokes.
- Dialysis access, in this case an arteriovenous fistula.

Don't forget: The 'obvious' physical sign

> The presence of an arteriovenous fistula is so obvious that some candidates may neglect to mention it. But many examiners may include it as a required physical sign in their calibration rubric. Candidates who neglect to present simple and obvious physical signs will lose marks!

Question and Answer

Suggested answer to the patient's concerns:

Mr Ezekiel, I suspect that your fractures may be related to kidney failure. You did mention that your kidney doctor has asked you to go for surgery of the parathyroid gland in your neck. Many patients with kidney failure have an overactive parathyroid gland and this causes the bones to be weak, leading to fractures. Poor control of phosphate levels also contributes to this situation. May I encourage you to revisit the discussion of parathyroid removal with your kidney doctor, and until this is done, it is important to take the afternoon dose of sevelamer as best as you can.

Suggested presentation to the examiner:

Mr Ezekiel presents with recurrent fractures and vascular calcifications on a background of kidney failure with long dialysis vintage and suboptimal compliance to phosphate binders. Physical signs include terminal phalanx resorption, genu valgum, and a left wrist arteriovenous fistula. The diagnosis is tertiary hyperparathyroidism; although neoplastic bone lesions such as myeloma must be excluded.

My investigations will include:

- Biochemistry – calcium, phosphate, PTH, and alkaline phosphatase (expect all four to be elevated in tertiary hyperparathyroidism, while calcium will be low or low-normal in secondary hyperparathyroidism)
- To exclude differentials:
    - Bone imaging (exclude bone tumours/myeloma)
    - May also consider testing for other differentials (e.g., thyroid hormone, sex hormone – may omit in practice if the diagnosis of tertiary hyperparathyroidism is clear)
- Abdominal X-rays often display aortic calcification

Management:

- Parathyroidectomy.
- May increase cinacalcet as a bridge to parathyroidectomy (this knowledge is not required in PACES).
- Optimise phosphate control – low phosphate diet, compliance to sevelamer.

Sample Marking Scheme

Attempt to craft your own marking scheme before referring to this sample!

Clinical communication	What key elements of history must a satisfactory candidate consider?
	– Fracture is atraumatic/pathologic
	– History of renal failure on haemodialysis
	– Non-compliance to phosphate binders
	– Patient was offered but not keen for parathyroidectomy
Physical examination	What key components of physical examination should a satisfactory candidate undertake?
	– Examination of hands
	– Examination of fluid status

(Cont'd)

Managing patient concerns	**How should a satisfactory candidate respond to the patient's concerns?** – Explain that his frequent fractures are likely a manifestation of poorly controlled mineral bone disease
Identifying physical signs	**What physical signs should a satisfactory candidate detect?** – Presence of a working arteriovenous fistula – Terminal digit resorption
Differential diagnosis	**What diagnoses should a satisfactory candidate consider?** – Tertiary hyperparathyroidism/renal bone disease – Reasonable differentials: malignancy, myeloma
Clinical judgement	**What key steps in management should a satisfactory candidate consider?** – Check serum biochemistry (at least calcium, phosphate, PTH) – Compliance to phosphate binder – Parathyroidectomy
Maintaining patient welfare	**Treats patient respectfully, sensitively, and ensures comfort, safety, and dignity.**

Colour Plates for Consultation Stations

Consultation 01

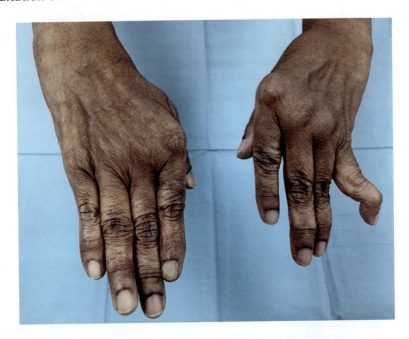

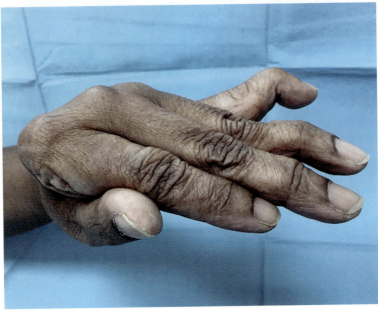

Clinical photo generously provided by Dr Stanley Angkodjojo, Sengkang General Hospital

Consultation 03

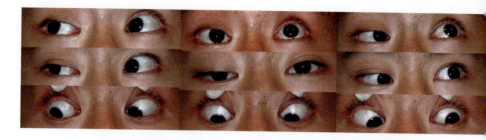

Clinical photo generously provided by Clin Assoc Prof Sharon Tow, Singapore National Eye Centre

Consultation 08

Photo 1

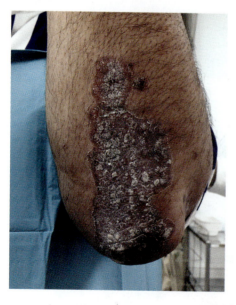

Photo 2

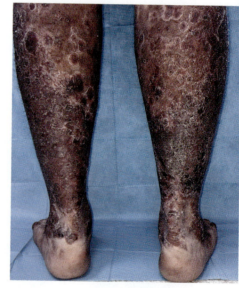

Photos 1 and 2 generously provided by Dr Stanley Angkodjojo, Sengkang General Hospital

Photo 3 (next page) generously provided by Dr Jon Yoong Kah Choun, Singapore General Hospital

Photo 3

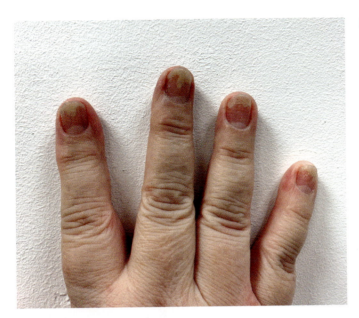

Consultation 09

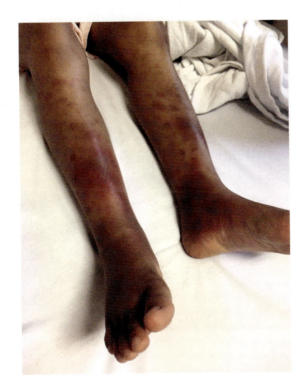

Clinical photo generously provided by Assoc Prof Derrick Aw, Sengkang General Hospital

Consultation 10

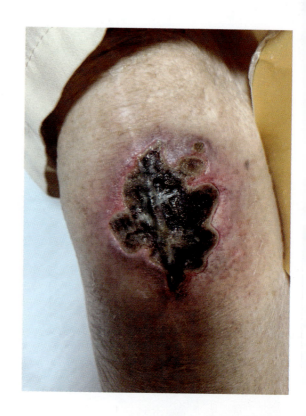

Clinical photo generously provided by Assoc Prof Derrick Aw, Sengkang General Hospital

Consultation 11

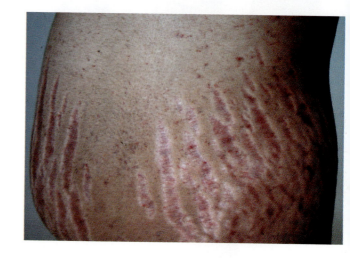

Reproduced with permission from DermNet NZ www.dermnetnz.org

Consultation 15

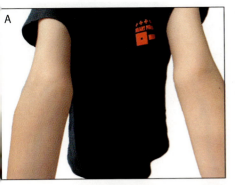
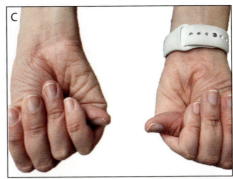
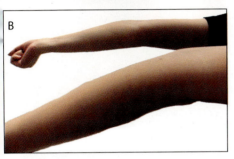
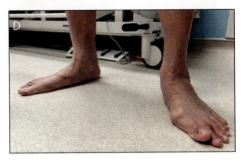

Clinical photo generously provided by Assoc Prof Tan Ju Le, National Heart Centre Singapore

Consultation 16

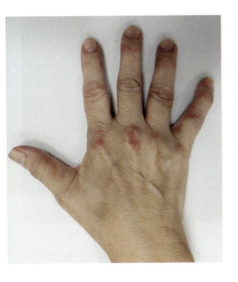
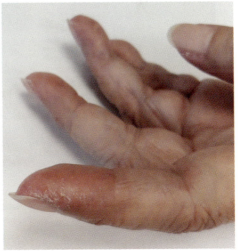

509

Consultation 17

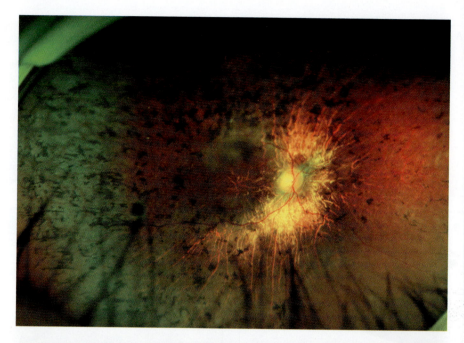

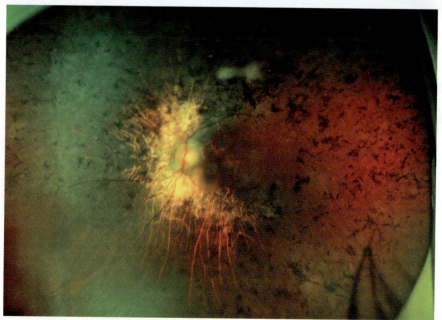

Clinical photo generously provided by Dr Nicole Chan, National University Hospital

Consultation 18

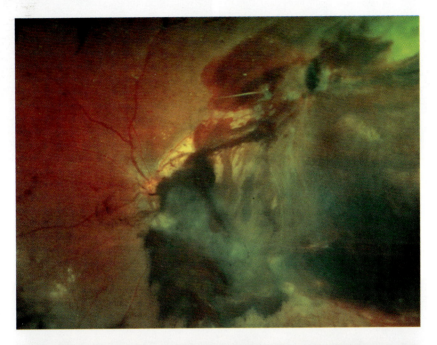

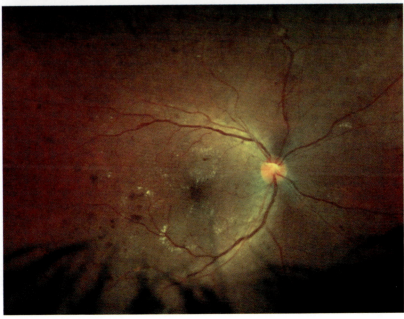

Clinical photo generously provided by Dr Nicole Chan, National University Hospital

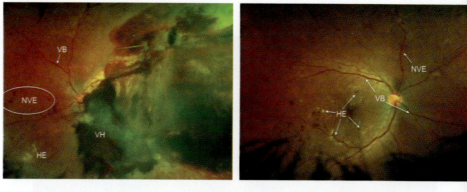

Findings annotated – HE: hard exudates; NVE: neovascularisation elsewhere; VB: venous beading; VH: vitreous haemorrhage

Consultation 19

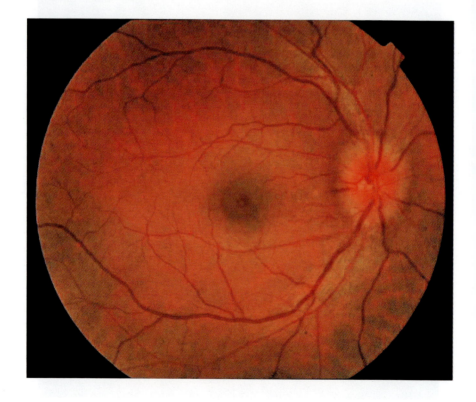

Clinical photo generously provided by Clin Assoc Prof Sharon Tow, Singapore National Eye Centre

Consultation 20

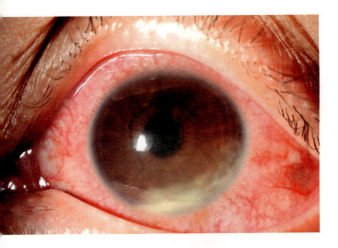

Clinical photo generously provided by Dr Jay Siak, Singapore National Eye Centre

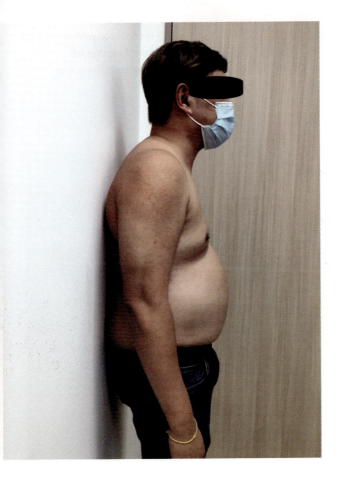

Clinical photo generously provided by Dr Stanley Angkodjojo, Sengkang General Hospital

Consultation 23

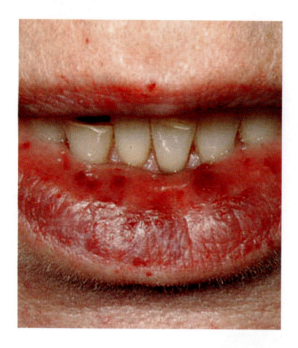

Photo by Raimo Suhonen.
Reproduced with permission
from DermNet NZ
www.dermnetnz.org

Consultation 26

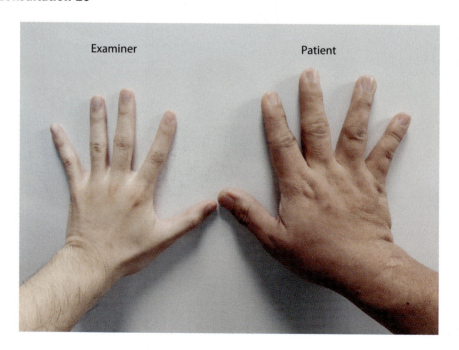

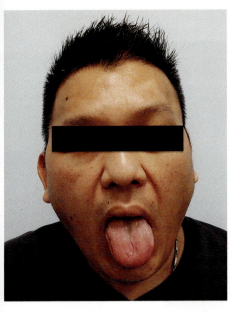
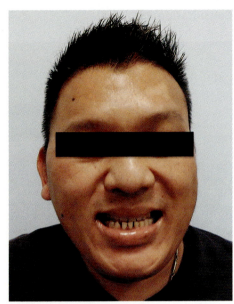

Clinical photos generously provided by Dr Loh Lih Ming, Singapore General Hospital

Consultation 27

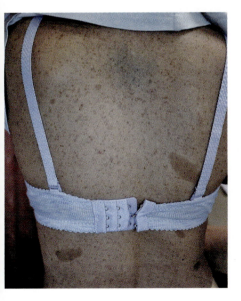
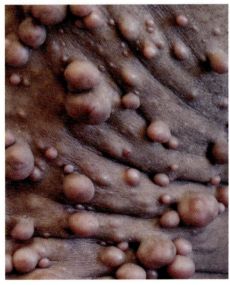

Clinical photo generously provided by Assoc Prof Mark Koh and Dr Cheryl Lie, KK Women's and Children's Hospital

Reproduced with permission from DermNet NZ www.dermnetnz.org

Consultation 29

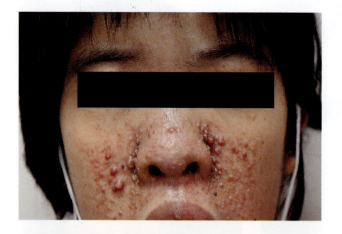

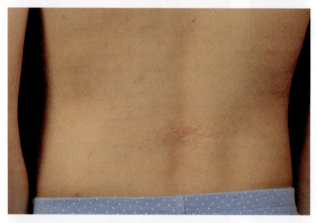

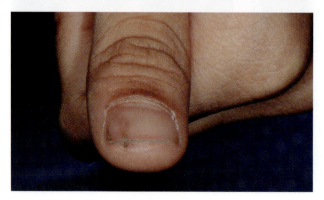

Clinical photos generously provided by Assoc Prof Mark Koh and Dr Cheryl Lie, KK Women's and Children's Hospital

Consultation 42

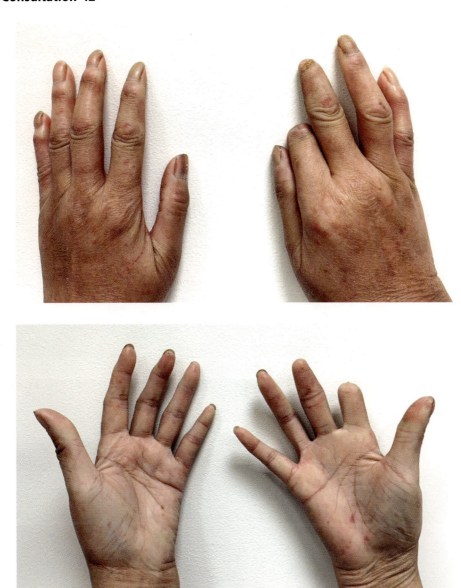

Clinical photo generously provided by Dr Jon Yoong Kah Choun, Singapore General Hospital

Consultation 49

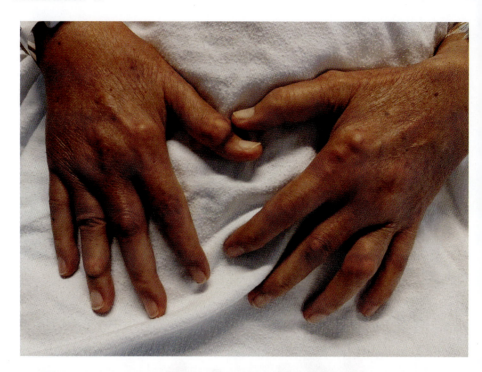

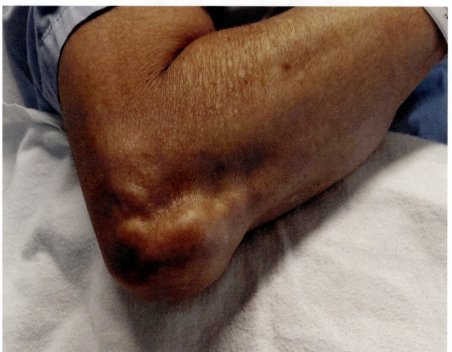

Consultation 50

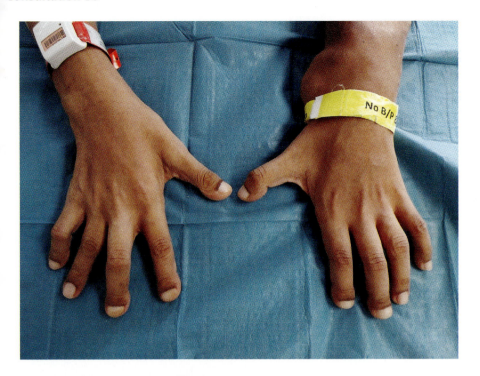

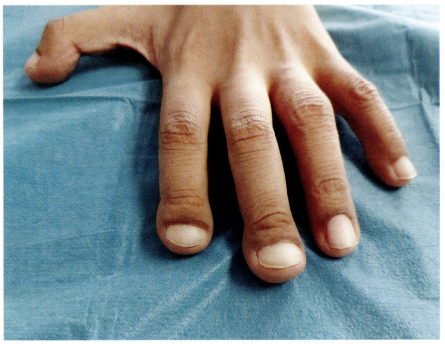

Section C: Communications

Communications

1 | Introduction and Walk-Through

The PACES communications station is a test of clinical maturity in dealing with tricky ethical and communications scenarios, and approximates real-life scenarios quite well.

Communication is not just about placating an angry patient or comforting a sad one. While these 'communications skills' are important, there is usually information that you must deliver and issues that you must address. By the end of your station, you must have provided enough information in an appropriate manner that empowers the patient to make an informed choice. You may also be required to formulate a workable plan and ensure that the patient (and those around him/her) is safe. To do so, you must often find out more about the patient, including his/her ideas, concerns, and expectations.

The communications station may also be a test of content knowledge in specific areas:

- Ability to explain disease conditions in a simple manner to the patient.
- Giving sound practical advice (e.g., fitness to drive, pregnancy).
- Negotiating a treatment plan.
- Knowledge of legal principles (e.g., those surrounding organ transplant, infectious disease, coroner's law, mental capacity, occupational health and industrial injury).
- Troubleshooting complex ethical dilemmas, particularly the tension between autonomy and beneficence/non-maleficence.

The best way to prepare for the communications station is to communicate well with real patients — whether breaking bad news (which we do all the time), dealing with angry patients (of which there are an abundance), or counselling on disease complications, compliance, and the like. Try to improve in all these interactions, learn good communication habits, and get feedback on how well you communicate. Under exam pressure, many of us revert to our 'baseline' at which we perform day to day, not to the 'ideal' which we practice for.

The new PACES format doubles the number of communications encounters, so this station must not be taken lightly.

The subsequent segments provide a run-through of the communications station and a discussion of appropriate strategy.

Planning and Suggested Framework

Use the time outside the room to identify what you must cover. The provided stem is often rather general (e.g., "inform Ms X about the diagnosis and address her concerns"). Apart from accomplishing the stated task, there may be additional hidden issues that you must address. These may only unfold during the course of the station, but can usually be predicted outside the room.

Example: consider the following vignette:

> Mr E, a 40-year-old odd job worker, was admitted for a seizure. He has a known diagnosis of epilepsy and has been admitted 4 times in the last 3 months for seizures. Your consultant is concerned that he does not seem to understand his condition. Please speak to Mr E and educate him about epilepsy.

This is a case of poorly controlled epilepsy. In addition to explaining the diagnosis of epilepsy, you must also:

1. Explore why his control is so poor:
   - Has he been compliant to medication? If not, why?
     - Has he suffered from medication side effects that need to be addressed?
     - What are the barriers to compliance? Can you offer any solutions?
     - Does he understand the risk involved? You need to convey in no uncertain terms that there is a risk of death associated with uncontrolled epilepsy.
   - Are there triggers that he needs to avoid?
2. Address the safety issue — in this case, driving.

Framework

We recommend the following framework to analyse a communications scenario.

1. What do I need to assess?/What information do I need to gather?
2. What do I need to convey?
3. What is the safety issue here?
4. What are the ethics and communications principles here?

1. **What do I need to assess?/What information do I need to gather?** Letting the patient talk more is often very important. Specific pieces of information that you need to gather may include:

- Finding out more about the patient, including his/her background, occupation, social setup, and daily life. This is particularly important if you are counselling the patient about a condition that affects his/her everyday living.
- In a patient who is not improving with treatment or is non-compliant to therapy, it is important to find out why the patient is non-compliant. This usually entails

Introduction and Walk-Through

delving into the patient's social background, what he/she values and might consider important, side effects and barriers to therapy, as well as unearthing misconceived ideas and expectations.

- How did the patient get this condition? In HIV diagnosis, for example, take a sexual history; in mesothelioma diagnosis, take an occupational history for asbestos exposure; if the patient has infective endocarditis, ask about known rheumatic heart disease and intravenous drug use.
- In a young lady, plans for pregnancy may be an issue.
- In an 'angry patient' scenario, find out how the patient has been doing *now* and address any immediate clinical need.

2. **What do I need to convey?** You must empower the patient to make an informed decision by providing all the necessary information in a clear but kind manner, tailored to the patient's need. For example:

- A patient who wants to discharge against advice/is non-compliant to treatment: "I am worried that you may die if you do not stay to receive treatment"; "You almost died from this attack of asthma and if you do not take steps to control your asthma, you are at a real risk of not surviving the next attack." Do not be vague or downplay the risks because that robs the patient of the chance to make an informed decision.
- In a very anxious patient whom you are informing of an unfavourable diagnosis, you have to be honest about the risks and potential outcomes, however bad. However, break the bad news kindly and empathetically, emphasising support or treatment that is available as well as any silver lining (if there is one).
- Do not give false hope – in a brain death or limitation of care scenario, you must state unequivocally that the patient is dead/has a poor prognosis. Any glimmer of hope (e.g., that the patient may still turn around or euphemisms that suggest perhaps the patient is not dead) will be seized upon and this will make it impossible to discuss limitation of care/organ donation/etc.
- In a disease counselling scenario, you are probably expected to give some information about the disease and come up with a holistic management plan.

3. **What is the safety issue here?** This is your responsibility to address and the patient surrogate may not specifically ask you about this.

- Clinical risk: in a new diagnosis of a condition, are there any clinical issues that the patient should be warned of? For example, in a patient newly diagnosed with polycystic kidney disease, you should counsel the patient on what to do if he/she suffers a sudden severe headache.
- Driving: if the station is about a condition that affects fitness to drive (e.g., stroke, transient ischaemic attack, hypoglycaemia, epilepsy), you must ask whether the patient drives, and if so, whether he/she does so vocationally. You may need to inform the patient that he/she is unfit to drive or refer him/her for a driving assessment to resume driving.

- Public health: any risk to public health needs to be addressed. For example:
  - Infectious disease: patients worked up for suspected HIV/diagnosed to have HIV must be counselled of the risk of transmission. You must inform the patient of the legal obligation to not 'recklessly spread' HIV (UK) or to inform all sexual partners regardless of whether a condom is used (Singapore). You should also explore testing of partners.
  - Patient diagnosed with mesothelioma: ask if the patient's spouse washes his/her clothes. If so, the spouse may also be at risk of asbestos exposure.
- Suicide risk/support strategy: in breaking bad news stations, the patient may become depressed and suicidal. It may not be necessary in every breaking bad news station but if the surrogate starts to sound depressed, you will need to assess and act on any suicide risk. Also assess the patient's social support (e.g., home alone) and whether he/she needs someone to look out for him/her.

4. **What are the ethics and communications principles here?** The PACES new format removes the 5-minute discussion with examiners in the communications station. While you will no longer be explicitly asked to describe the ethical principles in the encounter, it is still advantageous to be aware of these issues so that you can address them.

- Be aware of the communications framework that must be used (e.g., breaking bad news, angry patient, etc.).
- Understand the ethical tension in the scenario (e.g., between patient autonomy and risk to others; justice).
- Know the ethical bottom line – what you cannot give in to even if the patient tries to persuade you. For example:
  - You cannot divulge confidential patient information to a relative if the patient has explicitly denied consent for you to do so.
  - In a medical error scenario, you cannot give out the name of the person who made the mistake. Rather, you should direct the patient to the appropriate feedback channels and await results of official investigation.

During the Consult

The communications task is a conversation with the patient, so resist the urge to information dump or to talk over the patient. It is somewhat like peeling an onion — as the conversation develops, you peel off one layer at a time, allowing the patient to reveal to you his/her innermost concerns. Only then can you grasp the patient's agenda. You must address both the patient's agenda as well as the essential aspects that you must cover.

Tip 1: Begin with open-ended questions. Always establish what the patient already knows and has at the top of his/her mind. Do not be hasty to respond, but let the patient continue for at least a full minute. Only then, move to asking close-ended questions and probe for specific pieces of information you need.

Tip 2: Gather information. Let the patient talk more than you do. While you can guess the likely communications issue, you are provided with awfully little information about the patient's specific concerns. Consider:

> *Scenario: Patient has S. aureus bacteraemia from an infected tunnelled dialysis catheter. The line has been removed and he is scheduled for 2 weeks of antibiotics.*
>
> *Patient: "I don't care, let me go home now."*

Resist the urge to preach to the patient right away. Instead, pause to gather information — find out why the patient wants to go home. He may very well reply, "My 90-year-old bedbound mum is home alone and if I don't go home, nobody will feed her and she will starve to death." If so, then you must find a solution — make an arrangement that allows his mother to be cared for (e.g., call in social services, get a relative to help, arrange for home leave or outpatient antibiotic therapy if appropriate) while allowing the patient to complete his antibiotics! Subsequently, you can use his desire to care for his mum as a starting point: "I can see that you really love your mum. I am worried that if you do not complete your antibiotics, you might become very sick, stay in hospital for a long time, or even die. Has it come to mind how your mum would be cared for if something were to happen to you?"

Tip 3: Respond to the patient. Listen to the patient and do not just focus on your agenda! In particular, give the patient a chance to ask questions and answer his/her questions directly. Consider the following vignette:

> *Candidate: Mdm X, I'm afraid that the HIV test has returned positive. [Pause]*
>
> *Patient: I'm not surprised. I've had a hard life. Tell me, what do I do now?*

Many candidates respond by expressing empathy at the diagnosis and explaining all that needs to be done (including further tests, treatment initiation, informing partners, etc.). However, it would be far better to take up the lead that the patient dropped: "Why would you not be surprised?" This may reveal significant information that is of relevance to your counselling! Your PACES patient is a surrogate and must ask you the questions given in their briefing sheet, so they will lead you in the right direction.

Tip 4: Communicate clearly and sincerely. You must provide clear information that empowers the patient to make an informed decision. Avoid jargon and give information in bite sizes. Do not waffle around — if there is a risk of death, you must say so explicitly. At the same time, be kind. You can always offer a silver lining (e.g., "this is treatable" or "although we do not think that we can cure her, we will do everything we can to make sure that she does not suffer").

Tip 5: Dealing with emotion: mirror and meet the patient. Be sensitive to the patient's expressed emotions. Mirroring is a good tool to show empathy and that you are listening (e.g., Patient: "It doesn't matter because my life is a mess." Response: "It does matter. I care about you and I want the best for you"). Meet the patient where he/she is and match his/her emotional state. For example, if you have broken bad news and the patient is distraught, give him/her more time. On the other hand, if he/she is surprisingly alright and is pushing you with questions, do not harp on empathy statements.

Tip 6: Dealing with resistance: the techniques of motivational interviewing come in very handy here.

- **Roll with resistance**: Resist the urge to push back and get into a head on argument. Importantly, don't undermine the patient — show that you have heard what the patient has said. Explore the patient's point of view by trying to find out why exactly they say what they say. For example, if a patient complains about side effects of inhaled steroids, do not say, "No, the side effects are minor, you should still take them." Instead say, "Taking steroids must be very terrifying to you. Could you tell me a bit more about what you have heard about steroids or anything in particular you are concerned about?"
- **Develop discrepancy**: As you gather information about the patient, find out what the patient's wider goals and objectives are. Reflect back (in a non-confrontational way) how their views or short-term decisions might be discrepant from their expressed wider goals. For example, "I hear that you are really frustrated about your asthma control and in particular having to be admitted, which is really disruptive for your work. On the other hand, you don't really want to be taking these inhalers everyday because they are troublesome. The two things you want seem to be at odds here. Any thoughts on which of the two would be more important to you?" Another example: "I know that going back is very important to you and you don't want to stay in the hospital. If you go home without treatment and your disease worsens, would you be able to continue working?" Realise that to use this strategy, you need to find some reason for the patient to want the positive intervention. Become the patient's advocate and use his/her concerns against him/her.
- **Offer a solution**: Sometimes there may be a solution or compromise that will achieve both what the patient wants and what you want for the patient. Where you are faced with a binary choice, think of a 'third way' — for example, instead of a binary choice between discharge and inpatient care, consider offering outpatient antibiotic therapy as a compromise that marries the patient's desires with appropriate treatment.

Summarize and Formulate a Plan

The summary in the last 2 minutes is critical. You must:
1. Summarise the key points of your discussion and check if the patient has understood. Also state your reading of the patient's key concerns.
2. Explain the management plan going forward:
   a. The clinical management plan, such as tests you will do or treatment you will administer to address an issue (e.g., sick patient, medical error), as well as further tests or treatment for a new diagnosis.

b. The communications plan, such as referral to allied health counsellors, provision of patient information, and escalation of grievance to appropriate channels (e.g., patient liaison service, service quality, medical board).

c. If you are unable to completely address the communications issue, provide a follow up appointment to resume the conversation.

3. Reiterate safety issues, such as driving, red flag symptoms, and when to seek immediate medical attention.

Communications

2 | Worked Practice

This section provides deliberate practice for the PACES communications station. While they are in no way comprehensive, these cases are selected for their teaching points with a focus on challenging communication tasks and complex ethical and legal issues.

Each case includes information for the candidate and a detailed patient's brief. You should pair up to attempt these cases, rather than merely read through them! Each case is also accompanied by suggested planning notes (i.e., issues you should identify while outside the room) and a discussion of the relevant strategy, skills, and content knowledge.

Practice with a colleague or tutor. Use the pull-out 'candidate information' booklet, which gives the candidate's information for all practice scenarios, to blind yourself to the patient's brief and discussion.

2 Worked Practice

Communication Case 01

Missed Bleed

Use this case as practice! The pull-out booklet contains the candidate's information.

Information for the Candidate

Patient Details: Mdm Koh Ma, 80 years old

Your Role: Neurology Ward SHO

Information: Mdm Koh came to the Emergency Department yesterday evening complaining of headache and vomiting. She was diagnosed with migraine and sent home on analgesia.

This morning, her family members could not wake her up from sleep. She was brought back to the Emergency Department and a CT brain showed a massive subarachnoid hemorrhage. She is currently in the operating theatre undergoing decompression surgery.

Your task is to speak to Mdm Koh's daughter to update her of her mother's situation and address any concerns that she may have.

Planning (From the Stem)

1. **What do I need to assess?/What information do I need to gather?**
   - What does Mdm Koh's daughter already know?
2. **What do I need to convey?**
   - Break bad news and apologise for the error
   - Current management plan moving forward
3. **What is the safety issue here?**
   - Do not implicate a colleague
4. **What are the ethics and communications principles here?**
   - Breaking bad news
   - Dealing with medical error

Surrogate's Brief

You are a 55-year-old secretary. You are unmarried and stay with your elderly mum, with whom you have a close relationship. Mum is a sprightly 80-year-old whose only past medical history is hypertension. She spends her time volunteering at a local charity and playing mahjong with friends.

Yesterday morning, you brought Mum to the Emergency Department because she complained of sudden-onset severe headache and vomiting. The Emergency Department doctor said it was just a migraine and told her that she could go home. You understand that some basic blood tests were performed, but not a scan of the brain. You felt uneasy because Mum does not usually get migraines, but did not question the doctor then. Mum was fine when she went home and the pain subsided with medications.

To your horror, Mum could not be roused from sleep this morning. You even tried to splash cold water on her face, but she could not be roused. You immediately called for an ambulance which brought her back to the Emergency Department. It has been three hours and you have not been updated on Mum's condition. You are aware that Mum has been wheeled to surgery, but you have no other information on her condition except that it is serious. You are anxious and frantic.

If informed that Mum has a bleed in the brain, you will not take the news well. You are convinced that the diagnosis was missed yesterday when she first came to the Emergency Department. If a CT scan had been performed, perhaps Mum could have been operated on earlier and would not have had such a serious bleed. You believe that yesterday's doctor was incompetent and will like to seek redress for this error. You worry about whether Mum will ever wake up.

You have some specific questions for the doctor at this consultation:

- Why was she not scanned in the A&E yesterday?
- Tell me whose fault is this; give me the name of the Emergency Department doctor who saw her yesterday.
- Why are you talking to me; where is your consultant?

Case Discussion

Medical error and undesirable patient outcomes are classic PACES scenarios. While unpleasant and intimidating, they are among the easiest communications tasks to handle, rarely deviating from the standard communications playbook, requiring little content knowledge (which can trip you up in other stations), and containing few ethical dilemmas to navigate. 'Angry patient' scenarios are not actually difficult as long as you don't become frazzled — it is a test of patience and communication; be honest, empathetic, and clear.

Begin by breaking bad news as per the SPIKES framework (Table C5.1). Find out what the patient already knows — if the patient already knows that an error has occurred, go straight to the next segment. It is important to read the surrogate's verbal and non-verbal communication and respond accordingly — if he/she has no mood for gentle lead-ins, go to the point more quickly; if he/she is very distraught, give more space and time. Communicate clearly — one common error is to beat around the bush and not clearly explain, for example, that the patient is in a critical condition. This leaves the patient or caretaker confused and you with little time for the rest of the scenario.

Having broken the information in a neutral and factual manner, respond to the surrogate's anger by acknowledging, reflecting, and *validating* these feelings — for example: "I am so sorry that you are going through this, I can only imagine how you are feeling. I don't have all the answers for you now." Be mindful of non-verbal communication (see 'Pitfall') and avoid unhelpful messages (Table C5.2).

Table C5.1. 'SPIKES' – a template for breaking bad news.

Element	Key aspects/script
Setting	Introduce yourself
	Clarify the surrogate's name and relationship to patient
	Position yourself and the surrogate appropriately
	Ask if there is anyone else that he/she would like to join the conversation
Perception	"Before I begin, may I ask what you understand so far, so that I know where to start?"
Invitation	Warning shot and ask for permission to proceed, for example:
	"I need to tell you that Mum's not well… [pause]", or
	"I need to speak to you about Mum's condition. Is this a good time?"
Knowledge	Give information in bite sized pieces
	Check understanding as you go
Emotion	Acknowledge emotional response, including naming the emotion explicitly, for instance: "This is very sudden and very hard to bear. I can't imagine how upset you must be."
Strategy	Management plan going forward

Table C5.2. Unhelpful messages.

Theme	Examples
False empathy	"I understand" – an easy retort is "no you don't."
Limiting expression of emotions	"Do not worry" – this is as good as denying permission to talk about his/her worries.
	"You must be strong for your family"
Minimising losses	"You'll get over this" / "Time heals all wounds"
	"You must get on with life"
	"Others are worse off than you" / "At least she is still alive"
Religious cliché	"You must believe that God has a plan for this"
	"God never gives us more than we can handle"
	"Someday God will explain why this happened"
	"Only the good die young"
	(These themes may be appropriate if the patient/family first brings them up as a means of rationalising and coping)

Pitfall: Non-verbal communication

> Non-verbal communication is just as important as what you say! Practice 'angry patient' scenarios with each other and videotape yourself. You will be surprised how unaware of our mannerisms and body language we can be!

The delay in diagnosis of intracranial haemorrhage must be addressed.

- Avoid phrases like "the A&E made a mistake", "the A&E didn't think of XXX", or "the A&E should have done XXX." In this scenario, it is not clear that medical error has undeniably been committed. We do not know what information was available to the A&E physician at the time of the initial consult. There could very well have been no overwhelming clinical evidence of a sinister cause of headache that would prompt a CT brain then. You should not throw A&E under the bus.

  Note: For scenarios in which a clear medical error has been committed, you will need to acknowledge the error. Use neutral terms such as "there has been an issue" and state factually what happened. Be wary of legal terms such as 'negligent' because it is not your place to adjudicate the presence of negligence.

- On the other hand, you should not be overly defensive. For example, do not go out of your way to justify why the A&E did nothing wrong. You must demonstrate that you are trying to be open and do not have anything to hide.

- Explain that there will be an investigation or review process, for example: "Our hospital will conduct a full investigation into what exactly happened and once we have the full details, we can arrange another meeting to go through those findings with you." Explain that measures will be put in place to prevent a recurrence, if there indeed was a shortcoming and preventable error.

- If the surrogate/patient still has further grievances, refer him/her to appropriate channels (e.g., feedback unit, service quality, patient advisory and liaison) as per local practice.

Turn the focus to what you will do for the patient right now, for example: "You have every right to know what happened and we will keep you updated. Right now let me focus on doing everything I can for your mum." Explain the current clinical management plan, stating clearly that her condition is critical and requiring emergency surgery which is being arranged this very minute. Provide information about prognosis if this is available (e.g., likelihood of recovery after drug toxicity). In this scenario, you do not have prognostic information, so explain that you will update her after the operation is completed.

Her questions are commonly encountered both in PACES and in real life.

- *"Give me the name of the A&E doctor"*/*"Whose fault is it?"* The principle is not to implicate your colleague — it would be a clear 'fail'. A stock answer is: "I'm afraid I do not have this information right now. I cannot be giving you the wrong information. Many people have been involved in her care and we will need to review what happened and at what point. You will be updated about the outcome of the investigation and we will let you know exactly what happened, whether this could have been prevented, and if so, what steps will be taken." Note that the name of all physicians involved may eventually be provided, particularly if the patient pursues legal action, but it will have to be done only after careful review and not in the current setting.

- *"Why are you talking to me, where is your consultant?"* This is easier to deflect in PACES than in real life. Try: "The nurse told me that you are here and I did not want to keep you waiting, so I decided to speak to you first. My consultant was with another patient and he is making his way over right now. He should be here in 10 minutes, but let me answer as many of your questions as I can."

Communication Case 02

Brain Dead

Note: There are variations in organ transplant laws. How this scenario runs depends on where and when you take the exam. Use the relevant candidate information and refer to the further discussion in the worked answer.

Use this case as practice! The pull-out booklet contains the candidate's information.

Information for the Candidate

Patient Details: Mr Muhammad Bin Muhammad, 22 years old

Your Role: Intensive Care Unit SHO

Information: Mr Muhammad, a 22-year-old university student, was admitted 48 hours ago following a road traffic accident. He was crossing the road with the traffic lights in his favour, but was hit by a speeding truck and suffered massive intracranial haemorrhage.

Version (a) if taking the exam in Singapore, (b) if in the UK.

(a) **Singapore:** He has been pronounced brain dead by two independent consultants. Currently he is normotensive and in sinus rhythm. He is kept intubated and ventilated with the intention of facilitating organ harvesting. He is not known to have opted out of organ donation under the Human Organ Transplant Act.

(b) **UK:** He has been pronounced brain dead by two independent consultants. Currently he is normotensive and in sinus rhythm. He is kept intubated and ventilated with the intention of facilitating organ harvesting.

Your task is to update his parents about the diagnosis of brain death and approach the idea of organ donation.

Planning (From the Stem)

1. **What do I need to assess?/What information do I need to gather?**
   - What Mr Muhammad's parents understand about his condition.
   - Mr Muhammad's premorbid views on organ donation.
   - His parents' views on organ donation.
2. **What do I need to convey?**
   - Breaking bad news: Muhammad is brain dead.

- That Mr Muhammad is a suitable organ donor, and what this would entail.

3. **What is the safety issue here?**
   - Be clear that brain death = death.
4. **What are the ethics and communications principles here?**
   - Breaking bad news.
   - Justice – organ transplant and relevant legislation.

Patient's Brief

You are Mr/Mrs Muhammad (senior). Muhammad is your only son whom you love dearly. He was a bright young man and the first in your family to go to university. You are aware that your son has been involved in a traffic accident. You are not aware of the full extent of his injuries, but you notice that his heartbeat and breathing is intact. You believe that your son is still alive and will recover. You will react to bad news with shock and despair. You have never heard about the concept of 'brain death' and you struggle to grasp that your son is dead when he is still breathing and his heart is still beating.

Your entire family are practicing Muslims. You believe that the body must be buried immediately in its entirety and you are uncomfortable with organ donation — you are worried that it would disfigure the body, which might be unacceptable to Allah. You are unaware of any laws surrounding organ donation. While your son has never explicitly expressed his views on organ donation, he had always been actively involved in volunteer work and social activism, and you suspect that he might have supported organ donation. You may be persuaded to agree to organ donation on the basis that it might benefit others.

Note: If you are not convinced that your son is dead, you will not be willing to talk about organ donation.

You have some specific questions for the doctor at this consultation:

- Surely he can't be dead – his heart is still beating, is it not?
- Can he still wake up?
- Will organ donation delay his funeral and disfigure the body?

Case Discussion

This is a classic PACES station and one that is never easy in both PACES and real life.

Begin by gathering information (what does Muhammad senior understand) and breaking bad news using the SPIKES framework (Table C5.1). You have to be empathetic but firm in stating that Muhammad is dead and will not wake up. It is understandably difficult to grasp how he is actually dead when he is still breathing, so you must clarify that his heart and lungs are artificially maintained and he is not breathing on his own. Approach brain death as an established fact, not a decision that is negotiable.

State clearly that Muhammad has passed away — do not waffle around. You must not leave any sliver of hope that the patient could still be alive, or the surrogate will immediately cling on to it, leaving you in the unenviable position of trying to overcome the surrogate's doubts. It is far kinder and easier to be gentle but firm from the start. It will also be impossible to talk about organ transplant if you do not clearly establish that Muhammad is dead.

Next, transit to a discussion about organ donation. This transition can be tricky — one suggestion is: "There is one more thing I need to talk to you about. [Pause] Unfortunately I did not have the chance to meet your son, but I would like to find out from you as you know him best; if he were still able to speak for himself now, would he have wanted to save the life of someone else by donating his organs?" This lead-in directs the parent's focus to what Muhammad would have wanted, instead of eliciting the knee-jerk reaction of a parent to say no to something that is perceived to harm their child. Therefore, it is important to find out whether Muhammad had any known views about organ donation (e.g., if he said anything while he was still alive) and pay special attention to anything in the stem that might hint at Muhammad's character, in particular whether he would have wanted to help others.

You should be able to explain the process of organ transplantation (in particular that life support is kept 'on' to keep blood flowing to the organs, but is turned off immediately after organ harvesting). Emphasise the benefits of organ transplantation and how even in this loss, there is a chance that others may gain a new lease of life. There will be objections raised and you should address these, for example:

- Delay to funeral: acknowledge the delay which should be hours from the point of brain death. You will expedite the process.
- Disfiguring the body: organ harvesting will be like any other surgery. The wound will be closed up after harvesting, leaving a surgical scar. While there will be a scar, the body will not look disfigured.
- Emphasise that Muhammad will feel no pain or suffering (as he is already dead).
- Religious objection: the Islamic religious authorities in Singapore (MUIS)/Islamic scholars in the UK have issued *fatwas* declaring that deceased organ donation is permissible in principle. However, acknowledge that you are no expert on Muslim religious law and you will link him up with an Imam (Muslim religious authority) who may be able to clarify the religious position.

You will need to be cognisant of the legal position on deceased organ donation in the jurisdiction in which you are taking PACES. This is a developing area, so you must keep up-to-date on any changes occurring after the print date of this book.

- 'Opt-out' consent system. This is the case in Singapore (under the Human Organ Transplant Act) and in England from 2020. Under this system, individuals who do not opt out of organ donation are automatically organ donors. While organ donation can proceed regardless of family consent, you should not deal with organ donation as a matter of legal compulsion — that is, coldly stating that organ donation is compulsory and that the family has no say in the matter and no right to object. You must still demonstrate empathy, consideration for the human element, and advocate for organ donation.

- 'Opt-in' consent system. This is the case in the rest of the UK and in most other Commonwealth countries in which PACES is conducted. Under this system, organ donation can only proceed if the deceased has not expressed any objection, and if family members do not object. Family agreement is seen as critical — should the patient have opted in as an organ donor but the family subsequently objects, the practice is not to proceed with organ harvesting.

Depending on how surrogate is briefed, you may or may not be able to convince the surrogate to agree to organ donation — not being able to convince the surrogate does not necessarily mean that you have done badly. If you are able to convince them, follow up with an action plan, such as that a transplant coordinator will be in touch with them shortly and will explain the process in greater detail. If you are unable to, offer to have a transplant coordinator link up with them to provide further information, give them time to consider/discuss the matter, and set a time (e.g., 2 hours later) to meet again.

Think this through: Permutations to the scenario

> There are a number of permutations to this scenario including disagreements between family members (e.g., a spouse agrees but the parents do not). How would you deal with this?

Communication Case 03

Discussing Anticoagulation

Use this case as practice! The pull-out booklet contains the candidate's information.

Information for the Candidate

Patient Details: Ms Rebecca Clot, 30 years old

Your Role: Haematology Clinic SHO

Information: Ms Clot presented to the Emergency Department 2 days ago with right leg swelling. Compression venous ultrasound confirmed the diagnosis of deep vein thrombosis (DVT) involving the femoral and popliteal veins. The Emergency physician has started her on subcutaneous low molecular weight heparin (1 mg/kg) and given her a fast-track appointment to see you today.

You have determined that Ms Clot's DVT is likely provoked by use of a combined oral contraceptive pill. She does not have any other risk factor for DVT, no underlying medical illness, and no family history of thrombosis. There is no clinical concern for pulmonary embolism at the present moment.

Your task is to counsel Ms Clot about the management options for her condition.

Planning (From the Stem)

1. **What do I need to assess?/What information do I need to gather?**
   - If Ms Clot might be pregnant, or has any plans for pregnancy.
   - Risk of anticoagulation: bleeding risk, renal or hepatic impairment, or other drug use.
2. **What do I need to convey?**
   - Discuss therapeutic options in DVT – subcutaneous low molecular weight heparin (LMWH), direct oral anticoagulants (DOAC), or warfarin.
   - To stop oral contraceptive pills and consider other family planning methods that do not involve the use of oestrogen.
   - Symptoms of pulmonary embolism to watch for.
3. **What is the safety issue here?**
   - Ms Clot should receive anticoagulation. No treatment is not an advisable option.
4. **What are the ethics and communications principles here?**
   - Autonomy – shared decision making.

Communication Case 03

Patient's Brief

You are a 30-year-old lawyer. You went to the Emergency Department 2 days ago with a 3-day history of right leg swelling. The Emergency physician told you that you have a clot in your leg and started you on blood thinners via injection.

This diagnosis is frightening to you, and you have many questions about the treatment ahead. You have not had the chance to learn about your condition or the blood thinners you are taking. Your work schedule is hectic, you don't really like having to inject yourself each day, and you don't like the idea of having to return for frequent blood tests. If not taking any medicines at all is a feasible option, you would gladly go with that.

You do not have any significant medical history. You have never had problems with bleeding, easy bruising, or heavy periods. You do not have any weight loss, joint pain, breathlessness, recent illnesses, hospitalisation, surgeries, long flights, or kidney or liver problems. You have been taking the combined oral contraceptive pill daily for the past 5 years, but are otherwise not on any medications, including blood thinners, supplements, or herbal remedies. You have no family history of any blood disorder or clotting problems. You are certain that you are not pregnant as you are currently having your menses.

You are sexually active with your fiancé. You are planning to get married next month. You have not thought about when you might desire to have children — and would like to keep your options open for now and hear about treatment options for whether you are pregnant or not. You will not volunteer this information unless specifically asked.

You have some specific questions for the doctor at this consultation:

- Is not taking any medications an option?
- How long do I have to be on blood thinners for?
- I don't really like these injections. Are there any other blood thinners I can try?
- I've heard that blood thinners can cause bleeding. Will I bleed?
- Is there anything else I need to take note of?

Case Discussion

Discussing anticoagulation (whether for venous thromboembolism, atrial fibrillation, or prosthetic heart valves) is not only common in PACES but also likely to be a part of your daily clinical practice. Whereas other scenarios may emphasise communication skills with a difficult patient (e.g., non-compliance, refusal of anticoagulation), this scenario focuses on content knowledge and employs a cooperative if somewhat anxious patient.

The task is phrased in a rather non-specific manner ("counsel Ms Clot about the management options for her condition"); in such situations it is best to begin by finding out what the surrogate already knows and set the agenda upfront (i.e., ask the surrogate upfront what are his/her key questions).

The key communication principle in such a station is **shared decision making**. That is, you will need to provide information on the various options, their pros and cons, and come to a shared decision with the patient on the treatment plan. While you are explicitly asked NOT to take a history, and this stem helpfully provides you with a helpful amount of information, you will usually be required to elicit certain pieces of information — particularly, in this case, the consideration of pregnancy. Key points to cover are:

1. **Is anticoagulation necessary?**
   - Explain the diagnosis of DVT.
   - Note that there are some circumstances in which anticoagulation is not necessary (Table C5.3).
   - Outside of these scenarios, explain that anticoagulation is indicated to prevent clot extension and pulmonary embolism. Use layman language, for example: "If we do not treat you, the clot can grow bigger and cause more leg swelling and pain. A portion of the clot can break off and fly to the lung, which can cause you to be very breathless and in some cases can be very dangerous."
   - Drawing a diagram of the leg veins and how embolisation may occur can greatly aid your explanation (and demonstrate superior initiative and effort to the examiner).
   - Although you must simplify concepts, you cannot be inaccurate. For instance, it is not correct to say that anticoagulation will 'dissolve' the clot (it is not thrombolysis; resolution of existing thrombosis happens by physiological mechanisms and not because of anticoagulation).

Table C5.3. Circumstances in which no anticoagulation is favoured.

Circumstance	Comment
AF with CHA2DS2-VASc score = 0, or score = 1 for female sex alone	For AF with CHA2DS2-VASc score = 1 for other risk factors, either anticoagulation or none is acceptable
Asymptomatic distal (below knee) DVT	Follow up with repeat ultrasound to exclude clot progression
AF or VTE with high bleeding risk	Consider inferior vena cava filter if VTE with high risk of pulmonary embolism
Moribund patient	Patient not expected to benefit from anticoagulation

AF: atrial fibrillation; VTE: venous thromboembolism

2. **Which anticoagulation option to opt for?**
    - The three main options are:
        ○ Warfarin: requires dose adjustments based on frequent INR monitoring.
        ○ Low molecular weight heparin (LMWH): fixed-dose subcutaneous injections.
        ○ Direct oral anticoagulants (DOAC): fixed-dose and do not require injections but carries important contraindications.
    - The choice between warfarin, LMWH, and DOACs depends on the indication for anticoagulation, patient comorbidities, and patient preference (Table C5.4).
    - It is important to ask Ms Clot about pregnancy and plans for pregnancy as this will severely restrict anticoagulation options.
    - If she does not intend to get pregnant, then she would be a candidate for all 3 and you should explain all options and ask her for her preference.

3. **What duration of anticoagulation is required?**
    - Duration of anticoagulation in DVT depends on whether there is an identifiable risk factor that can be reversed. Note that the terminology of 'provoked' and 'unprovoked' DVT is less helpful (e.g., malignancy 'provokes' DVT but it is an irreversible risk factor).
        ○ DVT with reversible risk factors (e.g., recent surgery): 3 months anticoagulation, possibly extend to 6 months if there is extensive pulmonary embolism.
        ○ DVT with irreversible or persistent risk factors (e.g., malignancy on palliative therapy, congenital thrombophilia): long-term anticoagulation.
        ○ DVT without an identifiable risk factor: individualise decision. The 10-year recurrence rate off anticoagulation is 20–30%, so long-term anticoagulation is reasonable in a patient with low bleeding risk.
    - Ms Clot has oestrogen-associated DVT, which constitutes a reversible risk factor and therefore you should advise her to receive 3 months of anticoagulation and to stop oral contraceptive pills.

4. **Risks to counsel for**
    - Ask Ms Clot if she has any history of unusual bleeding (e.g., heavy periods) or if she is on any other blood thinners.
    - Advice Ms Clot of the risk of bleeding and safety precautions (e.g., avoid high-risk situations, when to seek medical advice).
    - Advice Ms Clot of symptoms of pulmonary embolism and when to seek medical attention.

Table C5.4. Factors in choosing anticoagulant options.

Factor	Choice	Comments
Indication for anticoagulation: Warfarin, LMWH, or DOACs are equally acceptable for most indications except –		
Valvular AF (severe mitral stenosis or mechanical valves)	Warfarin only	All other valvular lesions do not constitute 'valvular AF'
Antiphospholipid syndrome	Warfarin or LMWH	DOAC failure has been described
Patient comorbids		
Malignancy-associated VTE	LMWH Rivaroxaban Apixaban	Traditionally LWMH only, but recent trials show rivaroxaban, edoxaban, and apixaban as (at least) non-inferior[1]
Renal impairment (creatinine clearance < 30 ml/min)	Warfarin LMWH Apixaban	LMWH requires dose adjustment. Apixaban can be safely used with CrCl > 15 ml/min; use in end-stage renal failure is controversial[2]
Hepatic impairment (Child-Pugh B or C)	Warfarin LMWH	DOACs contraindicated as these patients were excluded from large trials
Pregnancy	LMWH	Warfarin is teratogenic. DOACs cross the placenta and are not studied in pregnancy
Breastfeeding	Warfarin LMWH	DOACs are not studied
Extremes of weight	Warfarin LMWH	Not well studied in DOAC trials and no specific monitoring parameter
Unstable INR despite compliance	DOAC	Unstable INRs predispose to thrombotic and bleeding complications
Patient preference		
Minimising blood-taking, injections	DOAC	Oral medication, no INR monitoring
Avoid initial parenteral therapy with LMWH	Rivaroxaban Apixaban	Warfarin, dabigatran, and edoxaban all require initial LMWH therapy

AF: atrial fibrillation; CrCl: creatinine clearance; LMWH: low molecular weight heparin; VTE: venous thromboembolism

---

[1] Pivotal DOAC trials in malignancy-associated VTE include edoxaban: HOKUSAI-CANCER (*NEJM* 2018), rivaroxaban: SELECT-D (*J Clin Oncol* 2018), and apixaban: Carravaggio (*NEJM* 2020).

[2] Apixaban undergoes hepatic metabolism and is thought to be safer in renal impairment. Patients with creatinine clearance as low as 15 ml/min were enrolled into trials of apixaban for atrial fibrillation. However, the FDA approval for apixaban in end-stage kidney disease is controversial as it is based on small pharmacokinetic studies; many clinicians are uncomfortable giving apixaban to such patients.

5. **Other management pointers**
   - You will need to do blood tests before starting anticoagulation (liver function, creatinine, blood count, coagulation studies) if these have not been done.
   - Specific to oestrogen-associated DVT:
     - OCPs or hormone replacement therapy is contraindicated. She should stop OCPs and use another form of birth control (e.g., barrier methods, progesterone-only pills, intrauterine/implantable devices).
     - Need for prophylactic anticoagulation (low molecular weight heparin) during pregnancy, as this is a physiological state with high levels of oestrogen.
   - If Ms Clot opts for warfarin, additional counselling points include:
     - Explaining INR, target range, and need for monitoring.
     - Dietary counselling including maintaining consistent dietary vitamin K intake.
     - Drug interactions (i.e., avoid supplements/traditional medicine and inform any doctor she sees that she is on warfarin).
     - Teratogenicity and therefore if she becomes pregnant, she will need to see a doctor immediately to switch to LMWH therapy.
   - Link Ms Clot up with a pharmacist for medication counselling.

Communication Case 04

Still Hypertensive

Use this case as practice! The pull-out booklet contains the candidate's information.

Information for the Candidate

Patient Details: Mr E. O. See, 30 years old

Your Role: Medicine Clinic SHO

Information: Mr See is the Chief Executive Officer of a fast-growing tech start-up. He recently sought to purchase a £2,000,000 term life insurance plan. Due to the high coverage amount, the insurance provider elected to send Mr See for routine health screening before extending the cover.

Mr See was found to be hypertensive with a blood pressure reading of 170/95 mmHg (average over two visits). As a result, the insurance company has rejected Mr See's application for life insurance.

The general practitioner who saw Mr See has started him on lisinopril 20 mg OM and referred him to your clinic for work-up of young hypertension.

Mr See's blood pressure today is 173/94 mmHg.

Your task is to discuss work-up of young hypertension with Mr See and address any concerns that he may have.

Planning (From the Stem)

1. **What do I need to assess?/What information do I need to gather?**
   - What is Mr See's understanding about his disease (hypertension)?
   - Mr See's blood pressure today is still high – has he been taking the lisinopril? If not, what are the barriers to compliance?
   - What is important to Mr See? When he sought to purchase insurance, who/what was he trying to protect?

2. **What do I need to convey?**
   - Provide information about the long-term cardiovascular implications of uncontrolled hypertension and empower Mr See to make an informed decision.
   - Discuss young hypertension work-up and further treatment.

3. **What is the safety issue here?**
   - As Mr See's blood pressure today is high, ensure that he has no symptoms of hypertensive urgency.

4. **What are the ethics and communications principles here?**
    - Patient autonomy (to not take the medication) vs. beneficence (to prevent complications of hypertension).

Patient's Brief

You are the high-flying Chief Executive Officer (CEO) of a fast-growing tech start-up, earning £500,000 a year (excluding bonuses and stock options). Your job requires you to travel weekly, and you have been worried about the recent spate of aeroplane crashes. This is why you decided to increase your life insurance cover so that, should you be involved in an accident, the financial needs of your homemaker spouse and 3 month-old child would be taken care of.

You went for health screening at the insurer's request, as is standard for high-coverage insurance plans, and you are surprised to hear that your blood pressure is high. You have no family history of high blood pressure and you eat healthily, exercise regularly, and do not smoke. You feel extremely insulted that you have been denied insurance cover and are angry with the general practitioner who performed your health screening. The general practitioner did explain to you that high blood pressure can lead to heart attack and stroke. You agree that these can happen in older people but right now, you feel completely well and believe that you are too young and too fit to have any heart or brain problems.

You were also given a blood pressure medicine (lisinopril 20 mg daily). You took this for a week but it gave you an irritating cough. Since then, you have not taken any medication. You feel completely well and believe that you are better off without medication and without the cough.

At the insistence of your wife, you agreed to attend today's clinic visit with absolutely no intention of doing any further tests or taking any other medication. However, you might be amenable to persuasion if you are convinced that tests/medication can help to protect your spouse and child.

You have some specific questions for the doctor at this consultation:

- You doctors are the bane of my life. I am completely fine. You doctors denied me insurance cover and gave me that terrible cough. Why should I even listen to you?
- How can it be that my blood pressure is high? I feel completely fine and I eat well, exercise regularly, and do not smoke.
- Can you promise that I won't have any further side effects?

Case Discussion

Recognise from the candidate information that Mr See's blood pressure has not improved — he may not be taking his medication. Some candidates (and physicians) will rush in to ask Mr See if he has been taking his medications, and if not, why he has been non-compliant. This is a suboptimal strategy as you have yet to accumulate the tools with which to persuade Mr See and, if not done well, risks turning confrontational (e.g., "It is important to take your medications." / "No doc, I am perfectly fine." / "But this is dangerous." / "But I am perfectly fine.").

Pitfall: Resist the urge to lecture the patient!

> Most of us encounter patients who do not comply with therapy. Lecturing the patient about his non-compliance is usually a poor strategy. Rather, try to find out more about why the patient has made such choices, including what he/she understands and believes to be in his/her best interest. Then you can try to align his/her interests with yours.

Begin the station by establishing rapport and finding out how Mr See has been. Given that his blood pressure is quite high, it will be due diligence to spend twenty seconds screening through symptoms of a hypertensive emergency. Next, explore Mr See's background, ideas, concerns, and expectations. You may begin with an open question such as: "What do you understand about your blood pressure?" and 'How do you feel about it?"

Mr See will quickly reveal that (1) he believes that hypertension will not affect him, (2) he is skeptical of the diagnosis of hypertension because he has made healthy lifestyle choices, and (3) the side effect of cough was a barrier to compliance with blood pressure medication. Each of these needs to be dealt with at both rational and emotional levels. Express empathy at the sudden diagnosis and being denied insurance cover. Point out that it is precisely because he is at increased risk of adverse health outcomes that the insurance company felt that he was too risky to cover unless his blood pressure is brought under control. Clarify his misconceptions and state in no uncertain terms that uncontrolled hypertension can and will affect him (e.g., stroke, heart attack).

The key to this station (and similar scenarios) is the principle that patients act in accordance with what they perceive to be in their best interests. Therefore, find out what Mr See believes to be in his best interest, then seek to align this with Mr See's treatment. Mr See is a CEO and will not take well to prescriptive advice. Instead, you must empower Mr See to make an informed decision and manage his ego carefully. Recognise that in seeking to insure himself, he must have something or someone in mind to protect — what might this be? An open-ended question to explore this could be: "What was your greatest concern when you were refused insurance coverage?" or "What most worried you when you heard that you had hypertension?"

Mr See will share that he purchased insurance to protect his family and his frustration at being denied insurance cover. Suggest how the control of hypertension is in his interest, for instance: "I know how much you care about your spouse and child, and how you wanted so much to protect them in case something untoward happens to you. I hear what the GP told you about the risk of stroke and heart attack with uncontrolled hypertension; I am wondering how you feel about that — would you feel that ensuring that these do not happen to you is a way of protecting your family as well?" This requires genuine concern and thoughtful suggestion — be careful not to guilt trip.

If Mr See can be convinced, the next step is to negotiate a work-up and treatment plan. The side effect of lisinopril-induced cough must be addressed, for instance by switching to an angiotensin receptor blocker. You cannot promise that there will be no side effects, but you can explain the principle of risk/benefit decision making (i.e., that the benefit of blood pressure control outweighs the risks and side effects) and offer support (i.e., that you will help to manage side effects, if any, including switching him to alternative classes of antihypertensives if necessary). You will also need to explain that hypertension is unusual at such a young age, thus further tests are necessary to determine if this is a sign of a more serious and/or treatable condition — this can be done in general terms as you will not be expected to delve deeply into the causes of young hypertension in a communications station.

If Mr See cannot be convinced, the overriding principle here is of patient autonomy. You will do your best to provide information so that he can make an informed decision, but the ultimate right of whether to accept treatment is his alone. The best option in this scenario is typically to provide additional reading material and schedule a follow up consult to discuss again.

Communication Case 05

Still Seizing

Use this case as practice! The pull-out booklet contains the candidate's information.

Information for the Candidate

Patient Details: Ms Vanessa Shake, 22 years old

Your Role: Neurology Ward SHO

Information: Ms Shake has been admitted for an episode of generalised tonic-clonic seizures. This is her third admission for seizure; she had her first seizure 1 year ago and a second seizure 3 months ago. She is otherwise stable with normal vitals.

Your task is to counsel her on the diagnosis and treatment of epilepsy.

Planning (From the Stem)

1. **What do I need to assess?/What information do I need to gather?**
   - Information about the seizures – how did they happen, were there any injuries, is she better now.
   - Why is she getting seizures? provocative events (e.g., sleep deprivation), compliance, drug interactions, dose changes.
   - Is she aware of her diagnosis and treatment plan?
   - Social history: personal background, relationship background, sexual history, intention for marriage and pregnancy.
2. **What do I need to convey?**
   - Diagnosis of epilepsy.
   - Uncontrolled epilepsy puts her at risk of brain damage, disability, and death.
   - Treatment of epilepsy → compliance to medication, avoidance of triggers.
3. **What is the safety issue here?**
   - Driving a car (or riding a motorcycle) and operating heavy machinery.
   - Pregnancy issues – teratogenicity of anti-epileptic drugs (AEDs), and AEDs which are enzyme inducers can decrease the effectiveness of oral contraceptive pills.
4. **What are the ethics and communications principles here?**
   - Aligning patient autonomy with beneficence.
   - Justice: public safety (if she drives with uncontrolled seizures).

Patient's Brief

You were admitted yesterday due to an episode of unconsciousness while driving, but managed to stop at the traffic junction. You could not remember what happened, but you woke up in hospital. You were told that your brain scans were normal and you did not suffer any injury. You are feeling much better and are looking forward to going home.

You are a final-year architecture student. Your sleep pattern is erratic due to the demands of your course, and because you have been driving for a ride-hailing service at night and on weekends to make ends meet. You do not like driving, but you have to support yourself as your parents are divorced and your family is in dire financial straits. You do not drink.

You do recall being told that you have had a few seizures before this episode and you were diagnosed with 'epilepsy'. However, you believe that these episodes of unconsciousness were 'minor' and did not think too much of it. You also believe that these episodes will not lead to any serious trouble should they recur. You are otherwise fit and well.

You have been told that you needed medication. However, you find it hard to be compliant to the doses, especially on days when you have dinner appointments but did not bring your medication along. You have been taking the same medication, and there were no recent changes to the dosage. You are currently taking an oral contraceptive pill (OCP), and no other over-the-counter drugs, supplements, or traditional medicines.

You have a boyfriend with whom you have regular sexual intercourse. You intend to get married soon after graduating, and you wish to have a child soon after your wedding.

You have some specific questions for the doctor at this consultation:
- What's the big deal with these episodes?
- Epilepsy? How does that affect me?
- Apart from taking medications, am I able to carry on with life as per normal?
- Should I get pregnant?

Case Discussion

Begin by gathering more information. Ask her about her background and what her hopes and dreams in life are. Ask her more about the current admission — circumstances leading to the admission, investigations that have been performed, insight into her condition, etc. You should also explore the circumstances surrounding the previous episodes. Assess her understanding about her recurrent seizures and if she has had prior counselling regarding both her condition and medications. Ask her if she had any suspicion of why she might be having repeated seizures.

Explain the diagnosis of epilepsy using the 'breaking bad news' framework. Should the patient fail to see the significance of having epilepsy, you will need to clearly state that "epilepsy is serious, and that severe and frequent seizures can potentially lead to brain damage, disability, and death." Discuss how she can avoid potential provocative triggers for seizures (e.g., ample rest), emphasise the important role her medications play in preventing seizures, and explain why compliance to her treatment is necessary. Assess her for difficulties in staying compliant (e.g., forgetting to take her medication) and offer feasible solutions (e.g., using a pill box, phone reminders, involving her family). You should also discuss how best to help her should she experience side effects from the medications (this may include discussion on switching AEDs, although this will not be necessary in this scenario).

The two relevant safety issues that regularly appear in the PACES communication station are pregnancy and driving.

Don't forget: Check for safety issues

> Driving and pregnancy are safety issues that you should always look for — the patient may not volunteer that he/she is driving a car or riding a motorcycle. You should also ask if they are vocational drivers (i.e., bus driver, taxi driver, etc.) and the type of vehicles they drive (e.g., pick-up truck, forklift, tractor-trailer) as these vary in the risk of potential harm to both the patient and the public.

Driving: You must express your concern that she is still driving a car, that she places herself and others at risk of injury, and that it is illegal for her to drive. Empathise with her financial situation and offer help (e.g., referral to a social worker for financial assistance, suggesting alternative jobs appropriate to her).

Tip: Driving guidelines

> Update yourself on the driving guidelines of the country in which you are taking the examination. You are not expected to recall all details, but should remain familiar with general concepts relating to the conditions commonly encountered by an internist.

Pregnancy: You must explore her sexual history and her desire for pregnancy. Pregnancy in patients with epilepsy is tricky as medications (such as valproate) have significant teratogenic potential.

A possible answer to the *"can I get pregnant"* question might be:
- I hear that you really want a child after marriage; that is a lovely desire and I want to help you get pregnant safely.
- Yes, you can get pregnant. However, there are important considerations we must discuss.
- Firstly, it is important that you become pregnant only when your epilepsy is well-controlled. Should you become pregnant when your epilepsy is not well controlled, you may be at risk of injury and complications.

- Secondly, you need to know that some anti-epileptic medications can cause birth defects, but there are some which have been shown to be safer during pregnancy. These include levetiracetam and carbamazepine. To further minimise the risk to your child, you will be monitored closely by a neurologist and an obstetrician during your pregnancy, and you will receive vitamins as part of your treatment.

Finally, you should recognise that she is using oral contraceptive pills, which can become less effective if taken together with enzyme-inducing epileptic medications (e.g., phenytoin and carbamazepine). Preferred contraceptive options in epilepsy include barrier methods, copper or hormonal intrauterine devices (Mirena), or birth control implants (e.g., Implanon).

Communication Case 06

Still Coughing

Use this case as practice! The pull-out booklet contains the candidate's information.

Information for the Candidate

Patient Details: Mr Hack, 30 years old

Your Role: General Medicine SHO

Information: Mr Hack has come to the walk-in clinic today requesting for cough syrup.

He was diagnosed with pulmonary tuberculosis 3 months ago and started on rifampicin, isoniazid, pyrazinamide, ethambutol, and pyridoxine. Sputum cultures have confirmed mycobacterium tuberculosis which is sensitive to all first-line anti-tuberculous therapy. Liver enzymes, fasting glucose, and a HIV test are normal.

Mr Hack has missed 2 review appointments to date. The records show that in the 3 months since his diagnosis, he has only collected 1 month's worth of medication. He is symptomatic with persistent cough.

Your task is to speak to Mr Hack about his non-compliance and formulate a treatment plan.

Planning (From the Stem)

1. **What do I need to assess?/What information do I need to gather?**
   - Current symptoms and how he feels about his symptoms.
   - Why has he not been compliant?
     - Medical barriers (e.g., drug side effects).
     - Social barriers.
     - Disease understanding.
   - Transmission risk – living arrangement, occupation, social background.
2. **What do I need to convey?**
   - Importance of compliance to tuberculosis treatment, particularly:
     - Risk of worsening disease and death.
     - Risk of multi-drug resistant tuberculosis.
     - Transmission risk to others.
3. **What is the safety issue here?**
   - Minimising risk of infection to others including direct observed therapy (DOT) and home isolation for 2 weeks.

4. **What are the ethics and communications principles here?**
   - Negotiating a treatment arrangement with the patient.
   - Risk to public health with untreated tuberculosis.

Patient's Brief

You have been coughing for the past 5 years. You had thought that this was a smoker's cough but 3 months ago, you started to cough out blood, so you went to see the doctor. You were told that you have tuberculosis, although you don't understand what this really means. You were given 5 different medications, which you find difficult to take because of the number of tablets and you tend to feel very nauseous after taking these medications. You find that you feel more sick when you take the medications, as compared to when you don't. You also noticed your urine turning orange after taking the medications — you suspect that the medication is injuring your kidneys. On the other hand, you find cough syrup much more helpful.

You have come to see the doctor today because you are still coughing. You will like to receive some cough mixture and you have no intention of going back on tuberculosis treatment. You will deny that you have been non-compliant unless specifically confronted. You do, however, recognise that you are unwell, having lost 6 kg in the last 3 months. Coughing out blood frightens you.

You come from a troubled family background, have had several run-ins with the law, and generally mistrust authority, especially if a paternalistic approach is taken. You are a waiter on the permanent night shift at a bar and you drink at least 5 shots of hard liquor per night. You stay alone in a basic single-room apartment in a run-down part of town. You do not have close friends or family and are socially isolated. You do not grasp the risk of transmission of tuberculosis. If asked to attend direct observed therapy, your main concern is that it is inconvenient because you sleep in the day. You also feel that the doctor is asking you to attend direct observed therapy because he/she does not trust you and looks down on you.

You have some specific questions for the doctor at this consultation:
- The medications are damaging my kidneys!
- If I get liver failure from these medications, are you going to be responsible?
- Doctor, do you trust me?
- Why are you telling me what to do? I know what is best for myself.

Case Discussion

The crux of this scenario is to identify the reason for Mr Hack's non-compliance and negotiating a solution that he can agree to.

Begin by asking Mr Hack how he has been. He will tell you about his cough and his request for cough mixture. Resist the urge to preach about tuberculosis treatment or confront him harshly. It is always far better to demonstrate empathy, concern, and find out more from the patient — let him tell you himself that he has been non-compliant. Ask Mr Hack if he is aware of any reason why he might be coughing incessantly. He will probably admit to having been told that he has tuberculosis — you must then clarify whether he understands what this means. If he claims ignorance, state that he had previously been given 5 drugs and ask if he knew what they were for. He may or may not confess to non-compliance — if he does not, you will need to explicitly state that the records show that has not collected his medications. You must come across as genuinely concerned about his cough and about him as a person, rather than as a naggy disciplinarian.

Assess why he is non-compliant. There are many possible reasons to explore for non-compliance — poor disease understanding (e.g., "I feel better, so why do I still need the medications?"), drug side effects, logistic difficulties with the many drugs and dosing regimen, social barriers, and embarrassment. Explore his social setup, which is relevant not just for compliance but also for transmission risk.

Mr Hack's main concern will be with drug side-effects. You should normalise his experience and inspire confidence that you have seen this a thousand times and are experienced in helping patients to overcome these side effects. For example, you can say, "I am sorry that you have had such a bad experience taking TB medication. These medications are notoriously difficult to take and many patients have had the same side effects. But stay with me — there are ways we can tackle the side effects and I will make sure we find something that works for you. If you have any problems, call me and we will deal with it. Don't stop taking the medications yourself." You must persuade him that the side effects are worse at the onset and he will soon feel much better with less cough and no more weight loss.

He has two specific questions relating to treatment side effects:

- *"The medications are damaging my kidneys!"* Find out why he feels that way. He will reveal that he is worried about the orange discolouration of his urine. Explain that orange discolouration of the urine is normal due to rifampicin (and it means that he has taken his medicine that day!). Reassure him that this does not mean there is kidney injury, but offer to check his kidney function anyway to be sure. Also warn him that his sweat and tears can be coloured orange.

- *"If I get liver failure from these medications, are you going to be responsible?"* State confidently that you will not let him develop liver failure because you will monitor his liver function tests regularly and catch any problem before liver failure develops.

Next, educate Mr Hack on the importance of tuberculosis treatment including life-threatening haemoptysis, death from untreated disease, and risk to family and friends.

- Explain the problem of non-compliance in terms that he can relate. For example, you may say, "The tuberculosis bug is stubborn and difficult to eradicate. Killing it takes 6 months of powerful antibiotics. Anything less, or if medications are not taken regularly, the bug won't die and it will become stronger and smarter. The next time you try to treat it, these antibiotics won't work anymore."

- Relate the effects of tuberculosis to the impact on his life, for instance: "Have the customers at your bar ever minded that you are always coughing?" Do not come from purely a public health perspective. He is aware that his symptoms are affecting his life and can be convinced that treatment of TB is needed for him to get better.
- Building a rapport with the patient is particularly important in this case. His concerns about *"do you trust me"* and *"I know what is best for myself"* have to be handled sensitively. A good strategy is to use the exact words he uses, for instance: "I trust you that you know your own body best. What I'm hearing is that you are so bothered about your cough that you are specially coming to see me when you could be sleeping at home after your night shift, and you are also scared by the blood in your phlegm. I take this very seriously. I know that you want to get better and I want to help you."

The final aspect is to negotiate a management plan. While the management of complex TB patients is a specialist-level topic, knowledge of basic strategies to reduce medication side effects and mitigate transmission risk is probably expected. The management plan should include:

1. Direct observed therapy (DOT). This can be a tough sell to someone who is suspicious of authority, but you should highlight the positives — you are enrolling him in DOT not because you do not trust him, but because you know how difficult taking TB medication is. With DOT, there will always be someone watching out for him if he develops side effects, he will not have to remember to collect and take the medications on his own, and it makes sure he gets better and minimises the risk of drug resistance. Explain that you will work out a DOT arrangement that fits in his schedule (e.g., immediately after work).
2. One strategy to improve tolerability is to start 2 drugs (rifampicin and isoniazid) first, add on ethambutol a week later, and finally pyrazinamide two weeks later (or not at all as it is not the backbone). This improves tolerability and enables the latest drug to be stopped if he is unable to tolerate it. It is possible to start one drug first and the next drug in close succession, but extended monotherapy must be avoided. Note that the standard 6-month duration of therapy may need to be extended if he is treated with less than 4 drugs.
3. Ask him to have a meal before coming for DOT to minimise gastrointestinal side effects. Give him some symptomatic medications (e.g., metoclopramide PRN on standby).
4. Advise complete abstinence from alcohol (or at least to reduce alcohol intake, if that cannot be achieved) due to the risk of drug interaction (liver enzyme inhibition or induction) as well as liver toxicity.
5. Consider repeating sputum cultures today to ensure that resistance has not developed.
6. Give 2 weeks of hospitalisation leave for home isolation — he will be considered infectious until 2 weeks of treatment have been completed, so he should not work until then.
7. Explain follow-up plan including monitoring of liver enzymes.

Additional note: You should not use it in this scenario, but be aware that in Singapore, there is a legal framework to compel a person to be treated for tuberculosis under the Infectious Diseases Act. No equivalent legislation exists in the UK — although TB is a notifiable disease and contact tracing will be done, the authorities are unable to compel a person to be treated.

Communication Case 07

Indeterminate Western Blot

Use this case as practice! The pull-out booklet contains the candidate's information.

Information for the Candidate

Patient Details: Mr C. Yolo, 42 years old

Your Role: Medicine Ward SHO

Information: Mr Yolo was admitted 4 days ago. He presented with a 2-week history of fever, rash, and sore throat after returning from vacation.

Your consultant has ordered several tests including a HIV test*. The laboratory has called to inform you that the HIV test is 'indeterminate'.

Your task is to speak to Mr Yolo about this result.

*Your laboratory uses a fourth-generation HIV assay, which is a combination test including the HIV antibody and p24 antigen. If this is positive, a confirmatory western blot is performed.

Planning (From the Stem)

1. **What do I need to assess?/What information do I need to gather?**
   - How Mr Yolo has been clinically.
   - What is Mr Yolo's exposure history – in particular, explore his travel history, sexual history, occupational exposures, intravenous drug use, blood transfusions.

2. **What do I need to convey?**
   - That Mr Yolo may have HIV infection.
   - Clinical management plan – Mr Yolo may have early HIV infection from very recent exposure. He will require further testing with either a repeat HIV test in 6 weeks or a HIV viral load (which can be performed immediately).

3. **What is the safety issue here?**
   - Mr Yolo should be counselled of precautions to avoid HIV transmission.
   - Suicide risk assessment if patient reacts poorly to the news.

4. **What are the ethics and communications principle here?**
   - Breaking bad news.

Patient's Brief

You are a 42-year-old insurance agent. In the last three weeks, you have been having fever, rash, and sore throat that did not seem to go away even after you saw multiple GPs. You came to the hospital 4 days ago and were admitted, and are at present still febrile and miserable. You feel frustrated that your doctors have not found out what is wrong after putting you through many blood tests and scans. You will open the conversation with: "Doctor, I want to be discharged. I'm sick and tired and nothing has been done for me these four days." However, you will be rapidly pacified once the candidate acknowledges your frustration.

You had just returned from Bangkok, Thailand approximately a week before the onset of fever. This was a fully sponsored incentive trip you earned for exceeding last year's sales targets. You went on this trip with several other insurance agents from your firm, with whom you did several 'boy things' such as visiting girly bars and having unprotected oral and vaginal intercourse with female commercial sex workers. You have never received any blood transfusions, undergone any surgery, or used any intravenous drugs. You are married with two children of primary school age. Apart from this episode and one or two casual relationships in your undergraduate days, you have only had sexual intercourse with your spouse. You have never had any other sexually transmitted diseases.

If informed that you may have HIV, you will react with surprise. You did not think much about this encounter as "everyone else did it too"; while you are aware of HIV, you do not think that it will happen to you. You will then seek to clarify whether you indeed have, or do not have, HIV — the information that you 'may' have HIV or that the test is 'indeterminate' makes you feel unsettled and confused. You are anxious and jittery. You will also seek to find out what you need to do next; if told that you need to repeat a blood test later, you will ask if there is any test that can be done now to confirm the diagnosis.

You have some specific questions for the doctor at this consultation:

- Doctor, how can this happen to me? It was just once and I have been faithful to my wife all along.
- I am confused. Do I have or not have HIV?
- Is there any way I can find out, right now, whether I have HIV?
- Can I be treated? Will I die?

Case Discussion

Apart from the standard breaking bad news and HIV counselling, this station requires some knowledge of HIV testing.

You should be able to identify from the stem that Mr Yolo likely has early HIV infection. Acute HIV infection presents with an infectious mononucleosis-like syndrome with fever, lymphadenopathy, sore throat, rash, myalgia, diarrhoea, and weight loss. While none of these symptoms are specific for HIV, suspicion is increased if symptoms are prolonged.

HIV testing begins with an initial screen using either a third-generation (ELISA) or fourth-generation combination assay (IgM and IgG antibody + p24 antigen). Positive screens require confirmatory testing with Western Blot[3]. The Western Blot tests for antibodies to HIV-1 viral proteins and may return negative or indeterminate in early HIV infection. Therefore, samples with a positive initial screening test but a negative or indeterminate confirmatory test are reported as 'indeterminate' — this may signify early HIV infection *and must not be misinterpreted as a negative HIV test*. Note also that the fourth-generation assay takes 15–20 days to turn positive following HIV infection; testing may be falsely negative if performed too early.

You will begin the station on the back foot after Mr Yolo informs you that he is frustrated and wants to be discharged. Acknowledge his frustration, apologise for the delay, and tell him that you have some results that you would like to discuss with him. Before proceeding any further, find out more about Mr Yolo. Specifically, explore his presenting symptoms and travel history. Ask if he has any suspicion what the diagnosis could be and if there was anything unusual on his recent trip.

Take a sexual history. Do not be squeamish — appear confident, professional, and non-judgemental. A good strategy is to begin with the least invasive questions. Pertinent points needed to stratify the risk of HIV exposure are outlined in Table C5.5.

Practice makes perfect: Taking a sexual history

> The sexual history is often poorly taken. Many candidates are squeamish and trained surrogates pick this up easily. It is important to not just identify 'positive sexual history' but to get a good sense of exactly how risky the patient's sexual behaviour is. Pair up with a friend and practice taking sexual histories from each other. Include scenarios such as positive commercial sex worker contact, homosexual/transsexual contact, and so on.
>
> In PACES, pay attention to stereotyped occupational histories such as long-distance truck drivers or travelling businessmen; while these may be unfair stereotypes, it is also often the question setter's hint that you should consider taking the sexual history.

---

[3] Some labs, particularly in the United States, perform a HIV-1/HIV-2 differentiation immunoassay as a confirmatory test in lieu of the Western Blot.

Table C5.5. A comprehensive sexual history template.

From the least to the most intrusive. Not every point may be relevant in every case.

No.	Item	Suggested words
1.	Opening statement	"There is a list of questions we usually ask everyone with prolonged fever. This includes a sexual history which is important to know how to get you better."
2.	Potential HIV exposure other than sexual intercourse	Ask about any blood transfusions, intravenous drug use, or surgeries in Thailand. This is both relevant and a good introduction to the more invasive questions.
3.	Marital status	"Are you married"? • If yes, patient is presumed to be sexually active. • If no, follow up with: "Are you sexually active?"
4.	Prior pregnancies (in ladies)	"Have you ever had a pregnancy, miscarriage, or abortion?"
5.	Sexual partners	"How many sexual partners have you had?" • If many, "How many have you had in the past month?"
6.	Regular vs. casual vs. paid partners	"Are these partners people you know well?" • If no, "Has there ever been paid encounters?"
7.	Use of barrier protection	"How often do you use a condom?" Note: Avoid using the word 'protection' as some take that to mean 'contraceptive pill'.
8.	Sexual practices	"Do you have sex with males, females, or both?" • Follow up with: "Do you engage in vaginal sex, anal sex, oral sex, or all of the above?" • For anal intercourse, find out if the patient is the insertive (male) or receptive (female) partner. Please do not ask: "Do you have 'normal' sex?"
9.	Previous sexually transmitted disease	"Have you ever had any sexually transmitted diseases?" "Have you previously been tested for HIV?"

Break bad news about the HIV diagnosis in the usual way (see Table C5.1), remembering to include pauses and giving Mr Yolo adequate space. Address his concern ("Will I die?") head on, for example: "It is true that one can die from HIV especially if it is untreated. But treatment is available and it is highly effective. People who are diagnosed early, treated early, and take their medications can live as long as everyone else."

You will need to explain that the HIV test can be 'indeterminate' in early infection and that a repeat confirmatory test is necessary. In such cases, we can repeat the HIV test in 6 weeks. However, given a high clinical suspicion for acute retroviral infection in Mr Yolo, it is ideal to perform a HIV RNA viral load which is typically high in early infection. This will allow prompt confirmation of the diagnosis and onward referral to an infectious disease physician for counselling and initiation of anti-retroviral therapy.

Finally, counsel on the risk of infection transmission, abstinence from sexual intercourse (including with his spouse), blood donation, and sharing of IV drug needles. If taking the exam in Singapore, you should also inform the patient that while he has yet to have a positive HIV test, Singapore law requires that a person "who has reason to believe that he has or has been exposed to a significant risk of contracting HIV Infection" not engage in sexual activity unless the partner is informed on the risk of HIV transmission and accepts the risk (Infectious Diseases Act 1976).

Communication Case 08

HIV Positive

Use this case as practice! The pull-out booklet contains the candidate's information.

Information for the Candidate

Patient Details: Ms Willy Wild, 36 years old

Your Role: Infectious Disease Clinic SHO

Information: Ms Wild is referred to the Infectious Diseases clinic for a 6-month history of cough and weight loss. A HIV test and confirmatory test are positive. She is married with a 3-year-old son.

Your task is to inform Ms Wild of the test result and address her concerns.

Planning (From the Stem)

1. **What do I need to assess?/What information do I need to gather?**
   - How Ms Wild has been clinically.
   - Ms Wild's exposure history – sexual history, intravenous drug use, and previous blood transfusions and surgeries, especially overseas. Try to assess whether HIV infection occurred before or after pregnancy and lactation – this has implications on vertical transmission to her son.

2. **What do I need to convey?**
   - The diagnosis of HIV infection.
   - Clinical management plan – initiation of treatment and that treatment is important.
   - Husband and son require testing and early treatment.

3. **What is the safety issue here?**
   - Inform of transmission risk and necessary precautions.
   - In Singapore, also inform of the legal requirement to notify sexual partners prior to sexual intercourse.
   - Suicide risk assessment if patient reacts poorly to the news.

4. **What are the ethics and communications principles here?**
   - Breaking bad news.

Patient's Brief

You are a 36-year-old inflight service manager/lead stewardess. You fly around the world to many top destinations, but are also often away from home. You frequently engage in both regular and casual sexual intercourse with 'boyfriends' and 'girlfriends' in various cities around the world. You have done so since becoming an air stewardess 15 years ago. You are usually careful to use a condom, but you occasionally forget. You do not do intravenous drugs and have never had a surgery or blood transfusion. You have never had any other sexually transmitted diseases.

You married your childhood sweetheart four years ago and gave birth to a boy one year after. You do not remember a HIV test done during the antenatal period. Your husband is a school teacher and is quite the prim-and-proper, 'goody two shoes' person (in fact he has recently been appointed the discipline master in his school). You love both your husband and son very much and are committed to them. He is absolutely unaware and unsuspecting of your sexual flings overseas — you live a double life.

You visited the GP two weeks ago complaining of a 6-month history of cough and weight loss, and performed some blood tests (including a HIV test) and a chest X-ray. The GP called you last week to arrange an appointment with the Infectious Diseases clinic. You suspect that your HIV test has come back positive; truth be told, you are hardly surprised and actually quite prepared for it. If informed that you are HIV positive, you will react by saying "I thought so, not surprised." You want answers about what is next for you.

You are aware that HIV is treatable and you want to start medicine immediately. You also understand the risk of HIV transmission and are prepared to abstain from sexual intercourse. If asked to inform your husband and son, you will not agree. Your husband has absolutely no idea that you have been having extramarital affairs and you believe that he probably divorce you if he found out. You do not think that it is necessary to inform them, and you will turn hysterical if the doctor mentions anything about 'contact tracing', 'infectious disease notification', or speaking to your husband. However, if informed that your husband and son are at risk of contracting HIV and that treating them is life-saving, you will relent and tearfully agree to tell them.

You have some specific questions for the doctor at this consultation:

- Does it mean that I can never have sex again?
- Do I need to tell my husband?
- Can I have your assurance that our consultation is confidential and that you will never tell my husband, family, or anyone else?

Case Discussion

Begin with the breaking bad news framework (Table C5.1). Spend time asking her about her background, why she did the test, and what she understands so far. When it becomes clear that she is not distraught and is in fact unsurprised, probe *why*. Move quickly from 'breaking bad news' to providing information and answers; do not dwell on providing emotional support when it is clear that the patient does not require this and instead wants answers. This is an exercise in learning to *read and respond to the patient*.

You will need to cover the following points:

1. **Sexual history**: Taking a sexual history to identify how she was infected and who else might be at risk of transmission (see Table C5.5).

2. **Clinical management plan**: Explaining the plan including:
   - Further blood tests (CD4 cell count, HIV genotype and resistance testing, serologies for possible opportunistic infections).
   - Initiation of antiretroviral therapy by an infectious disease physician (you will not be expected to know individual regimens in detail and should direct Ms Wild to your consultant who will make these decisions).
   - Importance of compliance.

3. **Transmission risk**: Informing Ms Wild of the risk of infection transmission and therefore the advice to abstain from sexual intercourse, IV drug abuse, and blood donation.

   Be aware of the regulations surrounding HIV:
   - Singapore: On confirmation of HIV-positive status, the attending physician is legally required to notify the Ministry of Health. The patient is also required to inform sexual partners of his/her HIV-positive status and of the risk of HIV transmission prior to sexual intercourse (regardless of whether a condom is used). You must counsel the patient about this requirement.
   - UK: HIV is not a notifiable disease, so people with HIV are not obliged to notify sexual partners. They will only run into legal peril if they 'recklessly spread' HIV. Reckless spreading constitutes (1) being aware of and understanding the diagnosis of HIV, yet (2) not informing partners of diagnosis and (3) not using a condom.

   Ms Wild's question, "Does it mean that I can never have sex again?" is an interesting one. The current understanding is based on the concept of 'undetectable = untransmissable'; that is, with good treatment and virologic suppression, the risk of transmission is minimal. Many people with HIV who achieve an undetectable viral load are able to have unprotected sexual intercourse with their spouses. However, this is still something that has to be agreed upon between the couple.

4. **Testing and treatment of husband and son**. The twist in this station comes when Ms Wild declares that she does not want to inform her husband and son. The strategy to deal with this is not to insist that she must inform her husband and son, but to explore *why* she is hesitant, as well as the relationship between her and her husband/son. She may be unaware that her husband and son are at risk of HIV and that early treatment is life-saving. Build on her love of her husband and son to convince her that this is necessary to start her husband and son on life-saving treatment. Note that a negative HIV test pre-pregnancy does not exclude HIV in

her son, because we do not know when she seroconverted (e.g., she could have transmitted HIV when breastfeeding).

If she refuses to tell her husband or son, this becomes quite problematic.

- Singapore: the legal obligation to inform sexual partners prior to intercourse means that Ms Wild is legally bound to inform her husband if they have sexual intercourse, but not if they do not engage in sexual activity. It is possible to leave testing of her husband/son to government contact tracers, but if her son proves to be HIV positive, the obvious question arises: "How did a pre-pubescent child get HIV?"
- UK: if Ms Wild refuses to tell her partner and son, there is no good way to prevent harm to them except by breaking confidentiality. This is generally not considered a justification to break confidentiality — it is not a 'Tarasoff rule' scenario whereby there is an immediate danger of violent harm to someone else. There is no easy way out and such a case is best escalated to an ethics committee.

Conclude the case by summarising the plan moving forward and offering support, such as support groups, psychologist referral, and offering to speak to the patient's husband/family to refute misconceptions (there are still people who believe that you cannot share a toilet seat with a HIV-positive individual).

Communication Case 09

Needlestick Injury

Use this case as practice! The pull-out booklet contains the candidate's information.

Information for the Candidate

Patient Details: Dr S. Suay, 23 years old

Your Role: Medical SHO-On-Call

Information: Dr Suay, the House Officer (FY1) with whom you are on call, comes to you distraught after sustaining a needlestick injury.

Your task is to calm the situation and advice Dr Suay on what she needs to do.

Planning (From the Stem)

1. **What do I need to assess?/What information do I need to gather?**
   - What is the risk of blood-borne virus exposure?
   - Dr Suay's background: sexual exposure, possibility of pregnancy.
2. **What do I need to convey?**
   - Immediate management of needlestick injury:
     - Test source patient and Dr Suay for blood-borne viruses.
     - If exposure is high-risk, post-exposure prophylaxis using a 'starter kit' available in most hospitals' A&E departments.
   - Follow-up plan including infectious disease/occupational medicine consult, interval HIV test.
   - Avoidance of sexual exposure and blood donation.
3. **What is the safety issue here?**
   - Ensure the HO is coping alright and not suicidal. She is no longer fit to continue the call and should be sent home.
4. **What are the ethics and communications principles here?**
   - Calming a distraught colleague.

Patient's Brief

You are a newly minted House Officer (FY1) and this is your 3rd ever night call.

Communication Case 09

You were called to clerk Mr Moo, a 45-year-old gentleman who has just been admitted from the A&E. He is known to be HIV positive but had defaulted on his follow-up and has not been prescribed any anti-retrovirals for 2 years. His presenting complaint was breathlessness and you suspect pneumocystis pneumonia.

As he had difficult venous access, you decided to perform a 'femoral stab' (i.e., drawing blood gases and a blood culture from his femoral artery using a green (18G) needle). Having performed the femoral stab, you unfortunately pricked your index finger while transferring the blood into blood culture bottles. You have performed first aid including squeezing out as much blood as you could and washing with soap and water. You feel quite dazed but are not overtly distraught.

You have a boyfriend with whom you are sexually active, although you are somewhat embarrassed to reveal this to a colleague. You have no other sexual partners and do not engage in intravenous drug use. You are on the oral contraceptive pill and do not use condoms. You are certain that you are not pregnant as you are currently having your period. You have been fully immunised against hepatitis B (as a prerequisite to medical studies). Your long-term professional interest is to be a GP and you have no intention to pursue a surgical, procedural, or A&E career.

You have some specific questions for the doctor at this consultation:

- Am I going to get HIV?
- What should I do now?
- If the HIV test is negative, does it mean that I am safe?
- If I get HIV, can I still work as a doctor?

Case Discussion

This is a reasonably standard needlestick injury case; more a test of content knowledge than of communication. Begin by setting an agenda. Find out more about what happened by assessing the risk of transmission of blood-borne viruses:

- Source patient: whether he/she is known to have or be at risk of having hepatitis B, C, or HIV.
- Nature of injury: whether the needle is clean or contaminated, whether it is a solid or hollow-bore needle.
- Victim: whether Dr Suay is vaccinated against hepatitis B.

As you do so, demonstrate empathy for what is a very traumatising experience. Offer appropriate support, remembering that you are helping her from a position of professional responsibility (as her senior on call). Do not 'downplay' the incident with platitudes (e.g., "calm down", "you'll be fine"); it is usually better to acknowledge her anxiety and fears and say that you will do your best to help.

It should become clear that this is a high risk exposure involving a HIV-positive patient who likely has high viral load, as well as a high blood inoculum (contaminated, large-bore needle). After establishing that she has performed appropriate first aid, immediate management will include:

1. Drawing bloods from Dr Suay to test for hepatitis B, C, and HIV. This establishes a baseline so that if seroconversion occurs, she will be eligible for work injury compensation.
2. Explain that you will seek consent to draw bloods from the source patient, Mr Moo (you should not ask her to do this, but instead offer to do so yourself).
3. Dr Suay should begin post-exposure prophylaxis with combination antiretroviral therapy. In most hospitals, this will be available as a 'starter kit' in the occupational medicine clinic (during office hours) or the A&E (after office hours). This must be done as soon as possible and should not wait until the next day. You would not normally be expected to know the drug regimen involved or the duration of prophylaxis required. However, you should verify that Dr Suay is not pregnant as this will have implications on the post-exposure prophylaxis regime offered. If you are unsure, you can say that you will contact the on-call infectious diseases physician to discuss.
4. Arrange a next-working-day appointment with the infectious diseases or occupational health physician. The post-exposure prophylaxis regimen may need to be modified if the source patient is known to have antiretroviral drug resistance (especially given that he is non-compliant).
5. Advise Dr Suay to abstain from sexual intercourse and blood donation until the confirmatory blood test is performed.
6. Tell Dr Suay that she should not continue with her call and you will arrange for appropriate cover.
7. A confidential incident report will need to be filed.

You must check that Dr Suay is coping with the incident. Offer support and counselling if she becomes distraught, and ensure that she is not suicidal before you send her home.

She will have a number of questions that must be answered correctly and handled sensitively. If you are unsure of the answer, it is better to offer to check with the infectious diseases physician rather than to guess.

- *Am I going to get HIV?* – "The chance of getting HIV is usually below 1%, even from a patient with known HIV. We can reduce the chance further by giving you post-exposure prophylaxis which you must take without fail in the weeks ahead."
- *If I test negative to HIV now, does it mean that I am safe?* – "Unfortunately not. We will only know for sure that you are safe when we do the subsequent blood tests in 6 weeks and 3 months. The HIV test now is a baseline. If you were to contract HIV from the needlestick injury, seroconversion will take 3–6 weeks, which is why we are giving you post-exposure prophylaxis to stop seroconversion from happening."
- *If I get HIV, can I still work as a doctor?* – "Generally yes, but you may face restrictions on performing exposure-prone procedures such as surgery. Routine blood drawing in the ward is OK. So if you are planning to be a GP, it should not be a problem."

Communication Case 10

Ascitic Drain

Use this case as practice! The pull-out booklet contains the candidate's information.

Information for the Candidate

Patient Details: Mr Gan Ying Hua, 53 years old

Your Role: Gastroenterology Clinic SHO

Information: Mr Gan, a 53-year-old Chinese gentleman, is on follow-up with the gastroenterology clinic for liver cirrhosis. He is hepatitis B positive and has a very strong family history of hepatitis B. In the past year, he has had two episodes of variceal bleed and one admission for hepatic encephalopathy. In the past two months, he has also been complaining of symptomatic ascites which has not improved in spite of maximal tolerated doses of furosemide and spironolactone.

Your consultant has just seen Mr Gan and decided to offer large volume paracentesis (therapeutic ascitic drain). This will be done today as an outpatient in the day procedure room.

Your consultant has tasked you to consent Mr Gan for this procedure and counsel him on further management of his cirrhosis.

Planning (From the Stem)

1. **What do I need to assess?/What information do I need to gather?**
   - Why has Mr Gan's cirrhosis decompensated? Why is he not responding to maximal doses of furosemide and spironolactone? Look for a precipitant, such as non-compliance to medication or salt restriction, new liver insults (drugs, alcohol, hepatitis A or C infection), constipation, intercurrent infections, or development of hepatocellular carcinoma.
   - What does he understand about his disease and its management?

2. **What do I need to convey?**
   - Explain the procedure of a therapeutic ascitic drain, including its indication, risks, and alternatives.
   - Explain other principles of management (e.g., salt restriction, avoidance of liver insults).

3. **What is the safety issue here?**
   - Risk of hepatitis B transmission with sexual activity.

4. **What are the ethics and communications principles here?**
   - Legal and ethical requirements for informed consent.

Patient's Brief

You are a 53 year-old Chinese gentleman. You are a small business owner and are married with two young children.

You were first diagnosed with hepatitis B in your 20s, when you volunteered to donate blood. You understand that you were probably 'born with' hepatitis B as both of your parents are carriers. Three years ago, a GP incidentally picked up that you had a big spleen and referred you to the gastroenterologist; further tests confirmed that you had cirrhosis. This has never really bothered you until the past year, during which you have been admitted 2–3 times for vomiting blood and once for confusion, which was attributed to your liver problem. You have had multiple scopes this year.

In the past two months, you have been having uncomfortable abdominal swelling. You have never had severe or sudden abdominal pain or any fever. Increasing doses of furosemide and spironolactone have not helped much. You take your medications regularly and are compliant to a very low salt diet. You do not take any traditional medications or supplements. You have not had any uncooked seafood or intravenous drug use. You have not been vaccinated for hepatitis A. You understand that your liver problem is getting worse and you are interested in finding out what can be done about this, in particular to stop the abdominal swelling from coming back.

You have been told that the 'water' in your belly can be drained and you will feel less uncomfortable after this is done. You have never had this procedure before but are enthusiastic to proceed. You will agree to proceed with the procedure after an explanation of its risks and benefits.

Only if asked – in the past year, you have taken approximately 3–4 shots of hard liquor each day. Your marriage is on the rocks and drinking provides you with something to do in the evenings. You need a beer most mornings when you wake up. While you know that patients with liver problems should not drink at all, you believe that 3–4 shots a day is a 'reasonable' amount. You have no intention to stop drinking and if pressed, you will at best promise to 'try' to cut down. You feel particularly irritated when your wife comments on your drinking.

Only if asked – You haven't really been going home and occasionally stay over at your secretary's place. You have had two instances of sexual intercourse without the use of condoms with your secretary. You do not know if your secretary is a hepatitis B carrier or if she has been immunised.

You have some specific questions for the doctor at this consultation:
- Is the procedure safe?
- Will the water in my abdomen come back after it is drained? How can I stop it from coming back?

Case Discussion

The first part of this encounter involves consent-taking, which most candidates will find somewhat routine — but be careful as many clinicians have run into medicolegal trouble with consent-related issues. As with all consent taking, you will need to explain the procedure (general principles hold regardless of the specific type of ascitic drain you are familiar with), indication (to relieve symptomatic ascites), risks (bleeding, infection, intestinal perforation, hypotension during drainage, re-accumulation of fluid, etc.), and alternatives (conservative management). You might earn brownie points for describing the use of IV albumin during paracentesis, which shows that you have truly 'been there, done that'.

Particularly for this patient who has a prior episode of hepatic encephalopathy, you should ensure that Mr Gan has the capacity to give valid consent (i.e., that he is able to retain information, understand information, weigh risks and benefits to make a decision, and communicate this decision to you).

The second half of the encounter is more interesting. While the given task ('counsel him on further management of his cirrhosis') is vague, remember that the first principle of the communications station is to 'find out more'. You will realise that Mr Gan had been well until he began to decompensate in the past year. This should prompt you to explore precipitants of decompensation in cirrhosis such as drug- or alcohol-induced liver injury, superimposed viral hepatitis, infections, and portal vein thrombosis.

This will uncover Mr Gan's alcohol use. Elicit the extent of his alcohol use, why he continues to use alcohol, and whether there is any component of addiction. The 'CAGE' questions are helpful in screening for addiction:

- Have you ever felt you needed to **C**ut down on your drinking?
- Do you feel **A**nnoyed when others comment on your drinking?
- Have you ever felt **G**uilty about drinking?
- Have you ever felt you needed a drink first thing in the morning (**E**ye-opener)?

Pitfall: Missing the 'hidden' issue

> Mr Gan's alcohol use disorder is easily missed by candidates. Unfortunately, there have been a number of similar PACES exam scenarios over the years; candidates who failed to uncover the 'hidden' issue did not pass the encounter. Remember that the first principle of the communications station is to 'find out more'. Exploring why a patient's chronic disease suddenly decompensated will lead you to the otherwise 'hidden' task.

Assess whether Mr Gan is ready to change. Prochaska and DiClemente's 'stages of change' model is useful here. This model describes various stages of change — pre-contemplation, contemplation, preparation, action, maintenance, and relapse. Mr Gan is firmly in pre-contemplation; he does not even recognise that he has a problem with regards to alcohol. On the other hand, he is symptomatic from ascites and recognises that his liver problem is getting worse — this could be a potential motivating factor to stop drinking. You must inform him in no uncertain terms that alcohol will worsen his condition and that no amount of alcohol is acceptable in cirrhosis.

The safety issue in this station is that Mr Gan has been having an extramarital affair with his secretary despite having a known diagnosis of chronic hepatitis B. While it is not your place to be judgemental about the extramarital affair, you must recognise that this poses a risk of hepatitis B transmission. You will need to counsel him of this risk and the use of barrier protection during sexual activity, as well as partner vaccination.

Other useful aspects of patient education to cover in this scenario, particularly to answer Mr Gan's question about how to slow the return of ascites, include:

- Compliance to salt restriction and medications.
- Vaccination against hepatitis A.
- Avoidance of exposure to hepatitis A (uncooked seafood) or C (IV drug use, sexual exposures).
- Avoidance of hepatotoxic drugs including supplements and traditional remedies.
- Counselling for liver transplant and transjugular intrahepatic portosystemic shunt (TIPS) as a bridge to transplant may be of benefit in this scenario, but this is beyond the scope of PACES.

Communication Case 11

Chronic Pain I

Note: Chronic Pain I and II share the same candidate information but are different scenarios.

Use this case as practice! The pull-out booklet contains the candidate's information.

Information for the Candidate

Patient Details: Mr Bo Kar, 27 years old

Your Role: Acute Care Clinic SHO

Information: Mr Bo walks in to the Acute Care Clinic complaining of worsening pain and requesting for a top-up of painkillers.

He had a right above-knee amputation 1 year ago after a road traffic accident in which he suffered popliteal artery injury and right calf compartment syndrome. He is able to walk with a prosthetic limb but has known phantom limb pain.

You note that he had just seen a GP 7 days ago and was prescribed with:

PO Tramadol 25 mg TDS PRN (for pain) — 3 weeks (63 capsules)
PO Lorazepam 1 mg ON PRN (for sleep) — 3 weeks (21 capsules)

Your task is to speak to Mr Bo and address his concerns.

Planning (From the Stem)

1. **What do I need to assess?/What information do I need to gather?**
   - Take a pain history – what is the nature of Mr Bo's pain and how severe is it?
   - Why is he asking for a top up/why has he run out so quickly? Note that he has finished a 3-week supply of tramadol and midazolam within 1 week.
   - Are there any drug side effects or toxicity?

2. **What do I need to convey?**
   - Empathy for the pain he is experiencing.
   - Need to create a management plan to achieve better pain control.

3. **What is the safety issue here?**
   - Suicide risk assessment.
   - Risk of drug dependence, overdose, and diversion (see discussion).

4. **What are the ethics and communications principles here?**
   - Patient safety.
   - Patient autonomy.

Patient's Brief

You are a 27-year-old. Your life was shattered 1 year ago after a freak traffic accident. It was none of your fault — a speeding Maserati ran the red light, knocked you down, and ran over your right leg. The doctors said that they had to amputate your right leg to save your life. You survived but barely, after a stormy hospital stay with multiple operations and infections. During this episode, you lost your job as a bartender and your fiancée left you. It stings that after trying so hard to walk with a prosthetic limb — and succeeding — your fiancée decided that she did not want a crippled husband and cancelled the wedding you had both been planning.

You have had right leg pain ever since the operation. You would describe this as a shooting sensation from your right thigh downwards, as if your leg were still there, being crushed by the vehicle tyre. The pain is severe, wakes you up from sleep, and keeps you from doing your daily activities — you can't do anything at all each day. The pain seems to be getting worse recently and it is all that is on your mind. Your amputation stump has healed well and there is no redness, swelling, lump, or wound problems.

Your usual painkiller is three 20 mg capsules of tramadol a day and a 5 mg tablet of midazolam to sleep most nights. In the past week, you have needed up to ten capsules of tramadol a day — the pain is just unbearable — and thrice the usual amount of midazolam before you can fall asleep. You have not opened your bowels in the past week and you know that this is likely a side effect of the tramadol. You feel tired and somewhat woozy, but you are still coherent and fully aware of the pain. You take no other over-the-counter medicine, prescriptions, or illicit substances.

You need pain control today and are impatient. If the doctor refuses to give you painkillers, you will react with extreme distress because you are in real pain. You will decline admission because the hospital brings back terrible memories.

You feel emotionally down, tired, and frustrated. In the entire consult, look down and avoid eye contact with the doctor. You feel that life is meaningless and that you can't carry on. You have had fleeting thoughts of suicide but no active intent or plan. You know that your mother will be distraught to lose you. You will accept any recommendation offered to you (e.g., to see a psychiatrist or psychologist).

You have some specific questions for the doctor at this consultation:
- Can you just give me the painkillers; I am really in pain. I am not lying.
- Am I getting addicted?
- Doctor, is there any hope for me?

Case Discussion

Reading the candidate's information should set off alarm bells in your mind. This is an unfortunate young man with chronic pain — how is he coping, medically, socially, and emotionally? Why has he run out of a 3-week supply of opioids and benzodiazepines within 1 week? The possibilities are that (a) he has lost the pills, (b) he is taking more pills than prescribed, (c) he is hoarding pills to commit suicide, or (d) he is diverting the pills (i.e., selling addictive medications on the black market).

As always, do not rush to confront him about these issues, but begin by seeking information. Open-ended questions like "what can I do for you today" are a good place to start. Mr Bo will tell you all about how bad his pain is. Respond with empathy and genuine concern for his pain. Set an agenda — tell him that you want to help him with this pain, but first you need find out more about the pain and how he has been.

Take a pain history — where is his pain, what is the nature of his pain, how severe is his pain, relief with analgesia, and the effect of his chronic pain on mood, sleep, and function. Consider briefly whether this is phantom limb pain or whether there are other complications such as stump infection, ischaemia, or pressure-related wounds (you should not take a detailed history in the communications station, but still adequately address the important aspects of clinical management). Distinguish between nociceptive and neuropathic pain — this will impact your management later.

Assess for medication side effects of opioids and benzodiazepines — ask specifically about drowsiness, nausea/vomiting, difficulty concentrating, and constipation.

Then turn your attention to the safety issues in this station. If Mr Bo has not volunteered the information yet, you will need to ask him about the discrepant pill count. Do so in a non-accusatory manner, for example: "I know you are doing your best in a really tough situation. May I just ask about the pills that you got from the GP last week? I understand that he prescribed a 3-week supply of pills but you have seem to run out early." In this scenario, he will reveal that he has been taking more than prescribed. Resist the temptation to lecture him for overdosing and instead empathise with the severity of his chronic pain.

"Am I getting addicted?" – "I hear that you are worried about the amount of painkillers you are taking. I don't think this is addiction, but I am concerned that your pain appears to be getting worse and you are getting side effects. This tells me that we need to adjust your pain medication regimen." (Opioid addiction is further discussed in the next station.)

You must assess for suicide risk. Depending on your surrogate's acting, you may be able to pick up depressive features from his body language. Respond to what your surrogate says, such as: "This sounds terrible. You are crying for help and some of the things you have said worries me. Sometimes when patients have such a low mood like you have at the moment, they think about harming themselves or others. Is this something you have thought about?"

Key questions to answer in the suicide risk assessment include (a full discussion of suicide risk assessment is beyond the scope of this guide[4]):

- Have there ever been previous episodes of attempted suicide or self-harm? If so, how lethal were these attempts?
- Is there active psychopathology? Search for depression, mania, hallucinations (mood-congruent vs. command), and delusions.
- Are there any predisposing factors for suicide? Apart from chronic pain and drug use/abuse, consider psychiatric history, medical history, and social factors.
- Is there any suicide ideation?
- If yes, is there seriousness of intent? Are there plans formulated?
- Are there any protective factors that will hold the patient back from suicide?

In this scenario, suicide risk is not high and can be managed outpatient (e.g., with a psychologist or psychiatrist referral). If suicide risk is high, you will need to admit the patient for inpatient psychiatric management.

Finally, you will need to manage the pain. Sending him home without opioids will be cruel. In this case, it is reasonable to give him a course of opioids to tide him through until he can see a pain specialist. Mr Bo will also benefit from the addition of non-opioid analgesia (paracetamol, NSAIDs), neuropathic pain agents (e.g., gabapentin), and laxatives. These are complex issues and you should refer him to a chronic pain expert — as PACES is an idealised setting, you can simply say you will arrange for the pain expert to see him on the same day (when this will be difficult in practice). Offer hope and demonstrate ownership: "I will not let you go home in pain today. If all else fails, I will admit you."

---

[4] For example, see Ng CW, How CH, Ng YP. Depression in primary care: Assessing suicide risk. *Singapore Med J* 2017 58(2):72–77.

Communication Case 12

Chronic Pain II

*Note: Chronic Pain I and II share the same candidate information but are different scenarios. **Please attempt Chronic Pain I first**.*

Use this case as practice! The pull-out booklet contains the candidate's information.

Information for the Candidate

Patient Details: Mr Bo Kar, 27 years old

Your Role: Acute Care Clinic SHO

Information: Mr Bo walks in to the Acute Care Clinic complaining of worsening pain and requesting for a top-up of painkillers.

He had a right above-knee amputation 1 year ago after a road traffic accident in which he suffered popliteal artery injury and right calf compartment syndrome. He is able to walk with a prosthetic limb but has known phantom limb pain.

You note that he had just seen a GP 7 days ago and was prescribed with:

PO Tramadol 25 mg TDS PRN (for pain) — 3 weeks (63 capsules)
PO Lorazepam 1 mg ON PRN (for sleep) — 3 weeks (21 capsules)

Your task is to speak to Mr Bo and address his concerns.

Planning (From the Stem)

1. **What do I need to assess?/What information do I need to gather?**
   - Take a pain history – what is the nature of Mr Bo's pain and how severe is it?
   - Why is he asking for a top up/why has he run out so quickly? Note that he has finished a 3-week supply of tramadol and midazolam within 1 week.
   - Are there any drug side effects or toxicity?
2. **What do I need to convey?**
   - Empathy for the pain he is experiencing.
   - Need to create a management plan to achieve better pain control.
3. **What is the safety issue here?**
   - Suicide risk assessment.
   - Risk of drug dependence, overdose, and diversion (see discussion).

4. **What are the ethics and communications principles here?**
   - Patient safety.
   - Patient autonomy.

Patient's Brief

You are a 27-year-old. Your life was shattered 1 year ago after a freak traffic accident. It was none of your fault — a speeding Porsche lost control and mounted the kerb, in the process running over your right leg. The doctors said that they had to amputate your right leg to save your life. You survived — you are a fighter. You have also learnt to walk with a prosthetic limb and returned back to work as a sales manager.

Open the consult with "I am in pain. Doctor, please give me more painkillers. I really need them." You have had right leg pain ever since the operation. You were told that this was called 'phantom limb pain' and you would need long-term painkillers. The amputation stump has healed well without problems. You have come to accept the diagnosis and it has become part of you. You are vague about the nature of pain, but you will admit that you feel no more than a mild nagging pain most times — thanks to the painkillers, which you find quite effective. Each tramadol capsule works for about 4–6 hours, but you take it every 1–2 hours. If asked, explain that the pills make you feel 'better'. If you do not take the pills, you start feeling anxious and irritable, your heart rate goes up, and you get a general sense of unease. You are not taking the pills in advance because of fear of the pain coming back. You are a little woozy at times and pass motion only once a week, but you are not troubled by this. You do not take alcohol, other drugs, or illicit substances. You do not give or sell your pills to anyone else.

You were previously prescribed three 20 mg capsules of tramadol a day and a 5 mg tablet of midazolam a night as required. You have been using similar painkillers for the past four months. You find yourself using up the prescriptions very quickly and needing to search for more supplies. You have been to many different emergency rooms and GPs with your old prescription, asking for refills of the same prescription.

Throughout the consult, insist that you need the painkillers. You are impatient and demanding but not anxious or in distress. Your mood is not low, and you have never had any thoughts about suicide. Your appetite and sleep are decent with the medicines. You do not like to be asked about psychiatric matters and will show impatience (e.g., "Doctor, just give me the medicines. I'm not crazy. Why are you asking so much?").

If the doctor refuses to give you the painkillers, you will react with distress and accuse the doctor of mistreating you and not caring about you. You are only mildly receptive to any counselling about the risk of opioid addiction. If the doctor treats you in an accusatory manner, say, "Doctor, I don't like how you are talking to me. Just tell me if you don't trust me, I'll go somewhere else." Your bottom line is that you need something for your pain today. You will accept any solution proposed as long as your pain is addressed, including a more limited prescription of painkillers. However, you prefer not to be admitted because the nurses will control the amount of painkillers you take.

You have some specific questions for the doctor at this consultation:

- Can you give me something stronger to take the pain away?
- So what are you going to do for my pain? I need something right now!

Case Discussion

Reading the candidate's information should set off alarm bells in your mind. This is an unfortunate young man with chronic pain — how is he coping, medically, socially, and emotionally? Why has he run out of a 3-week supply of opioids and benzodiazepines within 1 week? The possibilities are that (a) he has lost the pills, (b) he is taking more pills than prescribed, (c) he is hoarding pills to commit suicide, (d) or he is diverting the pills (i.e., selling addictive medications on the black market).

As always, do not rush to confront him about these issues, but begin by seeking information. Open-ended questions (e.g., "What can I do for you today?") are a good place to start. Mr Bo will tell you all about how bad his pain is. Respond with empathy and genuine concern for his pain. Set an agenda — tell him that you want to help him with this pain, but first you need to find out more about the pain and how he has been.

This scenario diverges from Chronic Pain I at this point. Issues discussed in Chronic Pain I are not repeated here. See how 'similar' scenarios can play out so differently!

Take a pain history and assess for medication side effects (as per Chronic Pain I). Recognise that (a) Mr Bo's pain is not actually severe, (b) he is taking additional doses of opioids in the absence of pain, and (c) he seems to get withdrawal symptoms if he *does not* take the pills. This is all suspicious for drug dependency.

This has to be handled with care. You have to raise your concern and will fail if you simply enable his behaviour by prescribing more opioids and benzodiazepines. On the other hand, you must acknowledge that he does have pain and a need for some analgesia, and you cannot take a confrontational stance. Try to come across from the perspective of trying to help him, and align his interest with yours. If he is experiencing side effects, you can use that to persuade him, but he is not bothered about side effects in this scenario. A possible line could be: "I want to help you. You are clearly in pain and I can't imagine how terrible it must be to lose a limb at your age. I know that the medicines help, but I am concerned about the number of tablets you are taking. What I am hearing makes me worried about your safety."

Assess for suicide risk (see Chronic Pain I), which is low in this case.

Propose a strategy to manage his pain. He will likely decline admission because his drug supply will be controlled inpatient. You should attempt to optimise non-opioid analgesia (paracetamol, NSAIDs, neuropathic pain agents) and refer him to a specialist in pain medicine. In PACES, you can say that you will get the chronic pain expert to see him on the same day. In real life this is unlikely, and you would have to tide Mr Bo through until his appointment with the specialist in pain medicine.

Managing opioid use in this case is complex and best managed by a specialist in pain medicine. Mr Bo will likely still need a controlled amount of opioid analgesia, but it should be supplied in the context of a patient-provider agreement (that he must attend follow ups, comply to dose limits, and not take opioids from other sources or multiple providers). Clear goals of therapy must be set (e.g., that pain will be manageable rather than that there will be no pain). Any reduction in opioid dose has to be done gradually as sudden cessation of chronic opioids could lead to withdrawal, pain crisis, and even suicidality.

If taking the examination in Singapore: Singapore's national guidelines for the safe prescribing of opioids[5] set out a practice boundary for medical practitioners who have not received formal training in pain management, guidelines on monitoring for signs of abuse, and legal requirements on the reporting of suspected drug addicts. It will be a reasonable expectation for the PACES candidate to be familiar with this guideline.

---

[5] Ministry of Health. 2021. National Guidelines for the safe prescribing of opioids. Retrieved 20 June 2021, from https://www.moh.gov.sg/docs/librariesprovider5/default-document-library/national-guidelines-for-the-safe-prescribing-of-opioids-2021.pdf

Communication Case 13

Drug Overdose

Use this case as practice! The pull-out booklet contains the candidate's information.

Information for the Candidate

Patient Details: Ms Theresa Downs, 35 years old

Your Role: Medical Ward SHO

Information: Ms Downs is a nurse working in your hospital. She was admitted to your ward two days ago after another nurse found her unconscious in the staff changing room prior to the start of her shift, and wheeled her to the Emergency Department. A drug screen for benzodiazepines has come back positive.

Your task is to speak to her about this episode and broach the topic of psychiatric review.

Planning (From the Stem)

1. **What do I need to assess?/What information do I need to gather?**
   - Circumstances surrounding the drug overdose – background psychiatric history, her mood at present, ongoing stressors, what drugs she took and where she obtained it.
2. **What do I need to convey?**
   - Your concern about her safety.
   - Refer for psychiatric review.
3. **What is the safety issue here?**
   - Was this a suicide attempt? – if so, you need a plan to keep Ms Downs safe.
   - Patient safety – Does Ms Downs pose a risk to patients? Is there a fitness to practice concern, or will she require additional supervision?
4. **What are the ethics and communications principles here?**
   - Patient autonomy vs. beneficence – convincing her to agree to psychiatric review and managing a situation in which she does not agree.
   - Confidentiality vs. justice (patient safety) – whether to inform her employer/ward nursing manager in view of potential harm to patients.

Patient's Brief

You are a nurse working at the same hospital to which you are now admitted. You have a history of depression, which has been stable on fluoxetine 10 mg ON for many years. In the last few months, however, you have been rather stressed at work as your ward is shorthanded. Your relationship with your husband has been poor for a while now, and you suspect that he is having an affair. Two mornings ago, you chanced upon a phone picture of your husband posing suggestively with a scantily clad lady, and you became extremely distraught. You remembered that your mother has some "calming pills" for her anxiety and put a bottle of them in your purse as you headed to work. In the spur of the moment, you took twelve of those pills just as you were clocking in for your shift. You did not intend to end your life but you wanted to take away these horrible emotions. You do not remember what happened after this.

You will initially deny taking any pills, but when confronted, you will admit to what you have done. You regret your actions and feel rather embarrassed about it. You did not think that twelve tablets would cause any adverse effect. You have never had, and do not currently have, any intention to end your life. You do not hear any voices. You have never attempted suicide or self-harm. You have never attempted to take medications or injections meant for the patients you care for. You have been otherwise well and feel completely well now. You have no past medical history.

Your main concern is that word about this event might get out. You do not want any doctors (other than those treating you now), colleagues, superiors, or family members finding out about what has happened. You want assurance from the candidate that none of these people will come to know about what has happened. You are also not keen for psychiatric review. If probed, explain that you are afraid that you will be spotted by colleagues or other hospital staff. However, you might be open to seeing a psychiatrist in a different hospital.

You are jumpy and suspicious. If the candidate says anything that has a whiff of suggestion that anyone else might come to know about your situation, you will get upset and agitated and even express feelings of being tricked into confiding in the candidate.

You have some specific questions for the doctor at this consultation:

- Can you not tell my husband that I took these pills please? It will make our relationship even worse.
- Please don't tell any one else, including the psychiatrist.
- Please promise me you will not tell my superiors. I'm not suicidal; I can go right back to work. Don't get me in trouble.

Case Discussion

This scenario is not straightforward. Begin by asking how she has been and what she understood has happened.

You will have to ask her about her drug overdose and such a confrontation is never easy. The key is to be supportive, non-judgemental, and non-accusatory. A possible way of phrasing this might be: "Ms Downs, you were found unconscious in the staff room earlier by your colleagues. As you know there are quite a few causes why someone might be unconscious including infections, strokes. Some drugs and toxins can also cause unconsciousness, and these can be taken intentionally or accidentally, such as in certain supplements bought online. Do you think any of this may have happened to you?" This will probably get her to open up and admit to having taken benzodiazepines. If not, you will have to explain that a routine urine test has come back positive for benzodiazepines and ask her if she has any idea why this might be so.

Thank her for confiding in you and offer empathy and support, and that you are here to help her and you want the best for her. If she is hesitant and not forthcoming, one useful strategy is to normalise her emotions, such as by saying that such emotions are common and many people face it at some point in their life. Assess her mental state and triggers, and perform a suicide risk assessment (see Case 11). Find out where she obtained the benzodiazepines, in particular, if she has ever taken any drugs from the ward that were meant for patients as this becomes a particular risk.

Formulate a management plan. The candidate information helpfully guides you to breach the topic of psychiatric referral (which you must do even if it were not stated for you). Explain your concern for her safety and that getting help is one way to bounce back quicker and stronger. When she resists the idea of seeing a psychiatrist, the correct strategy is to find out why she is hesitant, rather than simply persisting in explaining why you want her to see a psychiatrist. As it becomes clear that she does not want anyone in the same hospital to know that she is seeing a psychiatrist, offer to refer her to a psychiatrist in another hospital. Other aspects of management include giving her medical leave until her psychiatrist appointment due to concern of workplace safety (proximity to potentially hazardous medicines).

The confidentiality questions are ethically tricky. They juxtapose the tenet of protecting patient confidentiality against the risk of harm to others. These are also culturally sensitive, so the correct answer may differ depending on where you are taking PACES.

a) Telling her husband. This is quite clear — you should not breach confidentiality. You can explain that you will not speak to her husband about her condition except with her permission. Express empathy and your hope that they patch up.

b) Telling the psychiatrist/other medical professionals. You should do so on a 'need to know' basis — for example, to refer her to a psychiatrist, you will have to state what has happened so that she can be assessed appropriately. Express your understanding that she does not want too many people to know and that you will seek to mitigate this, for instance by not referring her to a psychiatrist in the same hospital. In the UK, the GP is an important part of continuity of care and should also be informed.

c) Telling her employer. You should encourage her to inform a trusted supervisor at work, but it becomes tricky if she refuses. We (the authors) have not found a clear consensus after consulting a number of senior clinicians and ethics board members in both Singapore and the UK. It is clear that if there is a risk to patients or a concern about fitness to practice, then you must tell the employer (or the regulatory body, for that matter). If there is no risk to patients, the best answer is probably context dependent — in Singapore, we would probably inform a trusted senior (e.g., the nurse manager) who must look out for her; in the UK, there might be greater emphasis on protecting patient confidentiality unless there is a risk of harm to others. You will have to make a decision and stand your ground. Alternatively, you could potentially side-step this by putting her on medical leave until the psychiatrist's consultation, leaving it to the psychiatrist's professional judgement whether to certify her fit to work and whether informing a trusted supervisor in the workplace will be a necessary condition for her to return to work.

Communication Case 14

Withdrawal of Dialysis

Use this case as practice! The pull-out booklet contains the candidate's information.

Information for the Candidate

Patient Details: Ms Elsa Queen, 77 years old

Your Role: Acute Medical Unit SHO

Information: Ms Queen is a 77-year-old with a past medical history of diabetes with diabetic nephropathy.

Three months ago, she presented in cardiogenic shock from an acute myocardial infarction. Emergency percutaneous coronary intervention was successful in stenting the left anterior descending artery. She had a stormy recovery with acute on chronic kidney disease requiring renal replacement therapy. She did not recover renal function and was discharged to community haemodialysis via a tunnelled dialysis catheter.

Since discharge, she has been readmitted thrice — once for dialysiscatheter infection, another for intra-dialytic hypotension, and most recently for methicillin-resistant *staphylococcus aureus* (MRSA) bacteraemia. Transesophageal echocardiography showed normal valves, no valvular vegetations, and an ejection fraction of 17%. She received intravenous vancomycin and a change of the dialysis catheter.

Ms Queen is currently admitted to your ward, having been referred by the dialysis centre for recurrent intra-dialytic chest pain and hypotension. Despite technical optimisation of the dialysis prescription, she has not been able to complete a full dialysis session since her last discharge. Ms Queen is breathless, acidotic, and hyperkalemic. Your consultant has decided to withdraw dialysis support as she is unable to tolerate dialysis.

Ms Queen's only child, who lives overseas, has flown back after hearing of the plan to withdraw dialysis.

Your task is to speak to Ms Queen's son, Mr Payne, and address his concerns. You may assume the necessary permissions to discuss the patient's confidential medical information with Mr Payne.

Planning (From the Stem)

1. **What do I need to assess?/What information do I need to gather?**
   - What does Ms Queen's son understand about the clinical situation?

- How has the patient been coping with haemodialysis, and what is her view on continuing dialysis?
- If her only child lives overseas, what is the patient's social setup like?

2. **What do I need to convey?**
   - That continuing haemodialysis is not in Ms Queen's best interest. The case vignette provides multiple reasons why this is so, including inadequate cardiac function to support haemodialysis, poor tolerability of dialysis, serious infective complications, etc.

3. **What is the safety issue here?**
   - That continuing haemodialysis does more harm than good. Do not capitulate to the patient's demands and offer haemodialysis.

4. **What are the ethics and communications principles here?**
   - Beneficence and non-maleficence, in not offering a treatment whose risks outweigh the benefits.
   - This may conflict with patient autonomy. However, should a patient insist on medical treatment that is not indicated or beneficial, the medical practitioner is not ethically required to provide such treatment.

Surrogate's Brief

You are Ms Queen's only child. You are stationed in China as the regional head of a large multinational firm and have lived and worked overseas for the past 10 years.

Yesterday, Dad called to say that the doctors have refused to dialyse Mum any further. Shocked and upset, you made arrangements to fly home immediately. You are well aware that Mum's kidneys have failed and that she will pass away without dialysis, so you cannot believe that the doctors would simply 'give up' on Mum. Furthermore, you are very perplexed by the move to stop dialysis when three months ago, doctors at the same hospital had told you that Mum needed dialysis or she would die; it was never really an 'option'. You would have understood the decision to stop dialysis if Mum were critically ill and too sick to be dialysed, but she currently appears quite well and the nurses have told you that her blood pressure and blood tests are normal. You cannot believe that the doctors, for all they say about saving lives, will consciously choose to let Mum die. Open your conversation with a statement to the effect of: "How can you let my mother die; do you not have a heart?"

You believe that you understand Mum's medical background well. You remember flying home in haste 3 months ago when Mum had a heart attack. You understand that her kidneys failed because of a contrast dye used during the heart 'balloon' procedure; you remain upset at this outcome and believe that Mum need not have suffered kidney failure had the doctors been more careful. You are not aware of any other hospital admissions since that episode. Over the phone, Mum has said that she found dialysis difficult to tolerate, describing it as 'four hours of torture' due to chest pain. At times she has asked whether she could stop dialysis, but you have encouraged her to soldier on. Mum has also had difficulty making it to the dialysis centre because she has become a lot weaker since the heart attack; Dad, whom she lives with, can't be of much help as he is himself a stroke patient. You know that Mum is not doing well at the moment. Nonetheless, in spite of these difficulties, you believe that continuing dialysis is preferable to letting Mum die.

Your aim in this conversation is to persuade the doctors to reverse the decision to withdraw dialysis. You feel a deep sense of betrayal by medical staff. Privately, you also feel a deep sense of guilt at having been overseas and away during your parents' twilight years. You want to do everything you can to keep Mum alive.

You have some specific questions for the doctor at this consultation:

- Did my mum's kidneys fail because of the heart stent procedure? I will sue the hospital!
- If we stop dialysis now, how long does my mum have to live?

Case Discussion

Grasp the clinical information in the scenario. Why is your consultant withdrawing dialysis? You must understand the clinical reasoning behind this decision before you can explain it to the surrogate. Ms Queen has heart failure with an ejection fraction of 17%. This is inadequate to support the haemodynamic demands of haemodialysis, which is why she is suffering intra-dialytic chest pain and hypotension. She is also encountering multiple infective complications. Can anything be done to improve the situation? Cardiac revascularisation has already been performed, and attempts to adjust dialysis settings have not resolved the issue (you will not be expected to know the technical details of dialysis prescription). Therefore, haemodialysis is unsustainable and may cause greater harm (sepsis, cardiac events) than good. The management of a patient who is unable to tolerate dialysis is complex and withdrawing dialysis is a last resort, but in this scenario the decision has been made for you.

The stem makes clear that Mr Payne is concerned about the plan to withdraw dialysis; he probably disagrees with it and may be unhappy. The correct strategy is not to preach to him or argue with him; rather, seek to probe his understanding of his mother's condition and guide him to a realisation that dialysis is not in his mother's best interest.

Mr Payne begins with an aggressive statement: "How can you let my mother die; do you not have a heart?" This is a difficult start, but resist the urge to rebut the statement or respond defensively. Instead, demonstrate that you hear his concerns — show 'listening' body language (e.g., learning into him, mirroring his posture), verbally acknowledge his concern/emotion, and state that you are here to fill him in on his mother's clinical condition and discuss the matter. Invite him to share what he understands so far and his thoughts on it.

Mr Payne is unaware of the dialysis-related complications Ms Queen has encountered and he believes that dialysis is the only way forward. Gently probe this, focusing not only on information-giving but also addressing his emotions, values, and personality. For example:

- Check understanding: "How has your mum been coping with dialysis?"/"What has your mum said about dialysis so far"? He will reveal that Ms Queen has been having difficulty with dialysis.
- Check emotional coping: "It must be very stressful for everyone"/"How is your family coping"?
- Values: "What does your mum value most?"/"What are your mum's worries/concerns?" He may even reveal that Ms Queen has actually expressed a desire to discontinue dialysis.
- Patient as a person: "Can you tell me more about Ms Queen as a person?"

It is important to respond to the information revealed in a manner that demonstrates that the medical team has been journeying with Ms Queen. For instance, when Mr Payne acknowledges Ms Queen's desire to stop dialysis, reflect these sentiments by saying, for instance, "Yes, she has been sharing this thought with us throughout her inpatient stay. Dialysis has been so hard on her." This builds trust by *showing* that the medical team's goals are aligned with Ms Queen's wishes, rather than by simply *telling* Mr Payne that the medical team has good intentions. Also do acknowledge how deeply Mr Payne loves his mum and validate his feelings that he cannot bear to lose his mum.

It may also be helpful to assuage his feelings of guilt about not being present for Ms Queen in the past, by redirecting his focus to his presence in the present. For example: "Ms Queen and the whole medical team are so glad you are finally here. Ms Queen has been telling us all about her only son whom she is proud of and loves very much. She has been looking forward to see you. Thank you for travelling all the way on such short notice to be here." This also further implies that the medical team has been journeying with Ms Queen, and is on his/Ms Queen's side.

Fill Mr Payne in with information on the episodes of line sepsis, and that Ms Queen's heart function makes her unable to tolerate dialysis. Be clear in explaining that dialysis will cause more harm than good. In particular, it can lead to life-threatening infections, dangerous episodes of low blood pressure, or trigger a heart attack.

Mr Payne's questions require some thought:

(1) Did my mum's kidneys fail because of the heart stent procedure? I will sue the hospital!
  - Explain that her kidney failure is multifactorial not only due to the contrast used, but also from underlying diabetic nephropathy and hypoperfusion from cardiogenic shock.
  - Explain that percutaneous coronary intervention, with its risk of contrast nephropathy, was unavoidable in the context of an acute myocardial infarction with cardiogenic shock — it was necessary to save her life.
  - If the surrogate continues to respond unfavourably and insists on suing, acknowledge his unhappiness and offer to direct the matter to the patient liaison service/service quality (or your local equivalent). Explain that legal action

is within his rights, but regardless of how he decides, your primary consideration right now is how best to take care of Ms Queen moving forward.

(2) If we stop dialysis now, how long does my mum have to live?
- If Ms Queen has no residual renal function (no longer passing urine), she is expected to pass away in about 2 weeks from cessation of dialysis.

This is a good juncture to transit into discussing Ms Queen's care moving forward. Explain the overarching goal to prevent suffering. Emphasise non-abandonment — that palliative care is not 'doing nothing' or 'letting her die'; rather, she will receive the best possible care to prevent suffering, including treatment of symptoms. Offer multidisciplinary team care including involvement of a palliative service

You or may not be able to persuade the surrogate to accept palliative management. Do not be pushy. If the surrogate is unable to accept palliative management, acknowledge that this is difficult and that he may need some time. Offer support and arrange a follow-up conversation. In real life, patients and families often need some time to accept scenarios like withdrawal of dialysis or terminal extubation.

Note: An additional consideration for the patient who cannot tolerate haemodialysis is whether peritoneal dialysis is a feasible alternative. This discussion is beyond the level expected of a PACES candidate. Similarly, detailed medical management of recurrent intradialytic hypotension is probably too advanced for MRCP PACES.

Communication Case 15

Supratentorial

Use this case as practice! The pull-out booklet contains the candidate's information.

Information for the Candidate

Patient Details: Ms Amy Dole, 42 years old

Your Role: Cardiology Clinic SHO

Information: Ms Dole is a 42-year-old lady with fibromyalgia, irritable bowel syndrome, and migraine on follow up with multiple specialists. Blood tests, multiple gastroscopes and colonoscopies, as well as a CT brain and CT abdomen are normal.

In the past six months, she has visited the Emergency Department seven times for chest pain; each time with normal ECGs, troponins, and chest X-rays. She has been referred to Cardiology and underwent further investigations including a treadmill stress test, echocardiogram, and 24-hour ECG monitoring, all of which were normal. She has been discharged from Cardiology follow up two weeks ago.

Ms Dole has walked in to clinic today, complaining of a two-day history of atypical chest pain. Her vital signs and clinical examination are normal. An ECG, full blood count, electrolytes, CRP, troponin, and D-dimer* are normal. Your consultant will like to refer Ms Dole for psychiatric consult for anxiety disorder.

Your task is to inform Ms Dole of her test results, offer psychiatric consultation, and manage her concerns.

*In patients with a low pre-test probability of pulmonary embolism and a normal D-dimer, the chance of a pulmonary embolism is approximately 0.1%[6].

Planning (From the Stem)

1. **What do I need to assess?/What information do I need to gather?**
   - Current symptoms – but be careful not to take a history.
   - What are Ms Dole's concerns? – there are likely to be very many, so it is helpful to gather all of them at the beginning and set an agenda.

---

[6] Bass AR, Fields KG, Goto R, Turissini G, Dey S, Russell LA. Clinical Decision Rules for Pulmonary Embolism in Hospitalized Patients: A Systematic Literature Review and Meta-analysis. *Thromb Haemost* 2017 117(11):2176.

- Is there any underlying psychological or social issue leading to multiple somatic complaints? Why does your consultant suggest psychiatric referral?

2. **What do I need to convey?**
   - Reassure Ms Dole that all test results are normal, there is no serious illness, and management is supportive.
   - At the same time, you must convey empathy and concern. Ms Dole must feel listened to; you must not downplay her symptoms.
   - Breach the topic of psychiatric consultation sensitively.

3. **What is the safety issue here?**
   - Appropriate use of diagnostic investigations.

4. **What are the ethics and communications principles here?**
   - Patient autonomy and empowerment.
   - Justice and responsible resource use – avoiding inappropriate over-investigation.

Patient's Brief

You have been in poor health for quite many years now. It started when your husband left you for a younger woman 5 years ago. Since then, you have been plagued by intractable tiredness, muscle aches, headaches, tummy aches, and episodes of diarrhoea. Despite seeing multiple specialists and doing many scans and tests, nobody can find out what is wrong with you. You have been told that it's all in your mind, but your pain is genuine; nobody understands you and nobody is listening.

You used to work as an accounts executive, but you have taken so many days of medical leave that successive employers have asked you to leave. You have been on social welfare for the past 6 months. It has been tough and you feel terrible about being a poor mother to your 8-year-old daughter.

Since losing your last job 6 months ago, you have been experiencing on-and-off chest pains. These seem to be a poking pain, alternately at the right and left sides of your chest. They come on at random times of the day and are not worse on exertion. Watching television dramas seems to help; stress makes it worse. You do not have any leg swelling, breathlessness, long-haul travel, or recent hospitalisations/surgeries. You take paracetamol and an antacid but no other medications, supplements, or contraceptive pills.

The Emergency Department has referred you to the heart doctors and you have done many tests; again, you have been told that your heart is completely normal. However, you have read online about a condition called 'pulmonary embolism', which affects young ladies and can present with chest pain. You know that the test for this condition is a special CT scan of the lungs, which you have not done. You are very worried about your health in general and about a pulmonary embolism in particular. You have not been able to sleep or eat well. You wonder what will happen to your daughter if you pass away from a pulmonary embolism.

You will open the consultation by informing the candidate of your chest pain. You are anxious; your speech is pressured and rapid. You are convinced that you need the special CT scan for pulmonary embolism. You will get upset if the candidate does not treat your pain seriously or dismisses your concerns. However, if listened to, you are reasonable and can be persuaded that you do not have a pulmonary embolism.

Your doctors have previously suggested psychiatric consultation but you have not been keen. You do not think that you are crazy and you will feel insulted by any suggestion to that effect. However, you are keen to find out what is wrong with you and you are motivated to get better. You are open to the possibility that your emotions may contribute to your symptoms and will consider seeing a psychiatrist/starting medicines for anxiety if you are convinced that this will help you get better.

You have some specific questions for the doctor at this consultation:
- Do I have a pulmonary embolism? I read that it can cause chest pain.
- Are you going to be responsible if I die from pulmonary embolism?
- What is wrong with me? Why can't anyone figure out what is wrong?
- What are you going to do for me?

Case Discussion

Ms Dole is a lady with multiple conditions with known psychosomatic links, who now complains of persistent chest pain despite normal investigations. All of us will have managed such patients with varying degrees of success; this encounter puts the spotlight on the communication skills required in the situation — good communication can be therapeutic in itself.

Open the scenario by listening to Ms Dole. Give her at least a minute to vent. Explain that you are here to help and ask her to list her concerns — she is likely to have many of them, so setting an agenda at the onset will aid your time management.

You must recognise that Ms Dole is very troubled by her symptoms. It is critical to show that you are listening and concerned, so as to gain her trust and establish a therapeutic relationship. Never downplay or dismiss a symptom no matter how psychosomatic you may think it is — it is real to the patient and any suggestion to the contrary will destroy any chance you have to persuade the patient of what you say.

After listening to Ms Dole, explain the test results (both the current encounter's and the normal treadmill, echocardiogram, and 24-hour ECG). Invite her to respond to the results.

Ms Dole is concerned about pulmonary embolism (PE). The candidate's information includes a footnote that a patient with low pre-test probability and normal D-dimer is unlikely to have PE. Such footnotes occasionally appear in MRCP scenarios (often added by a charitable question vetter who worries that candidates may not be familiar with a critical piece of information). The footnote suggests that you are expected to counsel her that the chance of PE is low — please take the hint! It is good practice to verify that she indeed has a low pre-test probability (e.g., no recent long-haul flight, no leg swelling), but do not spend too long here.

Her request for a CT pulmonary angiogram needs to be approached sensitively. You have to persuade her that CT is not necessary because the risk of PE is very low and the scan is not without radiation or cost, yet you cannot be seen as dismissing her concern. The question, "are you going to be responsible if I die from PE", is best defused by tackling her words head on, for example: "As your physicians we are of course responsible for you. I will do my best for you and I want you to get better." Shift the focus away from whether you will or will not do the CT scan. Instead, explore why she is worried about PE, which will reveal that online reading has made her anxious. Name this emotion — that she is anxious — and share how you come to the conclusion that PE is unlikely (i.e., clinical features inconsistent with the type of chest pain in PE, lack of risk factors + normal D dimer). Providing information about the decision-making process and making your thought process transparent is far more reassuring than a blanket denial of her request.

Ms Dole will reveal her frustration that she has persistent symptoms that nobody can figure out. The key here is in her psychological state and social stressors, both of which you must explore. One approach is to find out more about her background, how she is coping with social stressors, and gently suggest, "Is there anything in your life that you feel is making your health suffer?" Alternatively, acknowledge her symptoms and stressors, normalise it as a common experience, then ask her directly: "It sounds like there is a lot on your plate right now. Often people in your situation find that how stressed they are affects their physical health. Do you feel that the stress could be affecting your physical health?"

The topic of psychiatric consultation must not be raised out of the blue (e.g., "I think your chest pain is all in the mind, maybe you should see a psychiatrist"). It can only be raised if Ms Dole appreciates the possibility that her emotions may contribute to her symptoms, and that managing the emotions will help her symptoms or at least help her to cope better — only then will she agree to psychiatric consultation.

As you discuss the management plan, do manage expectations and set goals — she is unlikely to ever become pain-free, but the goal should be to minimise and cope with the symptoms, reassured by the knowledge that she is unlikely to have a serious medical condition. It will be good to craft a plan for the next time Ms Dole has chest pain (e.g., when to try analgesia at home, what are the red flags that require Emergency Department evaluation), and set a date for a follow-up consult. Find out what is important to her — align your interest with hers and set goals together. For example, a reasonable goal will be for Ms Dole to be able to cope well enough to return to work.

It is easy to run out of time in a scenario like this. You must ensure that you cover the task set — that is, if at the '2 minutes remaining' warning you have yet to discuss psychiatric referral, immediately move on to discuss this. If you are unable to address all of her concerns, wrap up and set a close follow-up visit to address her remaining concerns.

598   A STRATEGY TO AND WORKED PRACTICE FOR THE MRCP PACES

Communication Case 16

BRCA Testing

Use this case as practice! The pull-out booklet contains the candidate's information.

Information for the Candidate

Patient Details: Ms A. Jollie, 37 years old

Your Role: Medicine Clinic SHO

Information: Ms Jollie sees you in clinic to discuss BRCA1 testing. Her mother has recently passed away from ovarian cancer at 56 years of age. Her 38-year-old sister has just had her breast removed due to breast cancer.

Your task is to discuss BRCA testing with Ms Jollie.

Planning (From the Stem)

1. **What do I need to assess?/What information do I need to gather?**
   - Is Ms Jollie asymptomatic now?
   - Does her sister/mother have a known BRCA mutation?
   - Does she have a partner and is she planning pregnancy?
2. **What do I need to convey?**
   - Counsel on genetic testing, implications of positive and negative results, and the possibility of indeterminate results.
3. **What is the safety issue here?**
   - She is at high risk for breast cancer regardless of the result of BRCA testing and will require screening even if the result is negative.
4. **What are the ethics and communications principles here?**
   - Informed consent; pre-testing counselling in genetic testing.

Patient's Brief

You are a 37-year-old actress with a high-flying career. You have always been well with no medical conditions. You are still in shock that your mother passed away so young from ovarian cancer, and soon after, your younger sister has had to undergo mastectomy for a breast cancer. You were told that this was 'early stage'.

You have read about the BRCA mutation online and wonder if your family has the mutation. You will like to take control of your life and are keen to get tested. If you are positive for BRCA and are more likely than not to develop breast cancer, you wish to consider having your breasts and ovaries removed. You believe that BRCA testing will be able to give you a clear-cut "yes I will get breast and/or ovarian cancer" / "no I am not at increased risk of breast and/or ovarian cancer" answer.

Neither your mother nor your sister have been tested for the BRCA gene. Your sister is not keen to be tested. You do not know of any other family members who have had breast, ovarian, pancreas, or prostate cancer.

You currently have a partner. You do not have children yet but do hope to have children in the next 2 years. You are well-covered with many overlapping insurance policies, purchased by your managing agent the moment you began your acting career.

You have some specific questions for the doctor at this consultation:

- If I don't have the BRCA gene, does it mean that I am safe?
- If I have the BRCA gene, should I remove my breasts and ovaries?
- I don't have to involve my sister in this, do I?

Case Discussion

There is a lot to discuss in a short amount of time. A good strategy in such a situation is to let the patient guide the agenda – suss out what is important to this patient (and therefore what is on the marking sheet), so that you can provide necessary information but not overload her. You will be expected to know the basics of genetic counselling but not the full details.

Begin by expressing empathy for her mother's death and acknowledging her worry. Set an agenda — explain that you can't cover everything in 10 minutes, but will give her an overview and ask her what are the key questions that she will like you to cover.

Gather more information:

- Clarify that she is asymptomatic; that there is no breast lump, skin changes around the nipple, or nipple discharge.
- Find out more about her mother's and sister's cancer histories. In particular, ask whether any of them underwent BRCA testing or if they have any other cancers (in addition to breast cancer, BRCA is associated with increased risk of ovarian, pancreas, and (in males) prostate cancer).
- Ask her what she understands about BRCA testing.
- Ask her why she wants to be screened and what she plans to do with the results. Take note of misconceptions identified (but clarify it later rather than interrupting her there and then).

The second half of the station is for you to explain BRCA screening. The starting principle is that she is at high risk of breast cancer regardless of the BRCA test result. She will require breast cancer screening starting immediately (to start screening 5–10 years before the youngest case in family).

Explain what BRCA screening entails. BRCA testing is typically not done in isolation, but along with a panel of other genes that may cause hereditary breast cancer.

The ideal setting is when we know the family's mutation and this will require that we first test an index case known to have disease — that is, her mother or sister. Interpretation of results becomes trickier when we do not know the family mutation.

The BRCA result is not 'positive' or 'negative'. It is a gene and there are different variants of interest — some known to be associated with breast cancer, whereas others are indeterminate. Possible outcomes of BRCA testing are:

- If BRCA testing does not find any variant associated with breast cancer – based on family history alone she is still high risk and requires screening; this does not mean that she is 'safe'.
- If BRCA testing shows a variant known to be associated with breast cancer – she is definitely at high risk of breast cancer and ovarian cancer. In this situation, some patients would want to consider prophylactic mastectomy and oophorectomy after completing their family.
- If BRCA testing shows a variant of unknown significance – this is an indeterminate result and we are none the wiser. She remains high risk and requires screening.

BRCA testing carries implications including on insurance coverage, the potential for genetic discrimination, on family planning and potentially on bone health (if she decides on prophylactic oophorectomy, this will induce early menopause and require hormone replacement therapy). These must be discussed prior to doing the BRCA test. Some women with pathogenic BRCA mutations choose to complete their family earlier so as to minimize delay in having their ovaries and breasts removed.

Offer a plan moving forward. Explain that she does not have to make a decision immediately and you will like to arrange for her to meet a genetic counsellor and receive additional information about breast cancer screening. Schedule a follow-up appointment to continue the discussion.

Additionally, you should offer to meet her sister, who may also benefit from BRCA testing and prophylactic mastectomy/oophorectomy. There are therapeutic implications in that BRCA patients are treated differently in both the curative and metastatic settings.

Reference: NCCN guidelines (open access article):
Daly MB et al. CCN clinical practice guidelines in oncology (NCCN guidelines) genetic/familial high-risk assessment: breast, ovarian, and pancreatic. *J Natl Compr Canc Netw* 2021 19(1): 77–102.

Think this through: Other genetic diseases

Consider how pre-testing genetic counselling changes in the following scenarios:

a) Huntington's disease: a monogenic disease with 100% penetrance (all patients with the gene will develop disease) and good correlation between the number of trinucleotide repeats and age of disease onset. It is generally unnecessary to test the index case first as the mutation is known.

b) Familial adenomatous polyposis: even without genetic testing, disease manifestations may be quite obvious on colonoscopy (i.e., >10 colorectal adenomas).

c) If an adolescent requests BRCA testing.

Communication Case 17

Doctor Dangerous

Use this case as practice! The pull-out booklet contains the candidate's information.

Information for the Candidate

Patient Details: Dr Green, 25 years old

Your Role: Night-Duty SHO

Information: You are on night duty with Dr Green, the FY1/House Officer.

At approximately 2am, you were called to attend to a Code Blue involving Mdm Loh B. P., a 50-year-old lady admitted two days ago for pneumonia. Mdm Loh responded well to resuscitation and has been transferred to the intensive care unit. She appears to be alert with no permanent neurological sequelae.

While reviewing Mdm Loh's clinical notes, you noted that the ward nurses had called Dr Green at 8pm to inform that Mdm Loh was hypotensive and febrile. Dr Green asked to give a pint of normal saline and some paracetamol, but did not physically review Mdm Loh.

Dr Brainchild, the on-duty medical registrar, is concerned about Dr Green's actions leading up to Mdm Loh's Code Blue and has asked you to speak to Dr Green while he stabilises her in the intensive care unit.

Your task is to speak to Dr Green about his unsafe clinical management.

Planning (From the Stem)

1. **What do I need to assess?/What information do I need to gather?**
   - Why did Dr Green neglect to review Mdm Loh – was he overwhelmed, did he not grasp the significance of her hypotension, or something else?
   - What could be behind Dr Green's unsafe clinical management this night? Is there an underlying cause?

2. **What do I need to convey?**
   - That Dr Green's management of Mdm Loh was inappropriate and dangerous.

3. **What is the safety issue here?**
   - How to prevent further harm to patients due to Dr Green's management.
   - Is it safe for Dr Green to continue with his night duty? If not, should he be taken off duty immediately?

4. **What are the ethics and communications principles here?**
   - Patient safety – beneficence and non-maleficence.
   - Fitness to practice.

Surrogate's Brief

You are a 25-year-old FY1/House Officer. This is your first FY1 posting, having graduated from medical school 2 months ago. You have been in your current firm/hospital for 2 months and this is the 6th night duty you are performing.

You are surprised to hear that Mdm Loh had collapsed in the ward. You do recall receiving a call about Mdm Loh from the ward nurses earlier, informing you that Mdm Loh had a blood pressure of 80/42 mmHg. You looked through the electronic record and gathered that Mdm Loh had an established diagnosis of pneumonia and was on ceftriaxone. As she was already on appropriate treatment including antibiotics, all that was left for you to do was to give her some fluids. You did not deem it necessary to review her in person; besides, you had quite a lot of other patients to review (a long list — IV cannulae to set, patients with high blood glucose, patients whose fever spiked in the ward, patients with high blood pressure, and so on).

If told that you should have reviewed Mdm Loh, you become flustered and exasperated. You will respond defensively if the candidate tells you what you should have done — how would you have been expected to know this? You did what you thought was right. If her blood pressure did not pick up with saline, then the onus should have been on the nurses to call you again, which they did not.

You have been having a stormy time at work. It has been a drastic change from being a student. You have often felt unsure about patients and stressed about whether you are administering the right treatment. You find yourself quite slow in performing routine tasks such as drawing bloods or completing paperwork, and as a result often feel overwhelmed by the sheer volume of work. You dread doing night duties as the fatigue and incessant calls from nurses have been difficult to cope with. You have learnt not to ask for help because during your first week at work, a SHO treated you roughly and mocked you for asking for help to set an IV. You are aware that you have been assigned a clinical supervisor, Professor Golf, but have never met him/her.

You will readily open up about your personal situation if asked, but will not volunteer this information. Truth be told, you have been feeling quite distracted in the past week. Your father, who has a known history of lung cancer, was admitted to hospital (not the one you are working at) 5 days ago after a seizure. MRI scans showed brain metastases. You have been spending time at his bedside after work every day and feel exhausted. Your mother is in shambles emotionally and you are doing your best to be there for her, but feel anxious and overwhelmed yourself. The oncologist has quoted a prognosis of 3–6 months for your father and you do not know what to do next. You put on a steely front and come to work but this is just a façade. You will start to break down and tear up after talking about your father.

You have some specific questions for the doctor at this consultation:
- Why does everyone expect me to know things, but nobody teaches me?
- What should I do now?

Case Discussion

The overriding principle in this scenario is to ensure patient safety and to care for Dr Green.

Begin by finding out more about the event and why Dr Green made the clinical decisions he did. Beyond the immediate clinical incident, find out more about Dr Green in general so as to identify root causes behind Dr Green's unsafe clinical practice. It is important to take a non-confrontational tone and ensure that you do not come across as having pre-judged him.

Dr Green will reveal a number of worrisome issues:

1. Failure to recognise an unwell patient.
2. Poor clinical reasoning – that because Mdm Loh was already on antibiotics, nothing else needs to be done about her hypotension apart from a pint of saline.
3. Poor task prioritisation.
4. General inability to cope with FY1 work – this may be multifactorial due to inadequate clinical knowledge, unfamiliarity with the clinical environment, or the transition from a student to a position of responsibility.
5. Fear of asking for help or escalating to a senior due to a prior traumatising experience.
6. Personal life issues — father with end-stage cancer — affecting his work.

As Dr Green opens up about his fears, frustrations, and very personal matters such as his father, you must demonstrate genuine empathy and concern for him as a person. Thank him for sharing openly his struggles with you. Recognise that the transition from student to FY1 is not an easy one, and that it is important for him to seek help if he is struggling so that his seniors are aware and can help him.

These are not issues that you can solve within one conversation (or there and then at night, for that matter), but you need to craft a plan moving forward.

1. **Debrief Dr Green about his management of Mdm Loh**, in particular:
   - To recognise that Mdm Loh was unwell.
   - To review Mdm Loh in person.
   - To institute appropriate clinical management such as fluid challenge, escalation of antibiotics, and close review with a view to start vasopressors if persistently hypotensive.
   - To escalate to a senior appropriately.

   It is important to not come across as judgemental. Rather than highlighting personal lapses (second person phrasing such as "you should have assessed her in person",

or "you should have escalated to your seniors earlier"), maintain an objective tone focusing on the expected standard of care (third person phrasing such as "generally, a hypotensive patient should be assessed in person and close review after instituting a trial of treatment is important; if the blood pressure does not pick up then care must be escalated in a timely manner.") This is less likely to trigger a defensive response and help the trainee to receive the feedback better. It will also avoid discouraging a struggling trainee, which would be counterproductive in his reflection and growth from this event.

You will need to judge whether it would be appropriate to discuss these matters immediately or to arrange for another conversation later. If Dr Green becomes flustered or breaks down after talking about his dad, it may be wise to take the latter option (but state clearly that you will need to talk to him about Mdm Loh another day as this will likely be a marking point).

2. **Decide whether Dr Green should continue with his night duty**. If he is not in a good emotional state to continue, he should be sent home to rest. This is unlikely to be a decision you can make independently at your level, but you can suggest that you will consult the duty registrar to resolve this issue.

3. **A follow-up plan** is necessary to remediate the clinical difficulties Dr Green is facing. Apologise for Dr Green's bad experience the first time he attempted to escalate a problem to a senior and state categorically that this should not be the case. Explain that you will discuss with the department and/or his clinical supervisor, find people who are interested to mentor and walk with him, and ensure that he receives appropriate training such that by the end of his FY1 year he is in good stead to become a SHO. He may also require a temporary adjustment of workload or increased supervision. You will not be expected to have the details of such a plan ready, but merely to identify that a remediation plan will be necessary.

Communication Case 18

Send Her Home

Note: The tensions in this scenario are unlikely to play out in the UK National Health Service; it is more relevant in the Singapore context.

Use this case as practice! The pull-out booklet contains the candidate's information.

Information for the Candidate

Patient Details: Mdm Maria, 35 years old

Your Role: Medical High Dependancy SHO

Information: Mdm Maria is a 35-year-old foreign domestic worker from the Philippines with no known past medical history.

She was admitted for a 4-day history of fever, breathlessness, and altered mental state. Investigations revealed acute leukaemia with tumour lysis syndrome, which has caused renal impairment and pulmonary oedema.

Your consultant has discussed her case with the renal and haematology unit. The plan is to insert a non-tunnelled dialysis catheter, administer haemodialysis, and initiate chemotherapy urgently. Dual consultant consent has been obtained to proceed as Mdm Maria is confused and has been assessed to lack mental capacity. Your consultant expects that Maria will have a long and stormy hospital stay with multiple sessions of dialysis and a long course of chemotherapy. However, without treatment, Mdm Maria is expected to deteriorate and pass away within days.

Her employer, Mrs Blackheart, has made known that she objects to dialysis and chemotherapy, and requests to speak to a member of staff.

Your task is to speak to Mrs Blackheart and address her concerns. You may assume that Mdm Maria has consented to this conversation.

Planning (From the Stem)

1. **What do I need to assess?/What information do I need to gather?**
   - What does Mrs Blackheart understand of the situation? Why is she objecting to treatment?

2. **What do I need to convey?**
   - The seriousness of Maria's current condition and the urgency of treatment.
   - To address Mrs Blackheart's concerns and negotiate a workable treatment plan.

3. **What is the safety issue here?**
   - To ensure that Maria receives life-saving treatment.
4. **What are the ethics and communications principles here?**
   - Treatment of a patient without mental capacity in his/her best interest.
   - Interference in care by an interested third party.
   - Justice – treatment of the patient who is unable to afford care (and, as a foreigner, is not entitled to social assistance).

Surrogate's Brief

Maria has been your domestic helper for the past 2 years. You are generally happy with her work and have no complaints about her.

She has had a fever and breathlessness for the last 4 days, for which you have given her paracetamol. While you were out today, your neighbour found her lying outside the main door in a confused state and called for an ambulance. While you do not understand the details of her illness, your expectation is for the hospital to send her home with some oral tablets, so you are surprised to be told that she requires dialysis and chemotherapy.

You object to this treatment. While you purchased compulsory medical insurance for Maria, this will not be sufficient to cover the cost of dialysis and chemotherapy, and you are neither willing nor able to foot the bill. Your husband has recently lost his job, leaving you the sole breadwinner. You are financially strained with a mortgage to pay off, two children who are studying in overseas universities, and two dependent parents. You are aware that financial assistance/social help is not available to foreign nationals like Maria. While you would like to help Maria, taking care of your own family comes first.

Furthermore, you hired a domestic helper to perform household chores; now that she is seriously ill and no longer able to work, you intend to cancel her work permit and repatriate her to the Philippines immediately. While you do care for Maria and hope that she recovers, you do not believe it to be your duty to ensure that Maria has access to medical treatment—it will be for her and her family to seek treatment in the Philippines.

You are not aware that Mdm Maria may pass away within days without treatment. If informed of this fact, you will arrange for immediate repatriation so that she can be treated in the Philippines in a timely manner. You are alright to have Mdm Maria stay in hospital for a few days as the insurance will likely be sufficient for this. However, if the hospital insists on a full course of chemotherapy, you will refuse to pay for it.

You have some specific questions for the doctor at this consultation:
- Are you going to go against my wishes?
- She has cancer. I think you should just put a do not resuscitate order. That's what the hospital did when my grandfather had cancer.

Case Discussion

This is a difficult scenario. Your bottom line is to negotiate a solution that will enable Maria to receive life-saving treatment. Essentially, you need to inform Mrs Blackheart that she has no right to deny Maria life-saving treatment while listening to her concerns and avoiding an antagonistic confrontation.

As always, begin by gathering information. Find out what Mrs Blackheart knows about Maria's condition and why she is objecting to dialysis and chemotherapy. You will have to probe beyond the stated objections in a non-confrontational manner and assess what Mrs Blackheart sees as her deeper interest. This will reveal:

1. That Mrs Blackheart's does not grasp how sick Maria is — that dialysis and chemotherapy is not elective but actually emergent.

2. That Mrs Blackheart has genuine financial difficulty paying for Maria's treatment.

3. That Mrs Blackheart's deeper interest is to resolve the matter by repatriating Maria to the Philippines.

You will need to resolve these issues in turn. (1) is something you can immediately counsel Mrs Blackheart about — it will probably be sufficient to remove her 'objection' to the treatment itself, but insufficient for her to agree to foot the bill. You can also play on Mrs Blackheart's appreciation of Maria and some degree of care for Maria ("I can see that you do like Maria and you want her to recover"), although it will become clear that this care does not make Mrs Blackheart willing to inconvenience herself for Maria's sake.

Are you going to treat her against my wishes? This is a difficult question. Avoid a direct confrontation; that is: "Yes we will treat her and you have no right to object." It will be best to emphasise that "Mdm Maria is very sick and she may pass away within days if nothing is done. We will do what is necessary to save her life." This is something that few (notwithstanding the name *Blackheart*) can object directly to.

(2) and (3) are ethical dilemmas — should anyone be denied medical care because of inability to afford treatment, and if not, who should pick up the tab? In Singapore, there are financial assistance schemes for citizens and permanent residents that make the state the payer of last resort. Foreigners, however, do not have access to any government-run financial assistance schemes and have been denied medical care because of cost. Employers who hire foreign workers, including foreign domestic helpers, are legally obliged to purchase medical insurance for their employees. However, most of such insurance policies have a relatively low cap (SGD $15,000 to $30,000 at the time of writing) and will be insufficient to cover a prolonged hospital stay or course of chemotherapy.

The incorrect approach will be to guilt-trip Mrs Blackheart to pay or insist that she must pay for Maria's entire course of chemotherapy. Appreciate that she does have genuine financial difficulty and express appropriate empathy. Mrs Blackheart's proposal to repatriate Maria to her home country for treatment is a common and often inevitable outcome. However, that would only be suitable in an elective scenario where the patient can be repatriated safely. In this case, Maria's condition is life-threatening and she is in no state to return to the Philippines (barring aeromedical evacuation which would be even more expensive).

There is probably no feasible way for Maria to receive end-to-end cancer treatment in Singapore, but the bottom line is that she must not be denied life-saving treatment at the present moment. The best you can do is probably to negotiate a solution such as administering emergency treatment (e.g., dialysis) with the goal of stabilising Maria so that she can be repatriated to the Philippines for further treatment (e.g., chemotherapy). Other options include trying to seek charity funds for Maria's treatment. While it would not be wise to promise Mrs Blackheart that you will indemnify her of the cost of subsequent treatment, you must show that you appreciate her constraint and will update her the next day after seeking out various options and discussing with your team consultant. Maria's medical insurance will cover the cost of at least a few days' treatment.

Q: *She has cancer. I think you should just put a do not resuscitate order. That's what the hospital did when my grandfather had cancer.* Explain that every cancer patient is different and that 'do not resuscitate' is not always appropriate. It may have been appropriate for her grandfather if he had terminal cancer, failed multiple lines of treatment, or had serious comorbidities. As Maria is young and newly diagnosed with a curable cancer, advocating for a conservative treatment plan at the outset would be inappropriate — yet, paradoxically, it may well be what happens in her home country should she lack the means to afford treatment. You will also need to gently convey that do not resuscitate is a medical decision and not Mrs Blackheart's to make.

This case illustrates many ethical dilemmas, not least unequal access to healthcare for non-residents in Singapore, as well as global disparities in access to healthcare. Similar issues are encountered in many of the Commonwealth countries in which PACES is conducted. The UK National Health Service does well in ensuring that everyone can access healthcare regardless of ability to pay, but is not without its own set of problems. These challenges are complex and there are no easy solutions — certainly nothing that can be put forward in a 10-minute PACES communication scenario. Nonetheless, it is important to understand and be able to navigate these ethical issues in the local and national healthcare system in which you work (or where you are taking PACES).

Communication Case 19

Sacral Sores

Use this case as practice! The pull-out booklet contains the candidate's information.

Information for the Candidate

Patient Details: Mrs Park, 70 years old

Your Role: Acute Medical Unit Ward SHO

Information: Mrs Park was diagnosed with Alzheimer's dementia 15 years ago and has had a steady decline in function since then. In the last two years, she has become completely bedbound and dependent on others for her activities of daily living. She receives liquid feeds through a nasogastric tube.

Mrs Park was admitted through the Emergency Department yesterday for sepsis from unstageable sacral sores. She appears cachectic and hypovolemic. A sacral X-ray is significant for evidence of osteomyelitis and biochemical investigations reveal hyponatraemia, hypokalaemia, hypophosphataemia, and hypomagnesaemia. Your team has started her on IV antibiotics, IV fluids, electrolyte and thiamine replacement, and an appropriate feeding regimen.

This is Mrs Park's third admission for infected sacral sores in the past year. The social worker has highlighted several concerns about Mrs Park's care at home. In particular, although her husband, Mr Park, claims to pay for a home nurse service who visits three times a week, a call to the home nurse service reveals that Mr Park has been cancelling appointments and in the past month they have only come once.

Your task is to update Mrs Park's husband about her condition and convey your concerns about her care at home.

Planning (From the Stem)

1. **What do I need to assess?/What information do I need to gather?**
   - Mrs Park's family background – who is the main caregiver, are there any other children, and what the family dynamics are like.
   - How has Mrs Park been cared for at home – what is actually being done or not done?
   - Why have her care needs not been met – is the carer (Mr Park) not coping or is there intentional neglect?

2. **What do I need to convey?**
   - That Mrs Park's care has been inadequate and this has led to harm in the form of recurrent, preventable infections.
   - If the carer has not been coping, convey empathy that the care burden is high and acknowledge the burnout.
   - Find a solution – open a discussion about an alternative care arrangement.
3. **What is the safety issue here?**
   - Mrs Park is a vulnerable patient who cannot advocate for her own care and her main caregiver is unable to cope with her needs, leading to neglect.
4. **What are the ethics and communications principles here?**
   - Beneficence: you as Mrs Park's physician need to act in her best interests and advocate for an alternative care arrangement.

Surrogate's Brief

You brought your wife to the A&E yesterday because she was having a high fever that did not respond to paracetamol. You are worried about her condition and do not want her to pass away.

You are aware that she has sacral sores and have been taught by the hospital that she needs to be turned every 2 hours. However, you find it impossible to keep up with the 2-hourly turning. You do your best to administer her liquid feeds through the nasogastric tube, but each feed takes very long and you do forget sometimes. Nonetheless, you believe that you have been trying your best and you do not believe that anyone else can do better than you have done.

You are drained and burnt out after having been the sole caregiver for your wife, especially since she has become bedbound in the last 2 years. You love her deeply and are grieved that you can no longer recognise the woman whom you love, and neither does she recognise you. You have 1 married daughter who has moved out. You are not on good terms as both you and your wife did not approve of her marriage to a man who earns much less than her.

At the time of her last hospital discharge 4 months ago, you planned to engage a private home nurse to come by thrice a week to assist in Mrs Park's care. If confronted that you have been cancelling nurse appointments, you will admit that you have indeed done so because you did not have money to pay for the visit. As you are no longer working and do not have much savings to live on, you have run out of money to pay for the home nurse.

If accused of neglecting your wife, you will react with anger and become unhelpful. Conversely, if the candidate recognises that you are burnt out and offers support, you will open up. You would like Mrs Park to stay at home with you because you love her dearly, but you will be open to other care options including placement in a nursing home, if these mean better care for her.

You have some specific questions for the doctor at this consultation:
- Is my wife going to die?
- Is this all my fault?
- What should we do now?

Case Discussion

Begin by updating Mr Park about Mrs Park's condition. Do not jump into an accusation of neglect. Rather, probe gently about his thoughts on her condition ("I can see that you are worried... Could you share with me what is on your mind?") and what might have led to the sacral sores ("Are you aware that she has had sacral sores?"). He is likely to give away quite quickly the challenges he faces caring for her at home, which you can use as a starting point to assess how her care at home has been and how he has been coping.

The key to this scenario is to get on Mr Park's side rather than taking an accusatory tone. He is not intentionally abusing his wife or denying her care. Rather, he still loves his wife a great deal but is burnt out. He has some pride and will find it difficult to admit that the care he has provided is inadequate. You will need to offer a lot of empathy and affirmation that he really loves his wife and that it has been incredibly difficult to be the sole caregiver for such many years.

Next, transit into expressing your concerns about Mrs Park's care. The scenario is written such that you should specifically discuss (1) turning, (2) feeding, and (3) frequency of home nurse visits. Emphasise that you want the best for Mrs Park, just as he does. You acknowledge that he has tried his level best and you are not blaming him for these failings. However, inadequate care has led to recurrent, preventable infections, and as Mrs Park's doctor, it is your duty to see how her care can be improved so that she does not suffer these complications. You should also express your concerns about Mr Park's own health and the burden of full-time caregiving, and acknowledge his burn out. It may be necessary to refer him for caregiver support or even psychiatric care if indicated.

Open up the discussion about alternative care arrangements. You will only be able to do so if you get on Mr Park's side; conversely, he will not be agreeable if he feels threatened. Some options you can float are:

- Offering to have a family conference together with his sons to explain the situation (emphasise that you will not pin any blame on Mr Park) and garner their support/increased participation in Mrs Park's care.
- Having someone else be the full-time carer (e.g., a relative, domestic help if available in your country).
- Additional home help services such as a part-time nurse.
- Nursing home placement.

Involve a multidisciplinary team in planning Mrs Park's care, including getting the social worker to help with financial assistance or government-funded care (since this has been an issue) and involving the community nurse (e.g., district nurse, hospital-to-home care nurse, or equivalent in your country). Close by summarising the conversation and that having obtained his consent, you will explore Mrs Park's care plan and get back to him with a finalised arrangement.

Variation: A variation of this station is one in which Mrs Park suffers active neglect, or even abuse, at the hands of a carer who does not make any effort to care for her. Such a carer may be uncooperative and defensive. How would you tackle this scenario?

Communication Case 20

A Right to Know?

Use this case as practice! The pull-out booklet contains the candidate's information.

Information for the Candidate

Patient Details: Ms ABC, 35 years old

Your Role: Medicine Clinic SHO

Information: Several years ago, Ms ABC's father was diagnosed with Huntington's disease. Despite extensive counselling about the possibility that his children may inherit the Huntington gene, he firmly insisted that his children should not be informed. He was particularly concerned that his younger daughter, Ms ABC, who was pregnant at the time, would have an abortion should she be told. After much deliberation, his physicians opted not to override his confidentiality and inform his daughters of the diagnosis.

After childbirth, Ms ABC accidentally became aware of her father's diagnosis. She subsequently sought gene testing and was found to have the Huntington gene. It is not yet known whether her child is similarly affected because gene testing cannot be done until the child is 18 years of age.

Ms ABC wishes to speak to a member of staff about the failure to inform her of her father's diagnosis of Huntington's disease.

Your task is to speak to Ms ABC and address her concerns.

Planning (From the Stem)

1. **What do I need to assess?/What information do I need to gather?**
   - How the diagnosis of Huntington's disease has affected Ms ABC.
2. **What do I need to convey?**
   - Empathy at the diagnosis of Huntington's disease and how this has affected Ms ABC and potentially her child.
   - To explain why Ms ABC was not informed without being overly defensive.
3. **What is the safety issue here?**
   - N/A
4. **What are the ethics and communications principles here?**
   - The conflict between patient confidentiality (Ms ABC's father's refusal of permission for confidential information to be disclosed to his children) vs. the duty to inform a third party of potential harm.
   - Dealing with an angry patient.

Patient's Brief

Several years ago, your father shot and killed your mother. He was later assessed by the psychiatrists to have 'diminished responsibility' and sentenced to a hospital order in lieu of jail. You were pregnant at this time. You did not understand why he was deemed to have 'diminished responsibility'; neither were you told. You have a strained relationship with your father.

Sometime later, you accidentally found out that your father had Huntington's disease. You sought testing and were also found to have the Huntington gene, although you are currently asymptomatic. You understand that there is a 50% risk that your baby daughter may also have the disease, although she cannot be tested until she turns 18.

You are immensely upset that your father's doctors did not inform you of the diagnosis. Had you been informed, you would have sought testing, and if you were likewise found to have Huntington's disease, you would have sought a termination of pregnancy. You are a single mother and you did not want to become disabled and dependent on your daughter, or pass away and leave your daughter behind as an orphan. You also do not want to incur any risk that your child would inherit Huntington's disease.

You will enter the consultation with much anger and make it clear that you were denied an opportunity to prevent your daughter from suffering. You seek an answer as to why you were not informed, as well as restitution for the 'wrongful birth' of your child.

You have some specific questions for the doctor at this consultation:

- Why did nobody tell me? Does the incredible harm and suffering my daughter will have to go through not outweigh my dad's ego?
- If a patient says that he would take a gun and shoot someone he hated, would you not inform that someone to protect himself/herself, or at least call the police?
- I am going to sue. How is the hospital going to make amends now?

Case Discussion

This is an extremely challenging scenario, adapted from a real life case (*ABC v St George's Healthcare NHS Trust and Others*). At the time of writing, this case remains before the UK Court of Appeal, and as such the pertinent legal principle has yet to be firmly established.

The key ethical and legal dilemma is whether the duty to warn third parties known to be at risk of avoidable harm (i.e., Ms ABC) outweighs the duty of confidentiality to the patient (i.e., her father). The UK GMC considers non-consensual disclosure justified if "failure to do so may expose others to a risk of death or serious harm"[7]. The

---

[7] General Medical Council. Confidentiality: good practice in handling patient information. General Medical Council, 2017. https://www.gmc-uk.org/-/media/documents/gmc-guidance-for-doctors---confidentiality-good-practice-in-handling-patient-information----70080105.pdf

most famous exposition of this principle is the United States case of *Tarasoff*[8], in which a therapist was held liable for failing to inform a third party of a patient's expressed intent to murder the third party. Juxtaposed against this interest is the danger of damaging confidence in the doctor-patient relationship. The courts have at times ruled in favour of a 'weaker' obligation of disclosure — that the healthcare provider's duty is limited to warning the patient that his/her children should seek medical care (e.g., *Pate v Threikel*[9], a United States case). This is an evolving area and *ABC v St George's Healthcare NHS Trust and Others* is unlikely to settle the matter for good.

Keeping the ethical and legal background in mind, this communications task is essentially an 'angry patient' scenario. Begin by allowing Ms ABC to vent and demonstrate active listening, empathy, and genuine concern for how she and her daughter have been affected. Ms ABC wants answers as to why she was not informed — gently explain the ethical tension involved, but also acknowledge that she is likely to find this explanation unsatisfactory as the interest of someone else was prioritised over hers. You might attempt to point out that there is no agreement among doctors and lawyers as to what the right thing to do in the situation is, though this might not go down too well; to Ms ABC there was only one right thing to do, which was to have informed her. An alternative way to express this is to share that you are troubled by what has happened, and if you were the physician treating Ms ABC's dad, you would have felt trapped between a rock and a hard place. It is important not to sound overly defensive.

Ms ABC will express her desire to sue. Do not turn defensive, grovel, or beg her not to sue. It is her right to seek legal recourse and you should acknowledge this. Remain neutral, offer to facilitate her complaints (e.g., referral to the patient advice and liaison service, or equivalent), and state that regardless of her decision, the medical team will continue to treat and support her especially once she develops symptoms of Huntington's disease. Offer as much support as you can, such as to connect her to patient support groups, referral to a social worker to discuss care arrangements should she become disabled, and so on. Refrain from promising any form of compensation as it is not in your power to do so.

Further reading:
- Lucassen A, Gilbar R. Alerting relatives about heritable risks: the limits of confidentiality. *BMJ* 2018 361:k1409.
- *ABC v St George's Healthcare NHS Trust and Others* (2017) – this is the case on which this scenario is based.

---

[8] [1976] 551 P.2d 334 (Supreme Court of California)
[9] [1995] 661 So 2d (Supreme Court of Florida)

Index to Worked Cases

This index is a quick-search guide to look up key chapters to jog your memory (but please attempt the cases as practice before reading through them!).

Consultations: Diagnostic Approaches

This list of diagnostic approaches should be covered in the course of your PACES preparation. Use this as a checklist to ensure that you have gone over the necessary ground. Some approaches are not covered in this text; for your revision a reference is provided to the appropriate chapter of *Algorithms in Differential Diagnosis*[1] or the appropriate page of the *Physical Exam* section of this book.

Presenting Complaint		Case
Abdominal pain		39
Abnormal movements		40
Acute kidney injury		49
Altered mental state		43
Amenorrhoea		22
Anaemia		32
Arthritis		35
Back pain		14
Bleeding		23
Breathlessness,	chronic progressive	05
	fluid overload/cardiac failure	04
	in poorly controlled asthma	02
	in myasthenia gravis	03
	in rheumatologic disease	01
	with normal X-ray	07
Chest pain		15

---

[1] Fong N. 2019. *Algorithms in Differential Diagnosis: How to Approach Common Presenting Complaints in Adult Patients, for Medical Students and Junior Doctors.* Singapore: World Scientific.

Coagulopathy, prolonged aPTT		47
Constipation		*Algorithms* Chpt 14
Difficulty seeing,	acute and subacute	18, 19
	chronic	17
Diarrhoea		38
Double vision		see *Physical Exam* Syndrome 3.2
Dysphagia		34
Electrolyte imbalance,	hypocalcaemia	31
	hyponatraemia	33
	others	*Algorithms* Chpt 16–17
Eosinophilia		*Algorithms* Chpt 34
Epistaxis		23
Falls		30
Fatigue		25
Fever		41
Giddiness		41, 42
Jaundice/transaminitis		46
Haematuria		21
Haemoptysis		*Algorithms* Chpt 8
Hyperlipidemia		24
Hypertension		27
Leg pain		44
Leg swelling		*Algorithms* Chpt 47
Loss of consciousness,	syncope	28
	seizure	29
Muscle cramps		31
Numbness		26
Hand pain		13, 35
Palpitations		*Algorithms* Chpt 5
Polycythaemia		*Algorithms* Chpt 34
Polyuria		45
Proteinuria/nephrotic syndrome		24
Pruritus		37
Rash		08, 09, 10
Raynaud's syndrome		13
Red/painful eye		20
Stroke		41
Thrombocytopenia		48
Ulcers, mouth		36
Vomiting		*Algorithms* Chpt 12
Weakness		see *Physical Exam* section
Weight gain		11
Weight loss		16

Consultations: Conditions

Endocrinology	Case
Acromegaly	26
Adrenal insufficiency	25
Cushing's syndrome	11
Diabetes, complications of	07
Hyperthyroid, drug-induced	38
storm	04
Multiple endocrine neoplasia	45
Pituitary, adenoma	22
hypopituitarism	22
Post-thyroidectomy	31

Rheumatology	Case
ANCA vasculitis	02
Dermatomyositis	16
Giant cell arthritis	12
Gout	35, 49
Lupus	36
Raynaud's syndrome	13
Rheumatoid arthritis	01, 35
Systemic sclerosis	42
Takayasu arteritis	44

Dermatology	Case
Psoriasis	08
Erythema nodosum	09
Pyoderma gangrenosum	10

Ophthalmology	Case
Diabetic eye disease	18
Optic neuritis	19
Retinitis pigmentosa	17
Thyroid eye disease	20

Neurology	Case
Chorea	40
Myasthenia Gravis	03, 34
Normal pressure hydrocephalus	30

Haematology	Case
Antiphospholipid syndrome	47
B12 deficiency	32
CTEPH	05
Heparin-induced thrombocytopenia	48
Multiple myeloma	14
Polycythaemia vera	37

Syndromes	Case
Hereditary haemorrhagic telangiectasia	23
Marfan's syndrome	15
Neurofibromatosis	27
Tuberous sclerosis	29

Others	Case
Crohn's disease	39
HIV	06
Hypertrophic cardiomyopathy	28
Infective endocarditis	41
Multiple sclerosis	19
Nephrotic syndrome	24
Oncology patient	43
Polycystic kidney disease	21
SIADH	33
Wilson's disease	46

Communications

No.	Title	Synopsis	Core topic	Core skills
1	Missed bleed	A patient's headache is misdiagnosed as migraine. She returns with subarachnoid haemorrhage.	Medical error	Breaking bad news Angry patient
2	Brain dead	A young man suffers brain death. You are tasked to break the news and discuss organ donation.	Brain death Organ donation	Breaking bad news
3	Discussing anti-coagulation	A young lady with oestrogen-induced deep vein thrombosis sees you to discuss anticoagulation options.	Anticoagulation	Counselling: shared decision making
4	Still hypertensive	A young CEO is newly diagnosed with hypertension and is started on medication. At a follow-up visit, his blood pressure remains high.	Hypertension	Counselling: non-compliant patient
5	Still seizing	A young lady with epilepsy has recurrent seizures due to non-compliance to medicine. She is still driving and desires to conceive.	Epilepsy Fitness to drive Pregnancy safety	Counselling: non-compliant patient Awareness of safety issues
6	Still coughing	A patient defaults tuberculosis treatment because of drug side effects and fear of kidney damage.	Tuberculosis and public health	Counselling: non-compliant patient, managing side effects
7	Indeterminate Western Blot	A patient with recent high-risk sexual exposure has an indeterminate HIV test result.	HIV: test interpretation	Taking a sexual history
8	HIV positive	A HIV-positive patient refuses to tell her spouse and child, who may have been infected.	HIV: public health risk, confidentiality	Breaking bad news Counselling: unwilling patient.

(Cont'd)

Index to Worked Cases

No.	Title	Synopsis	Core topic	Core skills
9	Needlestick injury	Your House Officer/FY1 suffers a needlestick injury from a HIV-positive patient.	HIV: postexposure prophylaxis	Distraught patient
10	Ascitic drain	You are tasked to consent a cirrhotic patient for an ascitic drain and counsel him on management. He turns out to be struggling with alcohol addiction.	Alcohol-use disorder	Consent taking Identifying 'hidden tasks' Motivational interviewing
11	Chronic pain I	A young man asks for refill of painkillers. His pain is out of control and he has been taking more opioids than prescribed.	Chronic pain.	Recognising and assessing suicide risk
12	Chronic pain II	A young man asks for refill of painkillers. He has been taking additional doses of opioids even in the absence of pain.	Prescription drug abuse	Balancing patient's best interests vs. wishes
13	Suicidal nurse	A nurse ingests large quantities of sulphonylureas. She does not want anyone else to know.	Suicide attempt Confidentiality	Balancing patient's best interests vs. wishes
14	Withdrawal of dialysis	Your consultant plans to withdraw dialysis from an elderly lady who is unable to tolerate dialysis. Her son is upset that the doctors are 'heartless' and 'condemning mum to die'.	Medical futility	Discussing goals of care, limiting care
15	It's all in the mind	A lady has multiple somatic complaints. Your consultant will like to refer her to the psychiatrist.	Functional and psychosomatic disorders	Therapeutic communication and goal-setting
16	BRCA testing	A young lady seeks BRCA testing after her sister passes away from breast cancer.	Genetic testing Cancer screening	Counselling: pre-gene testing counselling

(Cont'd)

No.	Title	Synopsis	Core topic	Core skills
17	Doctor dangerous	Your night-duty House Officer/FY1 endangers patient safety. He has not been coping well and is distracted by his personal life.	Patient safety Fitness to practice	Leadership of a medical team
18	Send her home	A foreign worker is critically ill with acute leukaemia and has no mental capacity. Her employer wishes to repatriate her to her home country immediately.	Ethics in vulnerable patients: access to care	Management of a vulnerable patient
19	Sacral sores	A bedbound patient is admitted for recurrent sacral sores, raising concerns about neglect. Her family is unable to cope with her care needs.	Ethics in vulnerable patients: neglect	Advocating for your patient Managing conflict with a third party's interests
20	A right to know?	A patient with Huntington's disease refused to inform his daughter, who later finds out that she has the Huntington gene. She intends to sue the hospital for not informing her and for the 'wrongful birth' of her baby.	Genetic testing Patient confidentiality vs. third-party interest	Angry patient Managing a complaint

Candidate's Information for Practice Scenarios

This booklet gives the candidate's information for Consultations and Communications practice scenarios, for use during practice with colleagues or tutors. Refer to the respective scenarios for the patient's brief and a case discussion.

CONSULTATIONS

Consultation 01 — Mdm Ruby Toh, 37 years old

Your Role: Rheumatology Clinic SHO

Referral Letter:
Dear Colleague,

Thank you for seeing Mdm Toh who has been on your follow up. She has brought forward her appointment because she is short of breath.

Sincerely,

Dr Germaine Loo, GP

Vital Signs: BP 145/87 mmHg, HR 70/min, RR 16/min, SpO2 95% RA, T 37.0°C

Consultation 02 — Mrs Puff, 30 years old

Your Role: Respiratory Medicine Clinic SHO

Referral Letter:
Dear Colleague,

Thank you for seeing Mrs Puff for her asthma. I have stepped up her treatment to a Budesonide/Formoterol (Symbicort®) inhaler, but she still complains of persistent symptoms.

Thank you.

Dr Wilbert Ho, GP

Vital Signs: BP 155/95 mmHg, HR 70/min, RR 10/min, SpO2 99% RA, T 37.0°C

Consultation 03 — Ms G. Mao, 28 years old

Your Role: Emergency Department SHO

Referral Letter:
Dear A&E,

Thank you for seeing Ms Mao. She started having flu symptoms a few days ago, and on review today, she is complaining of difficulty breathing. Please assist to manage her.

Sincerely,

Dr Guo Weiwen, GP

Vital Signs: BP 110/60 mmHg, HR 81/min, RR 11/min, SpO2 95% RA, T 37.9°C

Consultation 04	Mdm Miles, 37 years old
Your Role:	Medical Admissions Unit SHO
Scenario:	Mdm Miles presents with breathlessness and nausea after returning from a holiday in New Zealand.
Vital Signs:	BP 155/91 mmHg, HR 161/min, RR 23/min, SpO2 94% RA, T 37.7°C

Consultation 05	Ms Chuan, 33 years old
Your Role:	Emergency Department SHO
Referral Letter:	Dear Colleague,
	Thank you for seeing Ms Chuan. She is complaining of worsening shortness of breath in the past month.
	Thank you.
	Dr Eugene Gan, GP
Vital Signs:	BP 125/80 mmHg, HR 81/min, RR 14/min, SpO2 95% RA, T 36.2°C

Consultation 06	Mr Freddie, 40 years old
Your Role:	Respiratory Medicine Clinic SHO
Referral Letter:	Dear Colleague,
	Mr Freddie has been complaining of cough and dyspnoea which did not respond to a course of clarithromycin. Could you please see him?
	Thank you.
	Dr Hutton, GP
Vital Signs:	BP 109/63 mmHg, HR 71/min, RR 13/min, SpO2 93% RA, T 37.2°C

Consultation 07	Mr Nafas, 49 years old
Your Role:	Medical Admissions Unit SHO
Referral Letter:	Dear Colleague,
	I will appreciate if you could kindly review Mr Nafas. He presents today with a 2-day history of dyspnoea and looks moderately unwell.
	Thank you.
	Dr Ed. Mitt, A&E Consultant
Vital Signs:	BP 128/70 mmHg, HR 100/min, RR 26/min, SpO2 100% RA, T 36.5°C
Investigations:	ECG: Sinus tachycardia
	Capillary blood glucose: 11.3 mmol/L
	Chest X-ray: Normal
	Blood investigations: Pending

Candidate's Information for Practice Scenarios 3

Consultation 08	Mr Ee Chee, 52 years old
Your Role:	Dermatology Clinic SHO
Referral Letter:	Dear Colleague,
	Mr Ee Chee presents with a 2-month history of rashes. Please see and manage.
	Thank you.
	Dr Lydia Chuah, GP
Vital Signs:	BP 146/87 mmHg, HR 57/min, RR 15/min, SpO2 99% RA, T 35.8°C

Consultation 09	Mrs S. Lump, 40 years old
Your Role:	Dermatology Senior House Officer
Scenario:	Mrs Lump complains of lower limb rash.
Vital Signs:	BP 100/70 mmHg, HR 50/min, RR 10/min, SpO2 97% RA, T 36.0°C

Consultation 10	Mrs C. Sweet, 35 years old
Your Role:	Dermatology SHO
Referral Letter:	Dear Colleague,
	Mrs Sweet is on follow up with me for diabetes mellitus. She has recently had an infected right lower limb wound. I have given two 1-week courses of co-amoxiclav without much improvement.
	Please help with her management. Thank you.
	Dr Nicholas Hong, GP
Vital Signs:	BP 130/83 mmHg, HR 67/min, RR 10/min, SpO2 97% RA, T 37.0°C

Consultation 11	Ms McDonald, 40 years old
Your Role:	Endocrine Clinic SHO
Referral Letter:	Dear Colleague,
	Ms McDonald was referred from the GP for bariatric surgery. I agree that this is strongly indicated, but could I please have you on board to optimise her diabetic control? Her latest hbA1c is still 8.2% despite three oral hypoglycaemic agents.
	Thank you.
	Dr Kentucky, General Surgery
Vital Signs:	BP 148/92 mmHg, HR 80/min, RR 13/min, SpO2 99% RA, T 37.1°C

Consultation 12	Mdm Grumps, 50 years old
Your Role:	Neurology Clinic SHO
Referral Letter:	Dear Colleague,
	I've been seeing Mdm Grumps for migraine. However, her headaches have gotten worse recently and doesn't respond completely to analgesia. Think it's best if you have a look at her.
	Thank you.
	Dr Linus Chua, GP
Vital Signs:	BP 120/80 mmHg, HR 70/min, RR 14/min, SpO2 99% RA, T 36.0°C

Consultation 13	Ms Ache, 28 years old
Your Role:	Neurology Clinic SHO
Referral Letter:	Dear Colleague,
	Thank you for seeing this pleasant lady who is complaining of painful hands but there doesn't appear to be an orthopaedic issue. Perhaps it could be a nerve problem?
	Thank you.
	Dr Carpenter, Orthopaedic Surgeon
Vital Signs:	BP 100/62 mmHg, HR 57/min, RR 14/min, SpO2 95% RA, T 37.0°C

Consultation 14	Mrs Potts, 60 years old
Your Role:	Medical Outpatients SHO
Referral Letter:	Dear Colleague,
	Thank you for seeing Mrs Potts. She has back pain that did not seem to improve with paracetamol. Will you please assist to manage her?
	Thank you.
	Dr Vivien Lee, GP
Vital Signs:	BP 135/82 mmHg, HR 87/min, RR 14/min, SpO2 97% RA, T 37.0°C

Consultation 15	Mr Pop, 23 years old
Your Role:	Respiratory Medicine SHO
Referral Letter:	Dear Colleague,
	Thank you for following up on Mr Pop. I saw him today for a non-traumatic pneumothorax, which resolved with supplemental oxygen. A chest X-ray prior to discharge was normal.
	Dr Darius Pan, A&E Physician
Vital Signs:	BP 115/85 mmHg, HR 67/min, RR 11/min, SpO2 97% RA, T 36.9°C

Candidate's Information for Practice Scenarios 5

Consultation 16	
Your Role:	Ms V. Slim, 60 years old
	Internal Medicine Clinic SHO
Referral Letter:	Dear Colleague,
	Thank you for seeing Ms Slim, who complains of a 2-month history of weight loss.
	Thank you.
	Dr Atkins, GP
Vital Signs:	BP 102/64 mmHg, HR 70/min, RR 12/min, SpO2 99% RA, T 36.2°C

Consultation 17	
	Mr A. Bocelli, 40 years old
Your Role:	Medical Outpatients SHO
Scenario:	Mr Bocelli complains of difficulty seeing.
Vital Signs:	BP 120/78 mmHg, HR 50/min, RR 10/min, SpO2 98% RA, T 36.3°C

Consultation 18	
	Mdm Kant Xi, 50 years old
Your Role:	Early Access Clinic SHO
Referral Letter:	Dear Colleague,
	Mdm Xi is in follow-up with this clinic for diabetes, which has been quite difficult to control. She has a new complaint of difficulty seeing. Will appreciate if you could see her.
	Thank you,
	Dr David Ng, GP
Vital Signs:	BP 130/89 mmHg, HR 60/min, RR 11/min, SpO2 99% RA, T 36.5°C

Consultation 19	
	Ms See, 30 years old
Your Role:	Medical Walk-In Clinic SHO
Referral Letter:	Dear Colleague,
	Thank you for seeing Ms See for difficulty seeing.
	Dr Benjy, GP
Vital Signs:	BP 120/88 mmHg, HR 70/min, RR 14/min, SpO2 98% RA, T 36.0°C

Consultation 20	Mr Hong Yan, 32 years old
Your Role:	Emergency Department SHO
Referral Letter:	Dear Colleague,
	Thank you for seeing Mr Hong Yan. He complains of redness and discomfort of the left eye, which did not respond to levofloxacin eyedrops.
	Warm regards,
	Dr Andrew Tan, GP
Vital Signs:	BP 107/63 mmHg, HR 74/min, RR 11/min, SpO2 98% RA, T 36.2°C

Consultation 21	Mr Pei, 45 years old
Your Role:	Medicine Clinic SHO
Referral Letter:	Dear Colleague,
	A pre-employment screening done for this patient 1 week ago identified blood 3+ and protein 2+ on urine dipstick. A repeat dipstick today showed persistence of these abnormalities. Please kindly assist with further investigation and management.
	Thank you.
	Dr Smily Lock, GP
Vital Signs:	BP 145/92 mmHg, HR 70/min, RR 14/min, SpO2 97% RA, T 36.5°C

Consultation 22	Mrs Childless, 34 years old
Your Role:	General Medicine Clinic SHO
Referral Letter:	Dear Colleague,
	Thank you for seeing Mrs Childless. She has missed her menstrual period for 3 months and is complaining of fatigue. A urine pregnancy test is negative.
	Thank you.
	Dr Stork, GP
Vital Signs:	BP 90/52 mmHg, HR 57/min, RR 11/min, SpO2 98% RA, T 37.0°C

Consultation 23	Ms Liu B. Xue, 30 years old
Your Role:	Internal Medicine Clinic SHO
Referral Letter:	Dear Colleague,
	Thank you for seeing Ms Liu. She has been seeing me for repeated episodes of nosebleeds. I have tried silver nitrate cautery, but this was only of limited effectiveness.
	Dr Sherilyn Liew, ENT Surgeon
Vital Signs:	BP 115/60 mmHg, HR 60/min, RR 12/min, SpO2 99% RA, T 36.2°C

Consultation 24

Mr A. M. Indra, 40 years old

Your Role: Cardiology Outpatients SHO

Referral Letter: Dear Colleague,

Mr A. M. Indra was diagnosed with hyperlipidemia on health screening 6 months ago. Despite Atorvastatin 40 mg ON, his low-density lipoprotein (LDL) levels remain at 5.6 mmol/L, from 5.7 mmol/L previously (normal < 4.1 mmol/L; optimal < 2.6 mmol/L). He is concerned about the risk of a heart attack and wishes to see you.

Thank you.

Dr Cheryl Lie, GP

Vital Signs: BP 125/82 mmHg, HR 57/min, RR 12/min, SpO2 99% RA, T 37.0°C

Consultation 25

Mdm Hashi, 36 years old

Your Role: Endocrine Clinic SHO

Referral Letter: Dear Colleague,

Mdm Hashi is on my follow up for hypothyroidism. She is complaining of persistent fatigue in spite of thyroxine replacement. Her latest free T4 is 12 pmol/L (normal: 11 - 21 pmol/L), and thyroid stimulating hormone is 3.0 mIU/L (normal: 0.5 - 5.0 mIU/L). Could you please see her?

Thank you.

Dr Moto, GP

Vital Signs: BP 91/52 mmHg, HR 42/min, RR 10/min, SpO2 100% RA, T 35.8°C

Consultation 26

Mr Rachmaninoff, 50 years old

Your Role: Neurology Clinic SHO

Referral Letter: Dear Neurology Colleague,

Mr Rachmaninoff is on my follow up for diabetes. He has been complaining of hand numbness. I wonder if you could have a look at him?

Thank you and warmest regards.

Dr Tung Lin, GP

Vital Signs: BP 155/92 mmHg, HR 77/min, RR 11/min, SpO2 99% RA, T 36.0°C

Consultation 27	Ms Kat, 30 years old
Your Role:	Medical Outpatients Clinic SHO
Referral Letter:	Dear Colleague, Ms Kat seems to be hypertensive at a rather young age, and her hypertension is difficult to control. Would you please see and manage her? Warm regards, Dr April Toh, GP
Vital Signs:	BP 175/91 mmHg, HR 80/min, RR 18/min, SpO2 98% RA, T 37.0°C

Consultation 28	Mr Kay, 30 years old
Your Role:	Medical Admissions Unit SHO
Scenario:	Mr Kay was brought to A&E after passing out at a charity fun run.
Vital Signs:	BP 120/80 mmHg, HR 70/min, RR 10/min, SpO2 100% RA, T 36.5°C

Consultation 29	Ms Oh, 30 years old
Your Role:	Medical Admissions Unit SHO
Scenario:	Ms Oh has been admitted after losing consciousness in public.
Vital Signs:	BP 105/62 mmHg, HR 111/min, RR 11/min, SpO2 99% RA, T 36.2°C

Consultation 30	Mr H. Dumpty, 70 years old
Your Role:	Geriatric Clinic SHO
Referral Letter:	Dear Colleague, Mr Dumpty was admitted for a right Colles' fracture which we have fixed. It seems that he has been having rather frequent falls. Could you please see him? Thank you. Dr Bone, Orthopaedic Surgeon
Vital Signs:	BP 132/71 mmHg, HR 70/min, RR 12/min, SpO2 97% RA, T 35.9°C

Candidate's Information for Practice Scenarios 9

Consultation 31

Ms Alice, 50 years old

Your Role: Emergency Department SHO

Referral Letter: Dear Colleague,

Thank you for seeing Ms Alice, who complains of persistent muscle cramps that did not resolve with rest and a muscle relaxant. She is on my follow-up for delusional disorder and is stable on risperidone 2mg daily. There have been no dose changes in the past 5 years.

Thank you.

Dr Aaron Tang, Psychiatrist

Vital Signs: BP 137/84 mmHg, HR 70/min, RR 14/min, SpO2 98% RA, T 37.0°C

Consultation 32

Mr White, 47 years old

Your Role: Medicine Clinic SHO

Referral Letter: Dear Colleague,

Mr White came for routine health screening and was found to be anaemic. Would you please see him for further management?

Thank you.

Dr Joyce Huang, GP

Vital Signs: BP 131/80 mmHg, HR 70/min, RR 11/min, SpO2 98% RA, T 37.0°C

Investigations:

Haemoglobin	9.8	g/dL	(13.0 - 17.0)
WBC	3.0	$\times 10^9$/L	(3.4 - 9.6)
Platelets	148	$\times 10^9$/L	(150 - 400)
Mean corpuscular volume	112	fL	(80 - 95)

Consultation 33

Mdm Na, 70 years old

Your Role: Emergency Department SHO

Referral Letter: Dear Colleague,

Mdm Na came to me last week complaining of lethargy. I decided to check her bloods and it turns out that she has rather significant hyponatraemia. Will you please see and manage her?

Thank you.

Dr Saw Tee, GP

Vital Signs: BP 130/70 mmHg, HR 72/min, RR 11/min, SpO2 98% RA, T 37.0°C

Investigations:

Na^+	119	mmol/L	(135 - 145)
K^+	4.0	mmol/L	(3.5 - 5.0)
Cl^-	88	mmol/L	(95 - 105)
HCO_3^-	23	mmol/L	(22 - 26)
Creatinine	72	umol/L	(normal)
Urea	10	umol/L	(normal)
Glucose	7.0	mmol/L	

Consultation 34

Your Role:	Mr E. Choke, 40 years old
	Gastroenterology SHO
Referral Letter:	Dear Colleague,
	Thank you for seeing Mr Choke for consideration of esophago-gastroduodenoscopy. He has been complaining of difficulty swallowing and has lost weight.
	Thank you.
	Dr Cai Jiashen, GP
Vital Signs:	BP 100/60 mmHg, HR 60/min, RR 13/min, SpO2 100% RA, T 36.2°C

Consultation 35

	Mr P. Philippe, 40 years old
Your Role:	Medicine Clinic SHO
Referral Letter:	Dear Colleague,
	Mr Philippe has been complaining of joint pains affecting both hands. I would appreciate if you could see him.
	Thank you.
	Dr Joshua Yeo, GP
Vital Signs:	BP 135/80 mmHg, HR 70/min, RR 11/min, SpO2 98% RA, T 37.0°C

Consultation 36

	Ms S. L. Ee, 33 years old
Your Role:	Rheumatology Clinic SHO
Scenario:	Ms Ee is on follow up for systemic lupus erythematosus. She has brought forward her appointment, complaining of mouth ulcers. She is worried of a lupus flare.
Vital Signs:	BP 115/66 mmHg, HR 67/min, RR 10/min, SpO2 97% RA, T 37.0°C

Consultation 37

	Mdm Yang, 49 year old
Your Role:	Dermatology Clinic SHO
Referral Letter:	Dear Dermatologist,
	I have been seeing Mdm Yang for a persistent generalised itch which does not respond to moisturiser creams or topical steroids. A trial of scabies treatment was also unsuccessful.
	Would you please see her? Thank you.
	Dr Shawn Lin, GP
Vital Signs:	BP 120/72 mmHg, HR 60/min, RR 12/min, SpO2 95% RA, T 37.0°C

Candidate's Information for Practice Scenarios 11

Consultation 38	Ms Poo, 47 years old
Your Role:	Gastroenterology Clinic SHO
Referral Letter:	Dear Colleague,
	Thank you for seeing Ms Poo. She has had a 1-month history of diarrhoea which does not resolve on symptomatic treatment.
	Thank you.
	Dr Loo, GP
Vital Signs:	BP 107/60 mmHg, HR 111/min, RR 12/min, SpO2 98% RA, T 37.0°C

Consultation 39	Ms L. Sai, 30 years old
Your Role:	Emergency Department SHO
Scenario:	Ms Sai, who is on follow up for Crohn's disease, complains of abdominal pain.
Vital Signs:	BP 100/60 mmHg, HR 111/min, RR 10/min, SpO2 99% RA, T 39.0°C

Consultation 40	Ms Jackson, 23 years old
Your Role:	Emergency Department SHO
Referral Letter:	Dear Colleague,
	Thank you for seeing this young lady with abnormal movements who is understandably very anxious.
	Thank you.
	Dr Wei Ting, GP
Vital Signs:	BP 103/60 mmHg, HR 71/min, RR 11/min, SpO2 98% RA, T 37.0°C

Consultation 41	Ms. Mabok, 34 years old
Your Role:	Emergency Department SHO
Referral Letter:	Dear Colleague,
	Thank you for seeing Ms Mabok. She complains of a one-day history of giddiness.
	Warm regards,
	Dr Hallpike, GP
Vital Signs:	BP 127/80 mmHg, HR 80/min, RR 14/min, SpO2 98% RA, T 37.0°C

Consultation 42	Ms Campbell, 41 years old
Your Role:	Rheumatology Outpatients SHO
Scenario:	Ms Campbell, who is on follow up for systemic sclerosis, brought forward her scheduled appointment because of giddiness and diarrhoea.
Vital Signs:	BP 180/108 mmHg, HR 90/min, RR 16/min, SpO2 95% RA, T 36.0°C
Investigations:	Haemoglobin 9.8 mg/dL, WBC 4.2×10^9/L, Platelets 90×10^9/L
	Creatinine 180 umol/L (baseline 70 umol/L)
	Urine dipstick – blood 1+, protein, and nitrites negative

Consultation 43	Mrs Drowsy, 64 years old
Your Role:	Oncology Unit Walk-In Clinic SHO
Referral Letter:	Dear Colleague,
	Mrs Drowsy is on home hospice support for metastatic ovarian cancer. We have found her to be intermittently confused over the past week. She is struggling to manage at home. Please kindly see her.
	Warm regards,
	Dr G. Reaper, Eternal Life Home Hospice
Vital Signs:	BP 125/82 mmHg, HR 77/min, RR 8/min, SpO2 96% RA, T 36.0°C

Consultation 44	Ms Claudia, 35 years old
Your Role:	Emergency Department SHO
Referral Letter:	Dear Colleague,
	Ms Claudia migrated from East Asia 2 years ago. She has been on my follow up since then for difficult-to-control hypertension. Today she came to see me with a new complaint of right leg pain. Would you please see her to exclude deep vein thrombosis?
	Thank you.
	Dr Dorothy Huang, GP
Vital Signs:	BP 155/82 mmHg, HR 48/min, RR 10/min, SpO2 99% RA, T 37.0°C

Consultation 45

Your Role: Internal Medicine SHO

Mr P. Pee, 30 years old

Referral Letter:
Dear Colleague,

Thank you for seeing Mr P. Pee who complains of frequent urination. He is too young to have a prostate problem.

Thank you.

Dr S. Shee, Urology

Vital Signs: BP 120/70 mmHg, HR 55/min, RR 13/min, SpO2 99% RA, T 37.0°C

Investigations:
Urine microscopy – normal
Fasting glucose 5.0 mmol/L
Uroflowmetry – normal

Consultation 46

Mr Kuning, 32 years old

Your Role: Gastroenterology SHO

Referral Letter:
Dear Colleague,

Thank you for seeing Mr Kuning for abnormal liver function tests detected on health screening.

Regards,

Dr Kelly Chng, GP

Vital Signs: BP 120/70 mmHg, HR 60/min, RR 15/min, SpO2 95% RA, T 36.0°C

Investigations:

Bilirubin	30	umol/L	(3 - 17)
Alanine aminotransferase (ALT)	160	IU/L	(5 - 35)
Aspartate transaminase (AST)	334	IU/L	(5 - 50)
Alkaline phosphatase (ALP)	70	IU/L	(30 - 150)
Albumin	37	g/L	(35 - 50)

Full blood count, creatinine, electrolytes – normal

Consultation 47

Your Role: Medicine Outpatients SHO

Referral Letter:
Dear Colleague,

Thank you for seeing Ms Fairchild for raised aPTT.

She saw me to do a face lift. Unexpectedly, the routine pre-op work-up found an elevated aPTT. I am hoping that you will be able to investigate further and let me know whether I can proceed with the procedure.

Thank you,

Dr W. Wu, Plastic Surgery

Vital Signs: BP 110/62 mmHg, HR 65/min, RR 10/min, SpO2 99% RA, T 36.0°C

Investigations:

Prothrombin time (PT)	12.0 s (normal)
Activated partial thromboplastin time (aPTT)	80.2 s (30 - 50 s)
Full blood count	normal

Consultation 48

Ms Rachel Clot, 47 years old

Your Role: Haematology Clinic SHO

Referral Letter:
Dear Colleague,

Thank you for seeing Ms Clot early for thrombocytopenia.

She has a history of systemic lupus erythematosus, diabetes, and hypertension. She was admitted last week for exertional chest pain and underwent a coronary angiogram. This showed minor coronary artery disease which we will treat medically.

She made an unscheduled clinic visit today complaining of right thigh swelling. An ultrasound confirmed deep vein thrombosis of the right superficial femoral vein. Unfortunately, her platelets were low, so I was unable to start anticoagulation.

Would you please see her for further management?

Thank you.

Dr B. Loon, Cardiology

Vital Signs: BP 106/64 mmHg, HR 80/min, RR 10/min, SpO2 97% RA, T 37.0°C

Investigations:

Haemoglobin	12.2 g/L	(12 - 16)
White cell count	4.0×10^9/L	(2.5 - 10)
Platelets	40×10^9/L	(150 - 400), previously normal

Consultation 49

Your Role: Medicine Clinic SHO

Referral Letter: Mr Beer was found to have a creatinine of 242 umol/L on routine laboratory investigations, up from 128 umol/L two months ago.

Vital Signs: BP 150/83 mmHg, HR 75/min, RR 10/min, SpO2 98% RA, T 37.0°C

Consultation 50

Mr Ezekiel, 58 years old

Your Role: Ward SHO

Referral Letter: Dear Medical Colleague,

Mr Ezekiel has had two fractures this year (proximal humerus and distal radius). Is there anything you can do to reduce his risk of fracture recurrence?

Thank you.

Dr Saw, Orthopaedic Surgeon

Vital Signs: BP 165/80 mmHg, HR 73/min, RR 12/min, SpO2 98% RA, T 37.0°C

COMMUNICATIONS

Comms 01 — Mdm Koh Ma, 80 years old

Your Role: Neurology Ward SHO

Information: Mdm Koh came to the Emergency Department yesterday evening complaining of headache and vomiting. She was diagnosed with migraine and sent home on analgesia.

This morning, her family members could not wake her up from sleep. She was brought back to the Emergency Department and a CT brain showed a massive subarachnoid hemorrhage. She is currently in the operating theatre undergoing decompression surgery.

Your task is to speak to Mdm Koh's daughter to update her of her mother's situation and address any concerns that she may have.

Comms 02 — Mr Muhammad Bin Muhammad, 22 years old

Your Role: Intensive Care Unit SHO

Information: Mr Muhammad, a 22-year-old university student, was admitted 48 hours ago following a road traffic accident. He was crossing the road with the traffic lights in his favour, but was hit by a speeding truck and suffered massive intracranial haemorrhage.

Version (a) if taking the exam in Singapore, (b) if in the UK.

(a) **Singapore**: He has been pronounced brain dead by two independent consultants. Currently he is normotensive and in sinus rhythm. He is kept intubated and ventilated with the intention of facilitating organ harvesting. He is not known to have opted out of organ donation under the Human Organ Transplant Act.

(b) **UK**: He has been pronounced brain dead by two independent consultants. Currently he is normotensive and in sinus rhythm. He is kept intubated and ventilated with the intention of facilitating organ harvesting.

Your task is to update his parents about the diagnosis of brain death and approach the idea of organ donation.

Comms 03 — Ms Rebecca Clot, 30 years old

Your Role: Haematology Clinic SHO

Information: Ms Clot presented to the Emergency Department 2 days ago with right leg swelling. Compression venous ultrasound confirmed the diagnosis of deep vein thrombosis (DVT) involving the femoral and popliteal veins. The Emergency physician has started her on subcutaneous low molecular weight heparin (1 mg/kg) and given her a fast-track appointment to see you today.

You have determined that Ms Clot's DVT is likely provoked by use of a combined oral contraceptive pill. She does not have any other risk factor for DVT, no underlying medical illness, and no family history of thrombosis. There is no clinical concern for pulmonary embolism at the present moment.

Your task is to counsel Ms Clot about the management options for her condition.

Candidate's Information for Practice Scenarios

Comms 04

Mr E. O. See, 30 years old

Your Role: Medicine Clinic SHO

Information: Mr See is the Chief Executive Officer of a fast-growing tech start-up. He recently sought to purchase a £2,000,000 term life insurance plan. Due to the high coverage amount, the insurance provider elected to send Mr See for routine health screening before extending the cover.

Mr See was found to be hypertensive with a blood pressure reading of 170/95 mmHg (average over two visits). As a result, the insurance company has rejected Mr See's application for life insurance.

The general practitioner who saw Mr See has started him on lisinopril 20 mg OM and referred him to your clinic for work-up of young hypertension.

Mr See's blood pressure today is 173/94 mmHg.

Your task is to discuss work-up of young hypertension with Mr See and address any concerns that he may have.

Comms 05

Ms Vanessa Shake, 22 years old

Your Role: Neurology Ward SHO

Information: Ms Shake has been admitted for an episode of generalised tonic-clonic seizures. This is her third admission for seizure; she had her first seizure 1 year ago and a second seizure 3 months ago. She is otherwise stable with normal vitals.

Your task is to counsel her on the diagnosis and treatment of epilepsy.

Comms 06

Mr Hack, 30 years old

Your Role: General Medicine SHO

Information: Mr Hack has come to the walk-in clinic today requesting for cough syrup.

He was diagnosed with pulmonary tuberculosis 3 months ago and started on rifampicin, isoniazid, pyrazanamide, ethambutol, and pyridoxine. Sputum cultures have confirmed mycobacterium tuberculosis which is sensitive to all first-line antituberculous therapy. Liver enzymes, fasting glucose, and a HIV test are normal.

Mr Hack has missed 2 review appointments to date. The records show that in the 3 months since his diagnosis, he has only collected 1 month's worth of medication. He is symptomatic with persistent cough.

Your task is to speak to Mr Hack about his non-compliance and formulate a treatment plan.

Comms 07	Mr C. Yolo, 42 years old
Your Role:	Medicine Ward SHO
Information:	Mr Yolo was admitted 4 days ago. He presented with a 2-week history of fever, rash, and sore throat after returning from vacation. Your consultant has ordered several tests including a HIV test.* The laboratory has called to inform you that the HIV test is 'indeterminate'. **Your task** is to speak to Mr Yolo about this result. *Your laboratory uses a fourth-generation HIV assay, which is a combination test including the HIV antibody and p24 antigen. If this is positive, a confirmatory western blot is performed.

Comms 08	Ms Willy Wild, 36 years old
Your Role:	Infectious Disease Clinic SHO
Information:	Ms Wild is referred to the Infectious Diseases clinic for a 6-month history of cough and weight loss. A HIV test and confirmatory test are positive. She is married with a 3-year-old son. **Your task** is to inform Ms Wild of the test result and address her concerns.

Comm	Dr S. Suay, 23 years old
Your Role:	Medical SHO-On-Call
Information:	Dr Suay, the House Officer (FY1) with whom you are on call, comes to you distraught after sustaining a needlestick injury. **Your task** is to calm the situation and advice Dr Suay on what she needs to do.

Comms 10	Mr Gan Ying Hua, 53 years old.
Your Role:	Gastroenterology Clinic SHO
Information:	Mr Gan, a 53-year-old Chinese gentleman, is on follow-up with the gastroenterology clinic for liver cirrhosis. He is hepatitis B positive and has a very strong family history of hepatitis B. In the past year, he has had two episodes of variceal bleed and one admission for hepatic encephalopathy. In the past two months, he has also been complaining of symptomatic ascites which has not improved in spite of maximal tolerated doses of furosemide and spironolactone. Your consultant has just seen Mr Gan and decided to offer large volume paracentesis (therapeutic ascitic drain). This will be done today as an outpatient in the day procedure room. **Your consultant has tasked you to** consent Mr Gan for this procedure and counsel him on further management of his cirrhosis.

Candidate's Information for Practice Scenarios

Comms 11–12

Mr Bo Kar, 27 years old

Note: Cases 11 and 12 share a common candidate's information.
Please attempt Case 11 first.

Your Role: Acute Care Clinic SHO

Information: Mr Bo walks in to the Acute Care Clinic complaining of worsening pain and requesting for a top-up of painkillers.

He had a right above-knee amputation 1 year ago after a road traffic accident in which he suffered popliteal artery injury and right calf compartment syndrome. He is able to walk with a prosthetic limb but has known phantom limb pain.

You note that he had just seen a GP 7 days ago and was prescribed with:

    PO Tramadol 25 mg TDS PRN (for pain) — 3 weeks (63 capsules)
    PO Lorazepam 1 mg ON PRN (for sleep) — 3 weeks (21 capsules)

Your task is to speak to Mr Bo and address his concerns.

Comms 13

Ms Theresa Downs, 35 years old

Your Role: Medical Ward SHO

Information: Ms Downs is a nurse working in your hospital. She was admitted to your ward two days ago after another nurse found her unconscious in the staff changing room prior to the start of her shift, and wheeled her to the Emergency Department. A drug screen for benzodiazepines has come back positive.

Your task is to speak to her about this episode and broach the topic of psychiatric review.

Comms 14	Ms Elsa Queen, 77 years old
Your Role:	Acute Medical Unit SHO
Information:	Ms Queen is a 77-year-old with a past medical history of diabetes with diabetic nephropathy.

Three months ago, she presented in cardiogenic shock from an acute myocardial infarction. Emergency percutaneous coronary intervention was successful in stenting the left anterior descending artery. She had a stormy recovery with acute on chronic kidney disease requiring renal replacement therapy. She did not recover renal function and was discharged to community haemodialysis via a tunnelled dialysis catheter.

Since discharge, she has been readmitted thrice — once for dialysis catheter infection, another for intra-dialytic hypotension, and most recently for methicillin-resistant *staphylococcus aureus* (MRSA) bacteraemia. Trans-esophageal echocardiography showed normal valves, no valvular vegetations, and an ejection fraction of 17%. She received six weeks of intravenous vancomycin and a change of the dialysis catheter.

Ms Queen is currently admitted to your ward, having been referred by the dialysis centre for recurrent intra-dialytic chest pain and hypotension. Despite technical optimisation of the dialysis prescription, she has not been able to complete a full dialysis session since her last discharge. Ms Queen is breathless, acidotic, and hyperkalemic. Your consultant has decided to withdraw dialysis support as she is unable to tolerate dialysis.

Ms Queen's only child, who lives overseas, has flown back after hearing of the plan to withdraw dialysis.

Your task is to speak to Ms Queen's son, Mr Payne, and address his concerns. You may assume the necessary permissions to discuss the patient's confidential medical information with Mr Payne.

Comms 15	Ms Amy Dole, 42 years old
Your Role:	Cardiology Clinic SHO
Information:	Ms Dole is a 42-year-old lady with fibromyalgia, irritable bowel syndrome, and migraine on follow up with multiple specialists. Blood tests, multiple gastroscopes and colonoscopes, as well as a CT brain and CT abdomen are normal.

In the past six months, she has visited the Emergency Department seven times for chest pain; each time with normal ECGs, troponins, and chest X-rays. She has been referred to Cardiology and underwent further investigations including a treadmill stress test, echocardiogram, and 24-hour ECG monitoring, all of which were normal. She has been discharged from Cardiology follow up two weeks ago.

Ms Dole has walked in to clinic today, complaining of a two-day history of atypical chest pain. Her vital signs and clinical examination are normal. An ECG, full blood count, electrolytes, CRP, troponin, and D-dimer* are normal. Your consultant will like to refer Ms Dole for psychiatric consult for anxiety disorder.

Your task is to inform Ms Dole of her test results, offer psychiatric consultation, and manage her concerns.

*In patients with a low pre-test probability of pulmonary embolism and a normal D-dimer, the chance of a pulmonary embolism is approximately 0.1%.[1]

Comms 16	Ms A. Jollie, 37 years old
Your Role:	Medicine Clinic SHO
Information:	Ms Jollie sees you in clinic to discuss BRCA1 testing. Her mother has recently passed away from ovarian cancer at 56 years of age. Her 38-year-old sister has just had her breast removed due to breast cancer.

Your task is to discuss BRCA testing with Ms Jollie.

---

[1] Bass AR, Fields KG, Goto R, Turissini G, Dey S, Russell LA. Clinical Decision Rules for Pulmonary Embolism in Hospitalized Patients: A Systematic Literature Review and Meta-analysis. *Thromb Haemost* 2017 117(11):2176.

Comms 17	Dr Green, 25 years old
Your Role:	Night-Duty SHO
Information:	You are on night duty with Dr Green, the FY1/House Officer.
	At approximately 2am, you were called to attend to a Code Blue involving Mdm Loh B. P., a 50-year-old lady admitted two days ago for pneumonia. Mdm Loh responded well to resuscitation and has been transferred to the intensive care unit. She appears to be alert with no permanent neurological sequelae.
	While reviewing Mdm Loh's clinical notes, you noted that the ward nurses had called Dr Green at 8pm to inform that Mdm Loh was hypotensive and febrile. Dr Green asked to give a pint of normal saline and some paracetamol, but did not physically review Mdm Loh.
	Dr Brainchild, the on-duty medical registrar, is concerned about the events leading up to Mdm Loh's Code Blue and has asked you to speak to Dr Green while he stabilises her in the intensive care unit.
	Your task is to speak to Dr Green about his unsafe clinical management.

Comms 18	Mdm Maria, 35 years old
Your Role:	Medical High Dependency SHO
Information:	Mdm Maria is a 35-year-old foreign domestic worker from the Philippines with no known past medical history.
	She was admitted for a 4-day history of fever, breathlessness, and altered mental state. Initial investigations revealed acute leukaemia with tumour lysis syndrome, which has caused renal impairment and pulmonary oedema.
	Your consultant has discussed her case with the renal and haematology unit. The plan is to insert a non-tunnelled dialysis catheter, administer haemodialysis, and initiate chemotherapy urgently. Dual consultant consent has been obtained to proceed as Mdm Maria is confused and has been assessed to lack mental capacity. Your consultant expects that Maria will have a long and stormy hospital stay with multiple sessions of dialysis and a long course of chemotherapy. However, without treatment, Mdm Maria is expected to deteriorate and pass away within days.
	Her employer, Mrs Blackheart, has made known that she objects to dialysis and chemotherapy, and requests to speak to a member of staff.
	Your task is to speak to Mrs Blackheart and address her concerns. You may assume that Mdm Maria has consented to this conversation.

Comms 19	Mrs Park, 70 years old
Your Role:	Acute Medical Unit Ward SHO
Information:	Mrs Park was diagnosed with Alzheimer's dementia 15 years ago and has had a steady decline in function since then. In the last two years, she has become completely bedbound and dependent on others for her activities of daily living. She receives liquid feeds through a nasogastric tube.

Mrs Park was admitted through the Emergency Department yesterday for sepsis from unstageable sacral sores. She appears cachectic and hypovolemic. A sacral X-ray is significant for evidence of osteomyelitis and biochemical investigations reveal hyponatraemia, hypokalaemia, hypophosphataemia, and hypomagnesaemia. Your team has started her on IV antibiotics, IV fluids, electrolyte and thiamine replacement, and an appropriate feeding regimen.

This is Mrs Park's third admission for infected sacral sores in the past year. The social worker has highlighted several concerns about Mrs Park's care at home. In particular, although her husband, Mr Park, claims to pay for a home nurse service who visits three times a week, a call to the home nurse service reveals that Mr Park has been cancelling appointments and in the past month they have only come once.

Your task is to update Mrs Park's husband about her condition and convey your concerns about her care at home.

Comms 20	Ms ABC, 35 years old
Your Role:	Medicine Clinic SHO
Information:	Several years ago, Ms ABC's father was diagnosed with Huntington's disease. Despite extensive counselling about the possibility that his children may inherit the Huntington gene, he firmly insisted that his children should not be informed. He was particularly concerned that his younger daughter, Ms ABC, who was pregnant at the time, would have an abortion should she be told. After much deliberation, his physicians opted not to override his confidentiality and inform his daughters of the diagnosis.

After childbirth, Ms ABC accidentally became aware of her father's diagnosis. She subsequently sought gene testing and was found to have the Huntington gene. It is not yet known whether her child is similarly affected because gene testing cannot be done until the child is 18 years of age.

Ms ABC wishes to speak to a member of staff about the failure to inform her of her father's diagnosis of Huntington's disease.

Your task is to speak to Ms ABC and address her concerns.